Adherence to Treatment in Medical Conditions

Adherence to Treatment in Medical Conditions

Edited by

Lynn B. Myers
University College London, UK

and

Kenny Midence
University of Wales, UK

harwood academic publishers
Australia • Canada • China • France • Germany • India • Japan
Luxembourg • Malaysia • The Netherlands • Russia • Singapore
Switzerland • Thailand • United Kingdom

Amsteldijk 166
1st Floor
1079 LH Amsterdam
The Netherlands

R
727
'43
A 34
1998

British Library Cataloguing in Publication Data

Adherence to treatment in medical conditions
  1. Patient compliance
  I. Myers, Lynn II.Midence, Kenny
  615.5

ISBN 90–5702–265–6 (Softcover)

Printed and Bound at Ajanta Offset, New Delhi, India

Contents

Preface

Adherence to treatment in medical conditions and its implications for clinical practice is an area of great interest amongst researchers and clinicians. It has generated a wealth of research studies, and publications, and our knowledge about the interdependence of factors involved in adherence is improving. Despite all this accumulated information, clinicians still find it difficult to persuade their patients to adhere to medical regimens, and some patients do not seem to follow medical recommendations despite the life-threatening consequences. It could be argued that researchers and clinicians know more about the theoretical, conceptual and methodological issues of adherence, than they do about patients' understanding of their treatment, and their decisions to adhere.

The present book brings together the expertise of various international professionals from different disciplines working in different settings and who encounter non-adherent patients in their clinical or research practice. We believe that there are basic conceptual and methodological issues, which need to be addressed by researchers and clinicians from different backgrounds. Therefore, in Chapter 1, Myers and Midence introduce the book by discussing important concepts and issues in adherence. This chapter highlights various problems in relation to the definition of adherence, measurement and assessment, and non-adherence in patients and health professionals.

The book is divided into four subsequent sections. The next section addresses general issues in adherence to treatment. In Chapter 2, Horne and Weinman provide an overview of several theoretical models (Social Cognition Models, Stage Models and Self-Regulatory Theory) which can be used to explain non-adherence in patients. Doctor-patient communication and its influence in adherence is addressed in Chapter 3, where Noble argues that adherence to treatment is not simply that patients have to do as they are told, but a complex issue which cannot be taken for granted. The importance of written information on patients' knowledge and adherence is discussed by Raynor in Chapter 4, who points out that information does not always result in knowledge which may lead to change in adherence behaviour. In Chapter 5, Ellis examines the importance of memory processes for successful medicine taking. Tones begins in Chapter 6 by examining the interrelationship of adherence and health promotion. The psychosocial and environmental factors which affect people's decision making in relation to health and illness are reviewed, and the implications for the delivery of interventions are discussed.

The chapters in the next section look at adherence in particular groups. In Chapter 7, Bryon reviews the research literature on adherence in children with chronic illnesses, and explores the reasons why some children show poor adherence even in the face of life-threatening diseases. Rosenblatt, in Chapter 8, addresses the implications of non-adherence at different stages of pregnancy, and the potential difficulties caused by health related behaviours, and medical complications. She also discusses non-adherence in obstetric, nursing and midwifery staff. Improving adherence in older adults is an important issue which is discussed by McElnay and McCallion in Chapter 9. They highlight the need to help this population because as the authors state, older adults are more likely to suffer adverse consequences from non-adherence. In Chapter 10, Sissons Joshi reviews the literature on adherence in ethnic groups with reference to South Asians.

The next section addresses issues of adherence in different treatments. Horne in Chapter 11 reviews the research literature on adherence to medication, and outlines the implications for clinical practice. In Chapter 12, Nicholson Perry, Rapoport and Wardle review the literature on adherence to dietary advice, explain the difficulties in adherence in this population, and suggest ideas for future research. Prescribing exercise to patients is one of the recent developments in the treatment for medical conditions. Chapter 13 reviews the limited research available, and outlines some of the approaches used to improve adherence to exercise. In this chapter, Jones, Harris and McGee point out the need to reduce obesity and high blood pressure, and emphasise the role of exercise to achieve these objectives. Sluijs, Kerssens, van der Zee and Myers review the available literature on adherence to physiotherapy in Chapter 14, and present preliminary findings of ongoing research in adherence to physiotherapy in The Netherlands.

The final section of this book presents issues related to adherence in specific conditions. In Chapter 15, Hand reviews recent literature on adherence and asthma, and investigates why some patients suffering from asthma fail to adhere to medication despite continuous medical advice. Hand also looks at non-adherence in health professionals, and provides suggestions for future research. In Chapter 16, Warren and Hixenbaugh address adherence and diabetes, and point out the serious difficulties and consequences that may arise as a result of non-adherence to treatment by people suffering from diabetes. They also highlight the importance of the psychosocial aspects of diabetes, including the patient's perspective, and attempt to raise awareness about some of the flaws in the diabetes literature. Schwartz begins in Chapter 17 by looking at the current research literature on adherence in paediatric renal disease and its treatment, and addresses issues of non-adherence in children with renal disease within a family framework and the healthcare system. In Chapter 18, Gidron reviews the challenges and difficulties associated with hypertension and coronary heart disease. He also addresses issues related to assessment methods and correlates of adherence in cardiovascular diseases, and examines the empirical research literature and strategies to improve adherence in these medical conditions. Finally, Chapter 19 by Elander considers ways in which adherence in methadone treatments of different types for opiate dependence can be improved and produce better outcomes. Elander suggests that treatment programmes and adherence are sometimes very difficult to differentiate in treatments for opiate dependence. His chapter attempts to clarify these two issues and examines the literature on adherence and aspects of the treatments.

This book will be of interest to all those health professionals, researchers and students who wish to understand adherence, and are looking for possible strategies and solutions to deal with this complex problem. It is impossible for any book to cover adherence issues in its entirety, but the book provides its readers with an up to date overview of theoretical and methodological considerations, and general issues in adherence in different treatments, in various populations, which may experience specific medical conditions.

We would like to thank John Weinman and Stan Newman for early encouragement. We are grateful to Jan Stygall for her invaluable assistance both for commenting on and proof reading the final draft of the book. In addition, we thank Jane Harrington, Lorraine Noble, Howard Myers and Liz Steed for their helpful comments. A special thanks goes to Mark Brumwell who as a non-psychologist, read and commented on many of the chapters. We also thank Mark for his never faltering encouragement throughout the process of producing this book.

Lynn B. Myers
Kenny Midence

Foreword

My fourteen year old daughter, Annie, was wondering aloud why her school holidays seemed to have gone so fast. "Perhaps", she said, "it was because I never got up before lunch time. I had decided that *this* holidays I was going to get up early each day, but when I awoke on the first morning, I sort of forgot I had made the resolution, and after that it didn't seem to matter". Her experience illustrates one of the most ubiquitous aspect of human experience – the difficulty in carrying out plans and intentions once the context in which the plan has been created has gone. This difficulty in adopting new habits when (if carried out) they would often be positively reinforcing, represents the flip-side of a puzzle discussed by behaviour analysts earlier this century, about why neuroses do not naturally extinguish. Psychologists referred to this failure to extinguish as the 'neurotic paradox', and there are good grounds for thinking that the 'adherence paradox' is every bit as puzzling.

I was reminded of the adherence paradox while listening to a news broadcast in March, 1997. A representative of the World Health Organisation (WHO) was describing DOTS – one of the main hopes for the treatment of tuberculosis. Eight thousand people a day are dying of TB, more than all other infectious diseases put together. "DOTS", he explained, "stands for Directly Observed Treatment

Short-course" – a combination of drugs taken for a few months costing, in all, little more than $30. The course of treatment had been found to cut the probability of death by half. The problem was that the whole course needed to be taken or it did not have this effect. The WHO had clearly taken the view that it was the Health-care Services in each country that had the responsibility to ensure adherence, hence the inclusion, in the title of the treatment, of the 'direct observation'. Not to observe whether the pills were being taken would constitute failure to administer the treatment on the part of the Health system.

This book illustrates that the adherence paradox raises its head in virtually every domain of medicine. For medical treatment is a collaboration between the person in need of treatment and the people in the Healthcare system who provide it. The chapters in this book show very clearly that even in the most severe medical conditions, in which failure to follow a treatment plan results in almost certain death, the collaboration may break down. Do patients fail to hear or understand what is said (a failure to encode), or do they forget once they are in another context (a failure of retrospective or prospective memory)? Do the patient and the health professional differ in their beliefs about what is causing or maintaining the problem? Or is it that patients' behaviour more powerfully depends on how they are feeling right now rather than on what has happened in the past or might happen in the future? Or is there a conflict of goals, between wanting to remain well (take the advice) and wanting to ignore their life threatening illness (forget the advice)? For those of us who are interested in understanding suicidal behaviour, this breakdown in the collaboration between the Health-care system and its users is reminiscent of the ambivalent attitudes to life and death we see in our suicidal clients. Feeling hopeless about the future and tired of struggling on against the odds, such people often seem to play Russian roulette with their lives, challenging the gods, as it were, to let them live or die. Is there any evidence of such an element in the failure to adhere to medical advice? Getting answers to these questions is extremely urgent, for lives depend upon them. This book comes at a critical moment for health systems all over the world. It is particularly important because there are no current books covering recent research and clinical efforts to understand and improve adherence. There has not been a book in the last ten years on these issues, yet much of the important research has been done over this period. This is the first British and European book on the topic. Many of the major contributors to the field are in Europe, and have contributed to the book. But most importantly, this book does not only discuss adherence in general terms. Instead, it explores the difficulties associated with specific patient groups, specific medical and non-medical treatments, and specific medical conditions. Myers and Midence have brought together expertise in cognitive, social, clinical and health psychology, together with Health education, primary care medicine, pharmacy and physiotherapy. For the first time it allows us to look across different specific problems and approaches for commonalities that will allow an integrative picture to emerge.

The authors examine in detail the questions raised by the adherence paradox, and the implications of these findings for communication and negotiation between health professionals and their patients (see Horne and Weinman''s overview and Noble's chapter on doctor patient communication). Raynor considers the impact of information in supporting such negotiation, raising the important issue of verbal versus written communication, and includes important practical advice arising from the research literature. Ellis's chapter embeds the adherence question in the broader field of prospective remembering, and addresses the attentional, memory and planning factors that facilitate or impair such behaviour. Tones considers health behaviour in the context of its wider psychological, social and environmental determinants, arguing for a health education x health public policy formula that brings about empowerment by combining *horizontal* programmes (that address fundamental causes) as well as *vertical* programmes (that address specific disease conditions).

Bryon's chapter on adherence in children addresses differences in adherence to different aspects of treatment, and whether it is the unpleasantness of the treatment, the interference with routines, the complexity of the treatment, the immediacy of change versus protection against longer term deterioration or the relationship with the health professional that determines adherence. Each of these may play a role, but child optimism and family coherence and support is also important. Health-enhancing or impairing behaviour during pregnancy is an important topic because of risk to the child, and Rosenblatt's chapter reviews the factors which may affect such behaviours as consumption of alcohol, smoking, fitness in general, adherence to medication, and the taking up of antenatal and perinatal care opportunities.

The increased health risks found in elderly people are considered by McElnay and McCallion, considering in particular the problem of older adults' increase in number and complexity of medication (which, incidentally, might defeat the prospective memory systems of many younger people), and what has and might be done about such problems. Sissons Joshi considers special issues that arise in ethnic minorities in the UK, including vocabulary of health and illness and its relation to distortions in diagnosis and treatment advice. The chapter points out that breakdown in communication between health professionals and members of ethnic minorities may go wider than this, especially when simple differences in use of 'please' and 'thankyou's' and in euphemisms for different body parts are interpreted as indifference or rudeness by the professional. Sissons Joshi also considers whether ethnic minorities have different actual or perceived risks for different diseases, factors that may powerfully affect their health-related behaviour.

Low rates of adherence to medication are found across the entire range of diseases including asthma, diabetes, heart disease, cancer, kidney disease, and even following organ transplantation. Why this is so is considered in detail by Horne. He points out the need for multifactorial models that include factors such as how the complexity of the regimen interacts with the individual patient's routine ('simple' is not always 'better'). Data suggest that a patient's knowledge does not always predict their medication use, so that the fact that a patient may forget much of what they are told in a consultation may not make the crucial difference, though patient satisfaction with the Healthcare professional may be important.

Nicholson Perry, Rapoport and Wardle consider adherence to lipid-lowering dietary advice. They review the outcomes of a number of large scale community dietary interventions side by side with the targeted interventions for high risk groups. As in other domains, research has focused on models such as 'stages of change', 'health-belief', and 'self efficacy' to understand why people find it difficult to implement or sustain dietary advice, and suggest that, where possible, individualised packages be used that take account of the nature of the problem, whether the person can meet the cognitive demands and other 'costs' of the programme. They also point out the importance of significant others' support and involvement in such programmes.

Similar issues are found in the literature on adherence to physical therapy and prescribed exercise. The chapter by Jones, Harris and McGee and that by Sluijs, Kerssens, van der Zee and Myers indicates that while research is in its infancy, therapist reports indicate that many patients fail to continue prescribed exercises once active treatment has stopped. Research is beginning to ask which exercises are most likely to give rise to problems, and what other factors are involved in non-adherence, so that advice about best-practice may be incorporated into training of therapists.

Finally, in a section on adherence in specific conditions, Warren and Hixenbaugh, Gidron, Hand, Elander and Schwartz examine the results from studies of diabetes, hypertension and coronary heart disease, asthma, opiate dependence and renal failure, respectively. These chapters illustrate all too well the point that ignoring the factors that enhance or damage adherence is sometimes to ignore the most important contributors to the outcome of patients. Sometimes (as with diabetes) it has been difficult to find the exact causes of non-adherence, but these difficulties do not undermine the fact that, with such chronic conditions, adherence may be crucial to health yet difficult to achieve, perhaps because of the enormous motivation and effort required of the patient. Gidron refers to non-adherence in hypertension and heart disease as constituting a problem 'of epidemic magnitude'. These chapters have important contributions to make in summarising what may be done to enhance adherence (for example, Hand's clear account of dealing with asthma, from the perspective of the family doctor, should leave no health professional in doubt where to begin in changing his or her practice).

Some authors refer in their chapters to the training of health professionals. It is clear that including specific training on adherence is relatively new in training courses in medical and health sciences, and remains sporadic and patchy. This book should become required reading for health professionals in training, as well as being a compulsory element in the continuing education courses of those already practising. Will such data be taken into account by health professionals? As with patients, whether professionals adhere to the advice emerging from this book will depend on a number of factors. Apportioning blame for non-adherence does not help in either case. Rather, the book challenges us to examine the aspects of the environment that affect our practice when we attempt to collaborate with our patients to bring about better health; and having examined these matters, and reflected on our practice, to change what we do so that the adherence issue is kept, where it belongs, at the centre of our concerns.

Professor Mark Williams
Director, Centre for Medical and Health Sciences,
University of Wales,
Bangor, UK

List of Contributors

Mandy Bryon
Clinical Psychologist, Department of Psychological Medicine, Great Ormond Street Hospital for Children, London, WC1N 3JH, UK

James Elander
PhD, Higher Scientific Officer, MRC Child Psychiatry Unit, Institute of Psychiatry, De Crespigny Park, London SE5 8AF, UK

Judi Ellis
PhD, Lecturer in Psychology, Department of Psychology, The University of Reading, Reading, RG6 6AL, UK

Yori Gidron
PhD, Researcher in Behavioural Medicine, Department of Sociology and Health, Faculty of Health Sciences, Ben-Gurion University at the Negev 84105, Be'er Sheeba, Israel

Christopher Hand
MSc, FRCGP, Associate Director for Postgraduate General Practice, Oxford and Anglia and Honorary Senior Lecturer, Health Policy and Practice, The School of Health, University of East Anglia, Norwich, NR4 7TJ, UK

Peter Harris
PhD, Lecturer in Social Psychology, School of Social Sciences, University of Sussex, Falmer, Brighton, BN1 9QN, UK

Paula Hixenbaugh
PhD, Head of Division of Psychology, University of Westminster, London, W1R 8AL, UK

Robert Horne
PhD, MRPharmS, Senior Lecturer in Clinical and Social Pharmacy, Department of Pharmacy, University of Brighton, Brighton, Sussex, BN2 4GJ, UK

Fiona Jones
PhD, Senior Lecturer in Psychology, Department of Psychology, University of Hertfordshire, Hatfield, AL10 9AB, UK

Jan J. Kerssens
PhD, Senior Researcher, Netherlands Institute for Primary Health Care, P.O. Box 1568, 3500 BN Utrecht, The Netherlands

C. Rosaleen McCallion
PhD, Research Fellow, School of Pharmacy, Queens University of Belfast, 97 Lisbuorn Rd, Belfast, BT9 7BL, Northern Ireland, UK

Laura McGee
Research Psychologist, Department of Psychology, Brunel University, Uxbridge, Middlesex, UB8 3PH, UK

James McElnay
PhD, MRPharmS, Professor and Director School of Pharmacy, Queens University of Belfast, 97 Lisbuorn Rd, Belfast, BT9 7BL, Northern Ireland, UK

Kenny Midence
MSc, Clinical Psychologist, Department of Clinical Psychology, University of Wales, Bangor, Gwynedd, LL57 2DG, Wales, UK

Lynn B. Myers
PhD, MRPharmS, Lecturer in Health Psychology, Department of Psychiatry and Behavioural Sciences, University College London Medical School, Riding House Street, London, W1N 8AA, UK

Kathryn Nicholson Perry
Clinical Psychologist. Health Behaviour Unit, Department of Epidemiology and Public Health, University College London, Torrington Place, London WC1E 6BT, UK. Current address: Richard Dimbleby Cancer Information and Support Service, Lambeth Wing, St Thomas' Hospital, SE1 7EH

Lorraine Noble
PhD, Dip. Clin. Psych, Lecturer in Communication Skills, Department of Psychiatry and Behavioural Sciences, University College London Medical School, Riding House Street, London, W1N 8AA, UK

Lorna Rapoport
Research Dietitian, Health Behaviour Unit, Department of Epidemiology and Public Health, University College London, Torrington Place, London WC1E 6BT, UK

D.K. Raynor
PhD, Head of Division of Academic Pharmacy Practice, School of Healthcare Studies, University of Leeds, Leeds LS2 9NS, UK

Deborah Rosenblatt
PhD, Lecturer in Psychology, Department of Psychology, The University of Reading, Reading, RG6 6AL, UK

Anthony Schwartz
MA, Clinical Psychologist, Paediatric Psychology Liaison, Child and Family Services, Alder Hey Children's Hospital, Liverpool, L12 2AP, UK

Mary Sissons Joshi
PhD, Senior Lecturer in Psychology, Psychology Department, School of Social Sciences and Law, Oxford Brookes University, Headington, Oxford, OX3 0BP, UK

Emmy M. Sluijs
PhD, Senior Researcher, Netherlands Institute for Primary Health Care, P.O. Box 1568, 3500 BN Utrecht, The Netherlands

Keith Tones
PhD, Professor of Health Education, Faculty of Health and Social Care, Leeds Metropolitan University Calverly Street, LEEDS, LS1 3HE, UK

Jane Wardle
PhD, Professor and Director of Health Behaviour Unit, Department of Epidemiology and Public Health, University College London, Torrington Place, London WC1E 6BT, UK

Laura Warren
Research Psychologist, Division of Psychology, University of Westminster, London, W1R 8AL, UK

John Weinman
PhD, Professor of Psychology as Applied to Medicine, Unit of Psychology, United Medical and Dental Schools, Guys Hospital, London SE1 9RT, UK

Jouke van der zee
PhD, Professor of Primary Health Care, Maastricht University and Director of Netherlands Institute for Primary Health Care, P.O. Box 1568, 3500 BN Utrecht, The Netherlands

Introduction

1

Concepts and Issues in Adherence

Lynn B. Myers and Kenny Midence

Patient adherence to medical conditions has become a topic of intense investigation, producing an enormous amount of research in the last few decades, and has also become an increasingly important aspect of health care. A literature search, (MedLine) indicates that in the last five years over four and a half thousand journal articles have been published in the area. This contrasts with 744 published between 1980–84, 810 published in the 1970s, 168 published in the 1960s and 25 published in the 1950s (Koltun and Stone, 1986). In addition, three major literature reviews were published in the 1970s and 1980s (DiMatteo and DiNicola, 1982; Haynes, Taylor and Sackett, 1979; Meichenbaum and Turk, 1987).

The cost of non-adherence is high. In the USA, for the year 1979, the cost of non-adherence in relation to ten drugs (ampicillin, benzodiazepines, cimetidine, clofibrate, digoxin, methoxsalen, propoxyphene, phenytoin, thiazides and warfarin) was estimated to be in the region of 396–792 million dollars (the Department of Health and Human Services, 1980).

Poor adherence to treatment is well recognised, and significantly contributes to treatment failures in medical interventions. It has been suggested that non-adherence has a significant part to play in the re-emergence of drug-resistant organisms (Gibbons, 1992) including tuberculosis (e.g. Gourevitch *et al.*, 1996). Although the level of non-adherence in the general population varies depending on the patient population, medical condition, form of treatment, and the definition of adherence, estimates of non-adherence range from 15% to 93% (Kaplan and Simon, 1990) with an average of around a third of patients failing to adhere to the recommended therapeutic regimen (e.g. Blackwell, 1973; Davis, 1966; 1968; Stimson, 1974).

In a review of the literature, Sackett and Snow (1979) estimated the degree of non-adherence in different conditions. They concluded that "patients will keep approximately 75% of the appointments they make, but only about 50% of those made for them... Compliance with short-term regimens declines rapidly... about one-half of patients on long-term regimens are compliant".

DEFINITION – COMPLIANCE OR ADHERENCE?

Although the literature has produced a large amount of research, few researchers have tried to define what they mean by adherence, while others have used the terms adherence and compliance interchangeably. The classic and most cited description of compliance has been provided by Haynes (1979a), who defined it as "the extent to which a person's behavior (in terms of taking medications, following diets, or executing lifestyle changes) coincides with medical or health advice". Haynes' definition places the patient in a passive role, having to follow the medical advice as the standard. This potential problem is noted by Haynes: "the term compliance is troublesome to many people because it conjures up images of patient or client sin or serfdom".

The term compliance has traditionally meant that the patient has to do as he or she is told by the clinician without taking into account the patient's concerns. Unsuccessful treatment meant a non-compliant patient who failed to follow the clinician's advice (Varni and Wallander, 1984). The term may be used in a judgmental fashion: "non-compliance [can be seen] as deviant behaviour and ensures that the blame for it is directed largely towards patients. It is patients who fail to comply, intentionally or unintentionally, because they are ignorant or forgetful" (Donovan and Blake, 1992).

In contrast, the term adherence implies a more active, and collaborative involvement of the patient, working together with the clinician in planning and implementing the treatment regimen. Adherence places greater emphasis on the patient's role in deciding to carry out a particular treatment. Leventhal (1993) has suggested that "the conceptual shift from compliance to adherence represents an important first step in moving away from roles emphasising obedience to instructions toward models emphasising the independence, or self-regulatory activity of the patient". The new way of conceptualising adherence seeks to empower patients by broadening the choices they can make about the way they react to and cope with illness, and helping them to obtain information which allows them to decide between the available choices in an informed way. The use of adherence rather than compliance has further been rationalised as "it is held to be more respectful of the role that the patient should play in his or her own treatment. It suggests that the doctor is engaged in reasonable negotiation with the patient, rather than the perfunctory issuing of instructions...if clinical interactions between health professionals [HPs] and patients are to be successful they should be seen as partnerships" (Royal Pharmaceutical Society of Great Britain/Merck Sharpe and Dohme, 1996). The implications of different terminology for doctor-patient communication is discussed by Noble, Chapter 3. In line with this point of view, this book will use the term adherence in preference to compliance, whenever possible.

ASSESSMENT OF ADHERENCE

The assessment of adherence is a complex task, which requires a creative approach to measure the level of patients' adherence to treatment. The concept of adherence involves a variety of health-related behaviours, and different measures have been designed to measure adherence. The example of measurement of adherence to medication will be used as it has been widely researched (see, for example, Gordis, 1979). One of the major problems in studying medication adherence is in obtaining accurate measures of adherence behaviours. There are, however, a number of different ways in which adherence to medication can be evaluated.

Self-report

When patient reports have been compared to some objective measure of medicine taking, studies have tended to show that patients are accurate when they say that they have not taken their medication (e.g. Fletcher, 1989). However, for those who state that they have taken their medication as prescribed, often these verbal reports are not confirmed by objective records. For example, in a clinical trial involving nebulized medication for asthma (Spector *et al.*, 1986), adherence was measured by a patient diary and an electronic method which records each inhalation (Nebulizer Chronolog; Advanced Technology Products, Lakewood, Colorado). Results indicated that patients over-reported using their medication over 50% of the time. Similarly, Gordis, Markowitz and Lilienfield (1969) estimated childrens' adherence to penicillin by urine analysis and mothers' reports of adherence. They found that the former figure was significantly lower than the latter figure (42% vs 73%).

Ley (1988) discusses some of the probable reasons that patients might under-report instances of non-adherence: they might wish to intentionally deceive the researcher, they might not understand their regimen and therefore not realise that they are not adhering; or they might forget instances of non-adherence. The problem of overestimation of adherence by self-report does not make it a less popular method of assessing adherence, possibly as it is an easy method. Caron (1985) in a review of a sample of studies which had taken place between 1977 and 1983 noted that self-report were used as the sole measure, or in combination with other measures of adherence in 68% of the studies. However, different methods of self-report may yield different results. It should not be assumed that a questionnaire completed in front of a doctor who is responsible for the patient's treatment will yield similar results to longer structured interviews, which allow independent raters the chance to assess patient adherence. The different results obtained between questionnaire measures and independently rated semi-structured interviews has been noted in other areas of psychological research (e.g. Myers, 1994; Myers and Brewin, 1994; 1996).

Despite the general evidence about the unreliability of self-reports, it has been suggested that certain simple self-report measures can be used to assess and predict adherence (e.g. Kaplan and Simon, 1990; Morisky, Green and Levine, 1986). In an extensive review of the literature, Kaplan and Simon (1990) conclude that patients can be very accurate in reporting the likelihood that they will adhere to treatment if they are asked simply and directly. Morisky *et al.*(1986) reported a 4-item measurement scale to assess and predict the medication-taking behaviour of 290 hypertensive patients who had been receiving care for their high blood pressure over the last 6 years. Results of the medication adherence behaviour and blood pressure control at 2 and 5 years follow-up showed that patients who had scored high on the scale during baseline, were more likely to have their blood pressure under control than patients who scored low. The authors suggest that this simple new scale can be used to assess patients' levels of understanding and adherence behaviours, and identify specific problems which may affect adherence to the regimen.

Using the doctor's judgement

There is evidence that doctors are particularly bad at determining whether patient's have or have not taken their medication correctly and tend to substantially overestimate adherence (e.g. Brody, 1980; Caron and Roth, 1971; Mushlin and Appel, 1977). Doctors are inaccurate in their judgement of patients' adherence and they tend to overestimate any agreement between recommendations and patients' behaviour (Norell, 1981). It may be worth considering utilising other HPs judgements of adherence, as a recent study has suggested that nurses may be less biased at rating patient adherence (Edelman *et al.*, 1996)

Objective measures

The most widely used of these methods is pill counts i.e. measuring the number of pills left at a certain time (e.g. Putnam *et al.*, 1994). Although this method typically yields higher estimates of non-adherence compared with self-report measures (e.g. Park and Lipman 1964; Rickels and Briscoe, 1970), the problem with this method, apart from being intrusive, is that it does not give any indication of when the medication was taken or whether it was thrown away and thus may result in overestimation of adherence (e.g. Bergman and Werner, 1963; Ley, 1988; Roth, Caron and Hsi 1970).

Checking prescriptions

This may be achieved by checking if and when repeat prescriptions are collected from the general practitioner's surgery. However, the problem with this way of monitoring adherence is that the patient may pick up a prescription, yet not have the medicine dispensed. It has been estimated that 25–30% of repeat prescriptions are not dispensed (Bearden *et al.*, 1993; Levy, 1991). Alternatively, a check may be made on whether prescriptions are taken to a pharmacy for dispensing. Obviously, just because a patient has had a prescription dispensed does not mean that he or she is taking the medication.

Electronic measurement devices

Electronic measurement devices are becoming more widely used. There are a variety of devices which include the Unit Dose Monitor (DVA Medical Centre, St Louis, Missouri), which records the removal of tablets from a blister pack; the Medication Event Monitoring System (MEMS, Aprex Corporation, Fremont, California), which records opening of a bottle to remove medication; the Pill Box Monitor (Clinical Research Centre, Harrow) which records opening of a pill box; the Eye Drop Monitor (University of Washington, St Louis, Missouri), which records inversion of bottle to dispense liquid medication and the Nebulizer Chronolog (Advanced Technology Products, Lakewood, Colorado), for asthma medication. However, these devices still have disadvantages. Some of these devices look unobtrusive (e.g the Eye Drop Monitor), others do not (e.g. the Nebulizer Chronolog and the MEMS). This results in the probability that patients will be aware that their medication usage is being monitored. Consequently, patient behaviour may be affected. In addition, these devices can only measure that a unit of medication has been dispensed from the container, it does not necessarily mean that any medication has been taken. Devices such as MEMs are expensive. However, electronic monitors have been used in a grow-ing number of studies (e.g. Brun, 1994; Mason and Matsuyama, 1995; Wallen, Andersson and Hjemdahl, 1994; see Cramer and Spilker, 1991, for a recent review). Two recent studies compared adherence measured by self-report, pill count and MEMS (Matsui *et al.*, 1994; Walterhouse *et al.*, 1993). In both studies, self-reported adherence and pill count both indicated significantly higher adherence than MEMS, suggesting that electronic devices may be more accurate in measuring adherence than other methods.

Outcome Measures

These measures can be useful in identifying patients who fail to reach treatment goals, and the argument for using outcome as a measure is the assumption that if a patient adheres to his or her treatment regimen, they will respond better to treatment. A major difficulty, however, is the unclear relationship between adherence and outcome. Ley (1988) argues that, when investigating group differences, changes in outcome might not be particularly responsive to changes in adherence. For example, if a change in adherence needs to be around 25% for a measurable change in outcome, then this method will not be able to measure quite large differences in adherence. It has been reported that approximately 60% of patients who took their medication as directed did not achieve their optimal blood pressure and between 16–28% of patients who did not adhere properly did achieve the required blood pressure (Lowenthal *et al.*, 1976; Sackett, 1979). However, the inclusion of outcome measures in adherence studies can help determine the degree of adherence necessary to ensure optimal benefits of the therapeutic treatment. See Noble, Chapter 3 for further discussion of this issue.

Direct methods

Direct methods include measuring blood levels or urinary excretion of medication. However, as noted by Gordis (1979), these methods are fraught with difficulties. There are genetic differences in how individuals absorb, metabolise and excrete drugs. In addition, the form in which the drug is administered has a major effect on absorption, with aqueous solutions and syrups being the most rapid and coated tablets being the slowest. Blood and urine levels will only be assessed during clinic visits. Hence, Ley (1988) argues that it is conceivable that patients may take their medications as prescribed for a day or two before their appointment, leading to drug levels that suggest better adherence than is the case. Furthermore, direct methods may not be acceptable to patients and such measures are often expensive.

Direct observation

Direct observation of patients has seldomly been used, with the exception of antitubercular treatment, (see Gourevitch *et al.*, 1996). However, this is undertaken to increase adherence to the tuberculosis treatment rather than as an objective measure of adherence. Direct observation has been used to monitor adherence in children with diabetes (see Bryon, Chapter 7).

WHEN IS A PATIENT NON-ADHERENT?

Ley and Llewelyn (1995) note that adherence to medication has been defined in a variety of ways: "not taking enough medication, taking too much medication, not observing the correct interval between doses, not observing the correct duration of treatment and taking additional non-prescribed medication. Advice about lifestyle changes such as dieting and giving up smoking has used analogous definitions".

Who should be labelled as non-adherent during a course of treatment? Is someone who misses one dose of medication non-adherent? As in most aspects of adherence research, there is a lack of consensus. For example, Gordis *et al.* (1969) defined adherence to a course of penicillin when 75% of urine tested was positive for the drug. Mäenpää *et al.* (1987) defined good adherence as 85% by pill count. Black *et al.* (1987) defined adherence as patients having removed at least 80% of the prescribed tablets. Peterson, McLean and Millengen (1984) identified non-adherence to anticonvulsant therapy as at least one subtherapeutic plasma level of medication and having the prescription dispensed at least one week later than expected.

Donovan and Blake (1992), in a study of rheumatic patients, identified different forms of non-adherence. Some patients were totally non-adherent and stopped taking their drugs; some took fewer tablets than prescribed, either by reducing the dose or taking the tablets fewer times per day; and some took more tablets than prescribed, although this was less common. Similarly, Ried and Christensen (1988) in a study of antibiotic adherence noted that some patients finished their medication but missed at least one dose during therapy and others did not complete the course.

A recent report on the problems of non-adherence by the Royal Pharmaceutical Society of Great Britain noted that there is no recognised or accepted definition of non-adherence: "apart from failure to have medicines dispensed, most departures from adherence are partial, not total. Terms like *poor* or *incomplete* or *inadequate* adherence are probably better descriptive of the problems" (Royal Pharmaceutical Society of Great Britain/Merck Sharpe and Dohme, 1996).

In some medical conditions, adherence is very complex. For example, in diabetes treatment different aspects may include medication, glucose testing, diet and exercise (for a discussion of adherence in diabetes, see Warren and Hixenbaugh, Chapter 16). In a prospective study of outpatients with insulin dependent diabetes, Glasgow, McCaul and Schafer (1987) found few strong relationships between adherence in different areas of the regimen. Similarly, Kravitz *et al.* (1993) noted that most individuals with diabetes took their medication, over half followed their diet but only around a fifth engaged in regular exercise.

IS NON-ADHERENCE A PROBLEM IN SERIOUS CONDITIONS? THE EXAMPLE OF ORGAN TRANSPLANTS.

Is non-adherence a problem in conditions which are life-threatening, or is it confined to less serious conditions? A number of adherence studies in patients who have received an organ transplant indicate that these patients are just as likely to be non-adherent, even though non-adherence to the medical regimen can lead to rejection of the organ or death of the patient.

Didlake *et al.* (1988) reported non-adherence to be the third leading cause of renal transplant rejection. Kiley, Lam and Pollak (1993) report unpublished data suggesting that non-adherence to the treatment regimen is a common cause of renal transplant failure in approximately 78% of patients in their second year after transplant.

Most research studies on adherence to organ transplant have used outcome measures rather than direct measures (e.g. Dew *et al.*, 1996). However, there is some evidence that non-adherence to clinic appointments, blood tests, and diet and exercise regimes is more prevalent than non-adherence to medication intake (Erdman *et al.*, 1993).

Rovelli *et al.* (1989) assessed adherence to immunosuppressive medications in organ transplant recipients in two studies: a retrospective review and a prospective study. In the retrospective review of 260 patients who had received kidney transplants, they assessed whether patients kept follow-up appointments and whether they had been adherent in taking immunosuppressant medication. Medication adherence was measured by self-report by patient, family report and doctor's judgement. From our previous discussion, it may be assumed that using self-report and doctor's judgement as measures would probably result in an overestimation of adherence. With this limitation in mind, the researchers found that 18% of patients were considered to be non-adherent to both follow-ups and medication. Three months post-transplant, 91% of these patients either rejected or died compared with 18% of adherent patients.

Kiley *et al.* (1993) carried out a retrospective study which investigated the incidence of non-adherence in kidney transplant patients. Non-adherence to immunosuppressant medication was measured by self-report and blood level of the drug at clinic visits. Adherence to diet was measured by body weight and self-report. Twenty six percent of patients were classified as non-adherent to medication; 23% were classified as non-adherent to diet and 28% were classified as non-adherent to both diet and medication.

Rovelli *et al.* (1989) carried out a further prospective study which involved 196 patients in a pre-transplant education program, with a simplified post-transplant medicine regimen. Fifteen percent of patients were considered non-adherent, with 30% of non-adherent patients rejecting or dying compared to 1% of the adherent patients. The researchers noted that: "even when graft loss meant loss of life, such as in heart and liver transplantation, medication non-compliance occurred. In our heart transplant recipients, 2/38 (5%) were noncompliant: one died....after one week of taking no immunosuppression: one has chronic rejection. Three of nine (33%) liver transplant recipients were non compliant and 2 died". The authors conclude that "medication non-compliance is a major and often unrecognised cause of graft rejection and death".

More recently, Dew *et al.* (1996) followed up 101 patients for 12 months after heart transplantation. Adherence was assessed by self-report, and corroboration by family members and nurses at 2, 7, and 12 months after transplantation. Eight areas of adherence were assessed: medication intake, clinic appointments, blood tests and monitoring blood pressure, exercise, diet, smoking and drinking habits. Even though adherence was measured by self-report, non-adherence for the various aspects of post-transplant care was relatively high. For a year post-transplant, non-adherence was rated as 20 to 25% for medication, 37% for exercise; 34% for monitoring blood pressure, 19% for smoking and 18% for diet. Non-adherence in most areas increased significantly over time, and only 7% showed complete adherence in all areas at 12 month follow-up.

POSSIBLE REASONS FOR NON-ADHERENCE

"I went to the doctor with a bad cough which had come on after I had a bad cold and it just wouldn't go away. The doctor gave me antibiotic pills which I had to take three times a day for one week. I took them for three days and then I stopped because I felt better. A few days later my chest felt really bad again and I couldn't breathe properly, so I took the rest of the pills. But I still didn't feel well, so I went back to the doctor and he gave me some more antibiotic pills. I didn't tell him that I hadn't taken all of the first pills."

This was related to a community pharmacist. The example serves to illustrate a number of possible reasons for non-adherence.

Information

The information that the patient needed to take the whole course may not have been impressed on her. In the UK, the bottle label would say "complete the course", but possibly the patient did not or could not read it. (e.g. Ley, 1982; 1988; Ley and Llewelyn, 1995; see

Raynor, Chapter 4 for a discussion of the influence of written information on adherence).

Memory

It is possible that the doctor told the patient to take the course of medicine and the patient forgot (retrospective memory, see Park and Kidder, 1996, for a recent review). Alternatively, the patient may have had problems in remembering the intention to take the medicine (prospective memory is concerned with remembering to do something at an appropriate moment; see Park and Kidder, 1996 for a review, and Ellis, Chapter 5 for a discussion on prospective memory and medicine taking).

Doctor-patient communication

There may have been a breakdown in communication between doctor and patient (e.g. Heszen-Klemens, 1987; Ley, 1988; see Noble, Chapter 3 for a discussion of doctor-patient communication).

Patient's beliefs and cognitions

Maybe the patient had certain beliefs about the medication. Amongst a variety of patients' characteristics, beliefs and cognitions have been widely researched as possible predictors of adherence to treatment. The most common theoretical models of cognitive-motivational predictors of adherence are discussed by Horne and Weinman, Chapter 2.

ADDITIONAL REASONS FOR NON-ADHERENCE

Characteristics of the patient

The great majority of studies fail to find an association between adherence and patients' sociodemographic variables (for reviews see Haynes *et al.*, 1979; Kaplan and Simon, 1990; Meichenbaum and Turk, 1987). For example, there is no consistent pattern of an association between adherence and gender (e.g. Buchanan, 1996; Haynes *et al.*, 1979b) or age (Buchanan, 1996; Haynes *et al.*, 1979b; Ley, 1988, Owens, Larrat and Fretwell, 1991). For a discussion of adherence in children, see Bryon Chapter 7 and for a discussion of adherence in the elderly, see McElnay and McCallion, Chapter 9. Ley (1979), in a review of the literature, concluded that patients' socio-demographic and personality characteristics were not related to adherence. In a review of papers published between 1979 and 1988, Kaplan and Simon (1990) concluded that traditional measures of personality characteristics are poor predictors of adherence. For a discussion about patient characteristics in asthma and attendance at follow-up appointments, see Hand, Chapter 15.

Characteristics of the physician

Studies have indicated that physician characteristics are not related to adherence (DiMatteo *et al.*, 1993; Ley, 1979). However, DiMatteo *et al.* (1993) in a two year prospective study of physician characteristics in relation to adherence to medication, diet and exercise, found that adherence was related to physician job satisfaction. Adherence to medication was related to the number of patients seen per week, and whether physicians made definite future appointments (or telephone calls) for follow-up. The more tests the physician ordered at a screening visit, the more likely patients were to adhere to dietary recommendations. Adherence to exercise was related to the tendency of physician to answer patients' questions no matter how long it took.

Characteristics of the treatment

A review by Haynes (1979b) indicates that features of the disease are not important determinants of adherence except that increasing symptoms may be accompanied by decreasing adherence and increased disability may be associated with increased adherence. Correlations were found between adherence and the duration of therapy and the complexity of the regimen as assessed by the number of drugs for treatment which were involved. Attendance at referral appointment was related to time from referral to appointment and the likelihood of clinic attendance was correlated with waiting time. Cockburn *et al.* (1987) found an association between adherence and the complexity of the treatment. Patients who did not adhere tended to have a more complex treatment regimen, and found it difficult to fit the dosage schedule into their daily routine.

ADHERENCE AND HEALTH OUTCOMES IN CLINICAL TRIALS

Clinical trials are designed to test the efficacy of new treatment and adherence is extremely important in this respect. It would be expected that adherence would be important for patients who receive the active drug but would have no effect in patients who receive placebo. However, in a review of a number of randomised, placebo-controlled trials, Horwitz and Horwitz (1993) concluded that "patients who adhere to treatment, even when the treatment is a placebo, have better outcomes than poorly adherent patients". For example, the Beta Blocker Heart Attack Trial (BHAT; 1982), was a multicentre randomized, double-blind trial comparing propranolol, a beta blocker, with placebo in patients who had survived an acute myocardial infarction. Horwitz *et al.* (1990) analysed the relationship between treatment adherence and mortality after a myocardial infarction amongst 2175 patients in the BHAT. Adherence was measured by pill count, and was defined as taking at least 75% of the medication. Adherent patients had a 1 year mortality rate of 2.2%, compared to 5.4% for non-adherent patients. This ratio was similar both for patients receiving the active drug (adherers 1.4%, non-adherers, 4.2%) and placebo (adherers 3.0%, non-adherers 7.0%). Results indicated that the differences in outcome between adherers and non-adherers could not be explained by the severity of the disease. One of the possible explanations for these results is that adherence may create the expectation that the treatment will be effective, hence patients will engage in other health behaviours which, in turn, will lead to better clinical health outcome (Horwitz and Horwitz, 1993; Kaplan, Sallis and Patterson, 1993). So, good adherers in the BHAT trial may have increased their exercise, lowered their stress levels and changed to a healthier diet.

ADHERENCE IN HEALTH PROFESSIONALS

In this chapter we have, so far, been discussing adherence in patients. However, there is an implicit assumption that HPs adhere to recommendations. Research indicates that this is not the case (see Ley, 1988 for a comprehensive review).

A number of studies indicate that physicians do not adhere to correct prescription protocols. For example, Schleifer *et al.* (1991) conducted a 26 week follow-up study of 170 women with a recent diagnosis of breast cancer, who were receiving chemotherapy. Fifty six percent of patients received unjustified changes to at least one of their medications. Cohen, Berner and Dubach (1985) noted that 50% of patients whose blood pressure indicated that they should receive treatment for hypertension were not treated. Two studies indicated that over 60% of patients received antibiotics in an inappropriate way (Sheckler and Bennett, 1970; Roberts and Visconti, 1972). Physician non-adherence can obviously have serious consequences. Peeters *et al.* (1988) reported that physicians' inability to adhere to the recommended protocol of therapy for treating children with lymphoblastic leukaemia was associated with a higher relapse rate of the disease.

Physician non-adherence is not confined to medication prescribing. Adherence rates of only 20% have been noted for infection control procedures (Miramontes, 1990) and for giving appropriate dietary advice to hypercholesterolaemia patients (Levin and Ornstein, 1990). For preventive care guidelines, only 36% of medical interns were found to adhere to recommended guidelines in diabetes (Nilasena and Lincoln, 1995). Physician adherence to USA annual mammography guidelines has been reported to be 57% (Costanza *et al.,* 1992).

Non-adherence has been noted in other HPs. In an early study (Hofling *et al.,* 1966), ninety five percent of nurses failed to adhere to an agreed protocol and accepted a telephone call for a medication made by an unknown physician. More recently, 50% of nurses did not adhere to infection control procedures (Miramontes, 1990). In a study of sixteen dental practices in the USA, it was reported that 66% of patients did not receive adequate shielding from x-rays. (Greene and Neistat, 1983). In a survey of 271 pharmacies by the Food and Drug Administration, 61% of pharmacists did not adhere to regulations to give Patient Packet Inserts (PPIs) when dispensing products containing oestrogens, if a PPI was not requested by the patient (Morris *et al.,* 1980). For a discussion of adherence in obstetric, nursing and midwifery staff, see Rosenblatt, Chapter 8.

CONCLUDING REMARKS

After more than thirty years of research, non-adherence remains a serious and widespread problem. At a very basic level, there is little agreement about terminology. Should we use the term compliance or adherence, as we have already discussed, or is it preferable to use one of the newer terms such as "co-operation" (Kaplan *et al.,* 1993) or "concordance" (Royal Pharmaceutical Society of Great Britain/ Merck Sharp and Dohme, 1997)? If clinicians and researchers cannot agree on suitable terminology on the topic they are investigating, how are they going to agree about anything else? Similarly, this chapter has highlighted a number of fundamental problems which are yet to be resolved e.g. "how should adherence be measured" and "what level of adherence is non-adherence?"

One of the reasons for a lack of consensus on these basic definitions may be that researchers and clinicians come from a wide variety of backgrounds and training e.g. doctors, dentists, pharmacists, psychologists, physiotherapists, nurses, dieticians and medical sociologists. Hence, different HPs will approach the problem from different perspectives. McGavock (1996) has rightly pointed out that "a fundamental problem is the absence of any co-ordinated research methodology; different researchers have looked at different factors, using different techniques and different experimental designs for different periods of study".

However, the diversity of backgrounds should be seen as a strength rather than a weakness. In future, it would be sensible for the many HPs tackling the problem of non-adherence to pool resources and approach the problem from a multidisciplinary point of view, leading to harmonised definitions and agreed research methods. In addition, we need closer collaboration between clinicians, researchers and *patients* in our efforts to develop effective methods to minimise the problem of non-adherence.

REFERENCES

Bearden, P.H.G., McGilchrist, N.M., McKendrick, A.D., McDevitt, D.G. and Mcdonald, T.M. (1993) Primary non-compliance with prescribed medication in primary care. *British Medical Journal* **307**, 846–848.

Bergman, A.B. and Werner, R.J. (1963) Failure of children to receive penicillin by mouth. *New England Journal Of Medicine* **268**, 1334–133.

Beta Blocker Heart Attack Trial Research Group. (1982) A randomized trial of propranolol in patients with acute myocardial infarction. *Journal of the American Medical Association* **247**, 1707–1714.

Black, D.M., Brand, R.J., Greenlick, M., Hughes., G. and Smith, J. (1987) Compliance to treatment for hypertension in elderly patients. *Journal of Gerontology* **42**, 552–557.

Blackwell, B. (1973) Patient compliance. *New England Journal of Medicine* **289**, 249–253.

Brody, D.S. (1980) An analysis of patients' recall of their therapeutic regimen. *Journal of Chronic Diseases* **33**, 57–63.

Brun, J. (1994) Patient compliance with once-daily and twice-daily oral formulations of 5-isosorbide mononitrate: a comparative study. *Journal of International Medical Research* **22**, 266–72.

Buchanan, A. (1996) *Compliance with treatment in schizophrenia.* London: Psychology Press.

Caron, H.S. (1985) Compliance: the case for objective measurement. *Journal of Hypertension (suppl. 1)* **3**, 11–17.

Caron, H.S. and Roth, H.P. (1971) Patients' co-operation with a medical regimen. *Journal of the American Medical Association* **203**, 922–926.

Cockburn, J., Gibberd, R.W., Reid, A.L. and Sanson-Fisher, R.W. (1987) Determinants of noncompliance with short-term antibiotic regimens. *British Medical Journal* **295**, 814–818.

Cohen, D., Berner, U. and Dubach, U.C. (1985) Physician compliance in the management of hypertensive patients. *Journal of Hypertension (suppl.3)* **3**, S73–76.

Costanza, M.E., Stoddard, A.M., Zapka, J.G., Gaw, V.P. and Barth, R. (1992) Physician compliance with mammography guidelines: barriers and enhancers. *Journal of the American Board of Family Practice* **5**, 143–152.

Cramer, J.A. and Spilker, B. (eds.) (1991) *Patient compliance in medical practice and clinical trials.* Raven Press: New York.

Davis, M.S. (1966) Variations in patients' compliance with doctors' advice: analysis of congruence between survey responses and results of empirical observations *Journal of Medical Education* **41**, 1037–1048.

Davis, M.S. (1968) Physiologic, psychological and demographic factors in patient's compliance to doctors' orders. *Medical Care* **6**, 115–122.

Department of Health and Human Services, (1980) Prescription drug products: patient packet insert requirements. *Federal Register* **45**, 60754–60817.

Dew, M.A., Roth, L.H., Thompson, M.E., Kormos,. R.L. and Griffith, B.P. (1996) Medical compliance and its predictors in the first year after heart-transplantation. *Journal of Heart and Lung Transplantation* **15**, 631–645.

Didlake, R.H. Dreyfus, K., Kerman, R.H., van Buren , C.T. and Kahan, B.T. (1988) Patient noncompliance – a major cause of late graft failure in cyclosporine treated renal transplants. *Transplantation Proceedings* **20**, 63–66.

DiMatteo, M.R. and DiNicola D.D., (1982) *Achieving patient compliance: the psychology of the medical practitioners role.* New York: Pergamon Press.

DiMatteo, M.R., Sherbourne, C.D., Hays, R.D., Ordway, L., Kravitz, R.L., McGlynn, E.A., Kaplan, S. and Rogers, W. (1993) Physicians characteristics influence patients' adherence to medical treatment Results from the medical outcomes study. *Health Psychology* **12**, 93–102.

Donovan, J.C.L. and Blake, D.R. (1992) Patient non-compliance: deviance or reasoned decision-making. *Social Science and Medicine* **34**, 507–513.

Edelman, R., Eitel, P., Wadhwa, N.K., Friend,R., Suh, H., Howell, N., Cabralda, T., Jao, E. and Aprileforlenza, S. (1996) Accuracy or bias in nurses ratings of patient compliance – a comparison of treatment modality. *Peritoneal Dialysis International* **16**, 321–325.

Erdman, R.A.M., Horstman, L., Van Domburg, R.T., Metter, K. and Balk, A.H.H.M. (1993) Compliance with the medical regimen and partner's quality of life after heart transplantation. *Quality of Life Research* **2**, 205–212.

Fletcher, R.H. (1989) Patient compliance with therapeutic advice: a modern view. *The Mount Sinai Journal of Medicine* **56**, 453–458.

Gibbons, A. (1992) Exploring new strategies to fight drug-resistant microbes. *Science* **257**, 1036–1038.

Glasgow, R.E., McCaul, K.D., and Schafer, L.C. (1987) Self-care behaviors and glycemic control in Type 1 diabetes. *Journal of Chronic Diseases* **40**, 399–412.

Gordis. L. (1979) Conceptual and methodologic problems in measuring patient compliance. In R.B. Haynes, D.W. Taylor, and D.L. Sackett (eds.) *Compliance in health care*. Baltimore: Johns Hopkins University Press.

Gordis, L., Markowitz, P.H.M. and Lilienfield, A.M. (1969) The inaccuracy in using interviews to estimate patient reliability in taking medications at home. *Medical Care* **7**, 49–54.

Gourevitch, M.N., Wasserman, W., Panero, M.S. and Selwyn, P.A. (1996) Successful adherence to observed prophylaxis and treatment of tuberculosis among drug-users in a methadone program. *Journal of Addictive Diseases* **15**, 93–104.

Greene, B.F. and Neistat, M.D. (1983) Behavior analysis in consumer affairs: encouraging dental professionals to provide consumers with shielding from unnecessary x-ray exposure. *Journal of Applied Behavior Analysis* **16**, 13–27.

Haynes, R.B. (1979a) Introduction. In R.B. Haynes, D.W. Taylor and D.L. Sackett (eds.) *Compliance in health care*. Baltimore: Johns Hopkins University Press.

Haynes, R.B. (1979b) Determinants of compliance: the disease and the mechanics of treatment. In R.B. Haynes, D.W. Taylor and D.L. Sackett (eds.) *Compliance in health care*. Baltimore: Johns Hopkins University Press.

Haynes, R.B., Taylor, D.W., Snow, J.C. and Sackett, D.L. (1979a) Annotated and indexed bibliography on compliance with therapeutic and preventive regimens. In R.B. Haynes, D.W. Taylor and D.L. Sackett (eds.) *Compliance in health care*. Baltimore: Johns Hopkins University Press.

Haynes, R.B., Taylor, D.W. and Sackett D.L. (eds.) (1979b) *Compliance in health care*. Baltimore: Johns Hopkins University Press.

Heszen-Klemens, I. (1987) Patients' noncompliance and how doctors manage this. *Social Science and Medicine* **24**, 409–416.

Hofling, C.K., Brotzman, E., Dalrymple, S., Graves, N. and Pierce, C.M. (1966) An experimental study in nurse-physician relationships. *Journal of Nervous and Mental Diseases* **143**, 171–180.

Horwitz, R.I. and Horwitz, S.M. (1993) Adherence to treatment and health outcomes. *Archives of Internal Medicine* **153**, 1863–1868.

Horwitz, R.I., Viscoli, C.M., Berkman, L., Donalson, R.M., Horwitz, S.M., Murray, C.J., Ransohoff, D.F. and Sindelar, J. (1990) Treatment adherence and risk of death after a myocardial infarction. *Lancet* **336**, 542–545.

Kaplan, R.M. Sallis, J.F. and Patterson, T.L. (1993) *Health and human behavior.* New York: McGraw-Hill.

Kaplan, R.M. and Simon, H.J. (1990) Compliance in medical care: reconsideration of self-predictions. *Annals of Behavioral Medicine* **12**, 66–71.

Kiley, D.J., Lam, C.S. and Pollak, R. (1993) A study of treatment compliance following kidney transplantation. *Transplantation* **55**, 51–56.

Koltun, A and Stone, G.C. (1986) Past and current trends in patient non-compliance research: focus on diseases, regimen programs and provider disciplines. *Journal of Compliance in Health Care* **1**, 21–32.

Kravitz,R. L, Hays, R.D., Sherbourne, C.D., DiMatteo, M.R., Rogers, H., Ordway L. and Greenfield (1993) Recall of recommendations and adherence to advice among patients with chronic medical conditions. *Archives of Internal Medicine* **153**, 1869–1878.

Leventhal, H. (1993) Theories of compliance, and turning necessities into preferences: application to adolescent health action. In N.A. Krasnegor, L. Epstein, S.B. Johnson and S.J. Yaffe (eds.) *Developmental aspects of health behaviour.* New Jersey: Lawrence Erlbaum Associates.

Leventhal, H., Diefenbach, M. and Leventhal, E.A. (1992) Illness cognition: using common sense to understand treatment adherence and affect cognition interactions. *Cognitive Therapy and Research* **16**, 143–163.

Levy, R.A. (1991) Failure to refill prescriptions. In J.A. Cramer and B. Spilker (eds.) *Patient compliance in medical practice and clinical trials.* New York: Raven Press.

Ley, P. (1988) *Communicating with patients.* London: Croom Helm.

Ley, P (1982) Satisfaction, compliance and communication. *British Journal of Clinical Psychology* **21**, 241–254.

Ley, P (1979) The psychology of compliance. in D.J. Oborne., M.M. Gruneberg. and J.R. Eiser (eds.) *Research into psychology and medicine. Vol. 2* London: Academic Press.

Levin, S.J. and Ornstein, S.M. (1990) Management of hypercholesterolemia in a family practice setting. *Journal of Family Practice* **31**, 613–617.

Ley, P. and Llewelyn, S. (1995) Improving patients' understanding, recall, satisfaction and compliance. In A. Broome and S.Llewelyn (eds.) *Health psychology: processes and applications. Second Edition.* London: Chapman and Hall.

Lowenthal, D.T., Briggs, W.A., Mutterperl, R., Adelman, B. and Creditor, M.A.. (1976) Patient compliance for antihypertensive medication: the usefulness of urine assays, *Current Therapeutic Research* **19**, 405–9.

Mäenpää, H., Javela, K., Pikkarainan, J., Mälköne, M., Heinonen, O.P. and Manninen, V. (1987) Minimal doses of digoxin: a new marker for compliance to medication. *European Heart Journal (suppl. 1)* **8**, 31–37.

Mason, B.J. and Matsuyama, J.R. (1995) Assessment of sulfonyurea, adherence and metabolic control. *Diabetes Education* **21**, 52–57.

Matsui, D., Hermann, C., Klein, J., Berkovitch.M., Olivier, N. and Oren, G., (1994) Critical comparison of novel and existing methods of compliance assessment during a clinical trial of an oral iron chelator. *Journal of Clinical Pharmacology* **34**, 944–949.

McGavock, H. (1996) *A review of the literature on drug adherence.* The Royal Pharmaceutical Society of Great Britain.

Meichenbaum, D and Turk, D.C. (1987) *Facilitating treatment adherence: a practitioners guidebook.* New York: Plenum Press.

Miramontes, H. (1990) Progress in establishing safety protocols on CDC and OHSA recommendations. *Infectious Control and Hospital Epidemiology (suppl. 10)* **11**, 561–2.

Morisky, D.E., Green, L.W. and Levine, D.M. (1986) Concurrent and predictive validity of a self-reported measure of medication adherence. *Medical Care* **24**, 67–74.

Morell, R.W., Park, D.C. and Poon, L.W. (1989) Quality of instruction on prescription drug labels: effects on memory and comprehension in young and old adults. *The Gerontologist* **29**, 345–353.

Morris, L.A., Myers, A., Gibbs, P. and Lao, S. (1980) Estrogen PPIs: an FDA survey. *American Pharmacy* **NS20**, 22–26.

Mushlin, A.I. and Appel., F.A. (1977) Diagnosing patient noncompliance. *Archives of Internal Medicine* **137**, 318–321.

Myers, L.B. (1994) Repressive coping: perceived parental attitudes and story recall. *Proceedings of the British Psychological Society* **2**, 44.

Myers, L.B. and Brewin, C.R. (1994) Recall of early experience and the repressive coping style. *Journal of Abnormal Psychology* **103**, 288–292.

Myers, L.B. and Brewin, C.R. (1996) Illusions of well-being and the repressive coping style. *British Journal of Social Psychology* **33**, 443–457.

Nilasena, D.S. and Lincoln, M.J. (1995) A computer-generated reminder system improves physician compliance with diabetes preventive care guidelines. *Proceedings of the Annual Symposium of Computing as Applied to Medical Care* **56**, 640–645.

Norell, S.E. (1981) Accuracy of patient interviews and estimates by clinical staff determining medication compliance. *Social Science and Medicine* **15**, 57–61.

Owens, N.J., Larrat, E.P. and Fretwell, M.D. (1991) Improving compliance in the order patient: the role of comprehensive functional assessment. In J.A.. Cramer and B. Spilker (eds.) *Patient compliance in medical practice and clinical trials*. New York: Raven Press.

Park, D.C. and Kidder, D.P. (1996) Prospective memory and medication adherence. In M. Brandimonte, G. Einstein and M. McDaniel (eds.) *Prospective memory: theory and application*. New Jersey: Lawrence Erlbaum Associates.

Park, L.C. and Lipman, R.S., (1964) A comparison of patient dosage deviation reports with pill counts. *Psychopharmacologia* **6**, 299–302.

Peeters, M., Koren, G., Jacubovicz, D. and Zipursky, A (1988) Physician compliance and relapse rates of acute lymphoblastic leukaemia in children. *Clinical Pharmacology and Therapeutics* **43**, 228–232.

Peterson, G.M., McLean, S. and Millengen, K.S. (1984) A randomised trial of strategies to improve patient compliance with anticonvulsant therapy. *Epilepsia* **25**, 412–417.

Putnam, D.E., Finney, J.W., Barkley, P.L. and Bonner, M.J. (1994) Enhancing commitment improves adherence to a medical regimen. *Journal of Consulting and Clinical Psychology* **62**, 191–194.

Rickels, K. and Briscoe, E., (1970) Assessment of dosage deviation in outpatient drug research. *Journal of Clinical Pharmacology* **10**, 153–60.

Ried, L.D. and Christensen, D.B. (1988) A psychosocial perspective in the explanation of patients' drug-taking behavior. *Social Science and Medicine* **27**, 277–285.

Roberts, A.W. and Visconti, J.A. (1972) The rational and irrational use of systemic anti-microbial drugs. *American Journal of Hospital Pharmacy* **29**, 1054–1060.

Roth, H.P., Caron, H.S. and Hsi, B.P. (1970) Measuring intake of a prescribed medication: A bottle count and a tracer technique compared. *Clinical Pharmacology and Therapeutics*, **2**, 228–237.

Rovelli, .M., Palmeri, D., Vossler, E., Bartus, S., Hull, D. and Shweizer, R. (1989). Compliance in organ transplant recipients. *Transplantation Proceedings* **21**, 833–844.

Royal Pharmaceutical Society of Great Britain/ Merck Sharpe and Dohme, (1997) *From compliance to concordance. Achieving shared goals in medicine taking.*

Royal Pharmaceutical Society of Great Britain/ Merck Sharpe and Dohme, (1996) *Partnership in medicine taking.*

Sackett, D.L. (1979) A compliance practicim for the busy practitioner. In R.B. Haynes, D.W. Taylor and D.L. Sackett (eds.) *Compliance in health care.* Baltimore: Johns Hopkins University Press.

Sackett, D.L. and Snow, J.C. (1979) The magnitude of compliance and noncompliance. In R.B. Haynes, D.W. Taylor, and D.L. Sackett (eds.) *Compliance in health care.* Baltimore: Johns Hopkins University Press.

Scheckler, W.E. and Bennett, J.V. (1970) Antibiotic usage in seven hospitals. *Journal of the American Medical Association* **213**, 264–267.

Schleifer, S.J., Bhardwaj, S., Lebovits, A., Tanaka, J.S., Messe, M. and Strain, J.J. (1991) Predictors of physician nonadherence to chemotherapy regimens. *Cancer* **67**, 945–951.

Schlenk, E.A. and Hart, L.K. (1984) Relationship between health locus of control, health value, and social support and compliance with diabetes mellitus. *Diabetes Care* **7**, 566–574.

Spector, S.L., Kinsman,R., Mawhinney,H., Siegel., S.C., Radhelesfsky, G.S., Katz, R.M. and Rohr, A.S. (1986) Compliance of patients with asthma with an experimental aerolized medication: implications for controlled clinical trials. *Journal of Allergy and Clinical Immunology* **77,** 65–70.

Stimson, G.V (1974) Obeying doctor's orders: a view from the other side. *Social Science and Medicine* **8,** 97–104.

Varni, J.W. and Wallander, J.L. (1984) Adherence to health-related regimes in pediatric chronic disorders. *Clinical Psychology Review* **4,** 585–596.

Wallen, N.H., Andersson, A. and Hjemdahl, P. (1994) Effects of treatment with oral isosorbide dinitrate on platelet function in vivo: a double-blind placebo-controlled study in patients with stable angina pectoris. *British Journal of Clinical Psychology* **38,** 63–70.

Walterhouse, D.M., Calzone, K.A., Mele, C. and Brenner, D.E. (1993) Adherence to oral tamoxifen: a comparison of patient self report, pill counts and microelectronic monitoring. *Journal of Clinical Oncology* **11,** 2547–8.

General issues in adherence to treatment

2

Predicting Treatment Adherence: an Overview of Theoretical Models

Robert Horne and John Weinman

Developments in health and social psychology have contributed several theoretical frameworks or models for explaining variations in health-related behaviours which can be applied to treatment adherence. These can be grouped under three broad categories: Social Cognition Models and Stage Models (see Conner and Norman, 1996) and Leventhal's Self-Regulatory Theory (Leventhal, Meyer and Nerenz, 1980). This chapter provides a brief outline of the salient features of these approaches and provides examples of where they have been applied to adherence.

SOCIAL COGNITION MODELS

Social Cognition Models (SCMs) are theoretical approaches to understanding health-related behaviour. They share a common assumption that attitudes and beliefs are major determinants of behaviour. Many use an expectancy-value approach in which behaviour in response to health threats or information arises from an active decision based on two types of cognition. These are: (1) expectancies or beliefs about the probability that a specific action (e.g. taking medication) will lead to a set of outcomes (e.g. improved health) and (2) the subjective value placed on them. Some SCMs, such as the Health Belief Model (e.g. Rosenstock, 1974) have been specifically developed to explain health-related behaviours, others, such as the Theory of Reasoned Action (Ajzen and Fishbein, 1980) are derived from general models of behaviour.

The Health Belief Model

The health belief model (HBM) was developed to explain why people failed to take up disease prevention measures or screening tests before the onset of symptoms (Rosenstock, 1974). The original model proposed that the likelihood of someone carrying out a particular health behaviour (e.g. attending for screening) was a function of their personal beliefs about the perceived *threat* of the disease and an assessment of the *risk/benefits* of the recommended course of action. Perceived threat is derived from beliefs about the perceived *seriousness* of the threat and the individuals perceived *susceptibility* to it. The individual then weighs up the perceived *benefits* of an action (e.g. screening will detect problems at an early stage) against the perceived *barriers* to the action (e.g. difficulty in finding time to attend screening). A further component was included by Becker and Maiman (1975) who stipulated that a *cue to action* or stimulus must occur to trigger the behaviour. The HBM has been modified several times to include additional variables such as general health motivation as shown in Figure 1. Thus, the HBM predicts that the likelihood of action is increased if the perceived threat of the disease is high, if the benefits of behaviour are thought to outweigh the barriers, and if certain cues are in place.

The original HBM is directed towards the individual's desire to avoid a specific disease threat. Several revisions have been made to this original model by including modifying factors as listed below:

• General health motivations which are seen as fairly non-specific
• Personal attributes which are stable across situation.
• Resusceptibility to an illness previously contacted and currently under consideration.
• General orientation towards medicine.
• Characteristics of the doctor-patient relationship.

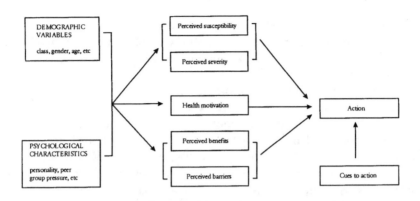

FIGURE 1 The health belief model (adapted from Sheeran and Abraham, 1996)

The HBM or its components have been utilised in a large number of research studies investigating health-related behaviours (see Sheeran and Abraham, 1996, for a useful review). Studies on adherence have included adherence to dietary recommendations (e.g. Caggiula and Watson, 1992; Urban *et al.*, 1992), breast self-examination (e.g. Calnan, 1984) and dental behaviour (e.g. Barker, 1994; Chen and Land, 1986). The HBM has also been used in studies investigating medication adherence across a range of illnesses including hypertension (e.g. Nelson *et al.*, 1978; Taylor, 1979), diabetes (e.g. Alogna, 1980; Bloom-Cerkoney and Hart, 1980; Brownlee-Duffeck *et al.*, 1987), kidney disease (e.g. Cummings, 1981) and psychiatric disorders (e.g. Budd *et al.*, 1996; Hogan, Awad and Eastwood, 1983; Kelly, Mamon and Scott, 1987; Pan and Tantum, 1989).

Although several studies have demonstrated the value of interventions based on the HBM in facilitating health-related behaviours such as attending for medical check-ups (Haefner and Kirscht, 1970) or using emergency care facilities in an acute asthma attack (Jones, Jones and Katz, 1987) few studies have applied this model to interventions to enhance medication adherence.

It is difficult to draw firm conclusions about the viability of the model because of differences in the way in which it has been operationalised and applied across studies. In the main, the HBM seems to work best when it is used as originally intended as a predictive model for preventive behaviours (Janz and Becker, 1984). A meta-analysis of studies relating the HBM to preventive health behaviours found that on average 24% of variation in behaviour was accounted for by combined HBM variables (Zimmerman and Vernberg, 1994). However, in more stringent perspective studies, HBM variables predicted much lower proportions of variance in health behaviours (see Abraham and Sheeran, 1997).

The available evidence supports the notion that our understanding of adherence may be enhanced by examining patients own ideas about their illness and treatment, and suggests that the cognitive variables specified in the HBM may be prerequisites of adherence in some situations. However, other cognitions are also likely to be salient. One limitation of the HBM is that it simplifies health-related cognitions into broad constructs such as "barriers" and "benefits", without specifying the beliefs underlying these constructs. A more detailed investigation of how individuals conceptualise these constructs may provide a fuller understanding of adherence decisions (Horne, 1997; Horne and Weinman, 1994). A further limitation of the HBM is that it fails to include an intention stage between beliefs and behaviour and does not specify the relationship between social factors, such as the desire for others approval, on health-related behaviour (Sheeran and Abraham, 1996).

The HBM also implies that health-behaviours arise from a single "one-off" rational decision based on a cost-benefit analysis. It is suggested that a more detailed theoretical framework may be necessary to explain adherence decisions, particularly those relating to the maintenance of treatment during chronic illnesses (Leventhal, Diefenbach and Leventhal, 1992; Sheeran and Abraham, 1996). This has recently been illustrated in relation to the adoption of "safer sex practices" (Abraham *et al,* 1996) and adherence to medication in chronic illness (Horne, 1997).

Theory of Reasoned Action

The HBM does not take account of social influences on behaviour or explain how perceived threat and the cost-benefit analysis are translated into action. Such issues are central to the Theory of Reasoned Action (TRA; Ajzen and Fishbein, 1980). The TRA was developed from research investigating relationships between attitudes and behaviour. It is not specific to health but has been widely used in this context (Stroebe and Stroebe, 1995). The central tenets of the TRA are that the formation of *intentions* precedes and predicts behaviour and that intentions are determined by *attitudes* towards the behaviour and *subjective norms* concerning the behaviour. Attitudes towards the behaviour are defined as the product of beliefs about the likely outcome (e.g. "following the doctors recommendations for using insulin will keep my diabetes under control") and the perceived value of the outcome (e.g. "keeping my diabetes under control is important to me"). The person's subjective norm comprises beliefs regarding others views about the behaviour (e.g. "my partner wants me to follow the recommendations") and the motivation to support these views (e.g. "I wish to please my partner by following the recommendations").

Theory of Planned Behaviour

Perceived behavioural control (PBC) and *perceived barriers* have been added to the TRA to form the Theory of Planned Behaviour (TPB; Ajzen, 1985), shown in Figure 2. These variables were added on the grounds that they appear to improve predictions of intentions and behaviour (Ajzen, 1991, Conner and Sparks, 1996). The TPB extends the TRA to encompass behaviours which may not be totally under the individual's volitional control. PBC describes the extent to which a person feels that behaving in a certain way is something that is within their control. This is dependent on control beliefs such as perception of both internal resources such as skills or information and external resources such as perceived barriers (Connor and Sparks, 1996). The concept is generally considered to be similar to Bandura's (1977) concept of self-efficacy (Ajzen, 1991; Schwarzer and Fuchs, 1996).

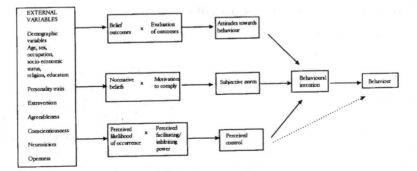

FIGURE 2 The theory of planned behaviour (adapted from Conner and Sparks, 1996)

In the TPB, attitudes and subjective norms exert their influence on behaviour indirectly via their effect on intention. PBC has both an effect on intention and a direct effect on behaviour. For example, given equally strong intentions, the person who is confident of their ability and perceives few obstacles is more likely to actually perform the behaviour.

Application Of Theory of Reasoned Action And Theory of Planned Behaviour

The TRA and TPB have been applied in studies investigating a range of health-related behaviours including giving up smoking (Godin *et al.*, 1992), engaging in an exercise programme (Godin, Vezina, and LeClerc, 1989; Godin *et al.*, 1991; Norman and Smith, 1995), initiating a healthy diet (Conner *et al.*, 1994) and using a condom during sexual intercourse (Chan and Fishbein, 1993). Some of the components of the TRA and TPB have also proved to be useful in predicting adherence to medication prescribed for the treatment of urinary tract infections (Ried and Christensen, 1988), bipolar affective disorders (Cochran and Gitlin, 1988) and hypertension (Miller, Wikoff and Hiatt, 1992; Ried *et al.* 1985). In the main, there is broad support for the assertion that behavioural intentions are influenced by attitudes and subjective norms although the strength of the relationship between intentions and behaviour varies across studies and between behaviours (see Connor and Sparks, 1996, for a more detailed review).

Beliefs About Cause And Control Over Illness

Attribution theory

Attribution Theory (e.g. Weiner, 1979) is concerned with the cognitive processes by which people explain the causes of events. Its application is based on the notion that a fundamental response to adverse events such as illness is the search for explanations about cause. Causal explanations are related to past experiences and can influence future response and adjustment to the illness.

Early research was mainly concerned with the extent of beliefs in *internal* causes (i.e. related to their own behaviour) or *external* causes (i.e. blaming fate or others) for causality of events. More recently, further dimensions have been added such as *stability* (i.e. whether the cause of the illness is long lasting or temporary), *globality* (i.e. global versus specific causes), *universality* (i.e. universal versus personal causal influences) and *controllability* (controllable versus uncontrollable influences). A number of studies have investigated the specific application of attribution theory to health problems including end-stage renal disease (Wright *et al.* 1990), and adherence to recommendations for life-style changes among pre-operative coronary patients (Naea De Valle and Norman, 1992). In addition to considering broad attributional dimensions such as internality, health psychology research has focused on the specific content (e.g. stress, lifestyle) of peoples' causal attributions for their health problems. From this work it is clear that causal attributions are related to beliefs about cure and can influence the patient's behavioural response and adaptation to illness. However, it has not been possible to identify one type of attribution which is universally adaptive. Certain attributions seem to adaptive in some situations but not others (Naea De Valle and Norman, 1992; Tennen, Affleck and Gershman, 1986).

Beliefs about control

The notion of *locus of control* was formulated by Rotter and operationalised in his 1966 scale. It arose from Rotter's (1954) social learning theory which states that the likelihood of a specific behaviour occurring in a given situation is a function of the expectancy that the behaviour will lead to a particular reinforcement in that situation and the value of that reinforcement to the individual. Rotter's (1966) locus of control scale was designed to measure generalised expectancy of reinforcement on a single dimension of internal vs. external locus of control of reinforcement. Hence locus of control refers to the extent to which the person feels that they have control over what happens in a situation (*internal locus i.e making internal attributions*) or that the situation is being controlled by other factors (*extremel locus i.e making external attributions*).

The concept of locus of control was applied to health by Wallston, Wallston, Kaplan and Maides (1976) who developed a measure of health locus of control (HLC). This categorised people according to whether they attributed control over their health to internal or external factors. Later, this measure was revised and extended to form the multidimensional health locus of control scale (MHLC; Wallston, Wallston and DeVellis, 1978), since research indicated that control beliefs should be assigned to three separate unipolar scales: an *internal* scale, and two external scales, *chance* and *powerful others* (Levenson, 1973a; Levenson, 1973b). The main prediction from the theory is that internals on the MHLC will be more likely to engage in health promoting activities, although during an acute or chronic illness it may be advantageous to believe in powerful others (see Norman and Bennett, 1996).

Empirical studies investigating the role of HLC beliefs in adherence are inconclusive. Some have found no association between control beliefs and adherence (e.g. Harvey, 1992; Harvey and Peet, 1991; Hazzard, Hutchinson and Krawiecki, 1990; West, Durant and Pendergrast, 1993) and in studies where associations were found, there is little consistency in the type of control which is associated with adherence (e.g. Bruhn, 1983; Wilson, 1995).

Many studies which have failed to demonstrate significant interactions between HLC and health behaviours have used a general measure of HLC, such as the MHLC, which is not condition-specific. These include studies of affective disorders (Harvey, 1992; Harvey and Peet, 1991), renal transplantation (Frazier, Davis Ali and Dahl, 1994; Kiley, Lam and Pollack, 1993) and in predicting intended adherence to an imaginary regimen in a study involving college students (McCallum, Wieb and Keith, 1988).

Measures of general health locus of control have been shown to be a fairly weak predictor of health behaviour (see Norman and Bennett, 1996). However, the use of disease-specific measures for assessing HLC improves the utility of this construct in explaining medication related behaviour (e.g. Beck, 1980; Georgiou and Bradley, 1992; Kohlman *et al.*. 1993; Johnson *et al.*, 1993; Reynaert *et al.*, 1995; Wallston *et al.*, 1991). Recently, Wallston, Stein and Smith (1994) developed a condition-specific version of the MHLC which further divides powerful others into two independent subscales: *doctors* and *other people*. A recent study utilised the condition- specific version of the MHLC to investigate adherence in adults with cystic fibrosis (Myers, personal communication). It was found that the doctors subscale of powerful others was strongly related to self-reported adherence, accounting for 33% of the variance.

Bradley and co-workers have developed condition-specific perceived control scales for use in diabetes which have been successful in predicting adherence to various aspects of diabetes self-care (e.g. Bradley *et al.*, 1984; 1990; 1994).

As one focuses attention on a specific behaviour (e.g. adhering to a prescription for the regular use of a steroid inhaler), beliefs about the degree of control one has over the behaviour may be closely related to other expectancies such as beliefs about ones competency in being able to perform the behaviour. These are self-efficacy beliefs and there is growing interest of their role as cognitions related to health behaviour.

Efficacy beliefs

In relation to adherence, at least two types of efficacy beliefs as important: *outcome efficacy* which concerns beliefs about whether the behaviour will result in an effective outcome (e.g. taking medication will reduce my blood pressure and so prevent renal complications) and *self-efficacy*, which covers the individual's beliefs as to whether they will be able to carry out the behaviour (e.g. I am confident that I will remember to take my medication every day). Individuals may acquire their sense of self-efficacy from their assessment of the outcome of their own behaviour, the behaviour of others and feedback about their own behaviour which they receive from significant others (Bandura, 1997). Several studies have demonstrated a relationship between perceived self-efficacy and adherence to recommended health-related behaviours such as giving up smoking (DiClemente, Prochaska and Gilbertini, 1985) or carrying out an exercise programme (Kaplan, Atkins and Reinsch, 1984). Efficacy and control beliefs are strongly influenced by the individual's past experience of success or failure in specific health-related domains, and should not be confused with unrealistic optimism (Schwarzer and Fuchs, 1996).

The inclusion of self-efficacy beliefs in SCMs such as the TPB has been shown to enhance their ability to predict various preventive health behaviours (Schwarzer and Fuchs, 1996), including adherence to medication for tuberculosis, in a study conducted in India (Barnhoorn and Adriaanse, 1992).

In general, self-efficacy beliefs are likely to be more salient for difficult behaviours, such as giving up smoking, than for behaviours such as adherence to a simple medication regimen (Flanders and McNamara, 1984). Beliefs about control over health and self-efficacy and outcome-efficacies may be influenced by previous experience and other cognitions.

LIMITATIONS OF SOCIAL COGNITION MODELS AS EXPLANATORY MODELS FOR HEALTH BEHAVIOURS

Limitations To Rational Decisions

One limitation of SCMs is that they cannot easily explain health-related behaviour which is apparently irrational, such as the patient who delays seeking treatment for a large and visible tumour. Several studies investigating health behaviour have found future behaviour to be more strongly predicted by past behaviour than by cognitions. The influence of past behaviour has been noted in relation to diet, exercise and smoking (Mullen, Hersey and Iverson, 1987), recreational drug use (Bentler and Speckhart, 1979) and wearing a seat belt (Sutton and Eiser, 1990). In considering this question, Norman and Connor (1996) draw attention to Ajzen's (1988) suggestion that the effects of past behaviour on future behaviour are mediated by variables included in the SCMs. According to Ajzen (1991) past experience of a behaviour may be an important source of expectations about and attitudes towards repeating the behaviour in the future. Relationship between past and future behaviour may predominate because key cognitions have not been considered or have been poorly operationalised. Also, the relationship may be inflated by congruence between the methods of measuring past and future behaviour. A further explanation is that some health behaviours become habitual or routine (e.g. brushing ones teeth before bedtime) and are not always preceded by a rational decision based on expectancy-value considerations.

Stages To Health Behaviour

The fact that cognitions and behaviour change over time has major implications for the validity of SCMs. Firstly, the notion that interactions between behaviour and cognition may be dynamic rather than static, leads us to question when inter-relations specified in the model are particularly salient. It has been suggested that health behaviour may proceed in stages and that different cognitions may be more important in particular stages than in others: for example the thinking underlying *initiation* of a particular behaviour may be qualitatively different from that involved in *maintenance* of the behaviour. Weinstein (1988) suggests that some of the cognitive components of SCMs – such as beliefs about personal susceptibility – are also best described in stages. He goes on to suggest that interventions to promote behaviour are likely to be more effective if they are targeted at the particular cognitions which characterise the particular stage that the individual has reached in their thinking about or implementation of the behaviour

Several stage models of health behaviour have been proposed in which health behaviours occur as the result of several stages of cognition. The Transtheoretical Model or Stages of Change Model (TM, e.g. Prochaska and DiClemente, 1983) suggests that the maintenance of health behaviour occurs in five progressive stages of change: pre-contemplation, contemplation, preparation, action and maintenance.

- Precontemplation. In this stage the person is not even thinking of change, possibly because they are not even aware of the need, or they refuse to think about the risks, or they think they may not be capable of changing.
- Contemplation. This is defined as the stage at which the person is thinking about changing their behaviour, but is not yet committed.
- Preparation. The person intends to take action in the near future and is likely to have a clear plan of action.
- Action. Active attempts are made to change behaviours.
- Maintenance. This is the stage which is characterised by attempts to characterised prevent relapse.

Progress through stages may not be linear but is likely to take a cyclical route characterised by many brief or partially successful attempts before behaviour change is established. This framework has been successfully applied to a variety of situations, including smoking (DiClemente *et al.* 1991; Velicer *et al.*, 1992), dietary modification and weight control (Curry, Kristal and Bowen 1992; McCann *et al.*, 1996; Suris-Rangel, DiClemente and Dunn 1988) and exercise (e.g. Marcus *et al.*, 1992).

Other stage models include the health action process approach (HAPA, Schwarzer, 1992); the precaution adoption process (Weinstein, 1988) and goal setting theory (Bagozzi, 1992) Norman and Conner (1996) discuss the overlap between the various stage models. For example, (1) stage models have a temporal theme and follow the basic pattern from a pre-contemplation stage through a motivation stage to the initiation and maintenance of behaviour and (2) they assume that different cognitions are important at different stages.

One of the criticisms of stage models (and SCMs) is that they do not fully address the issue of how motivation to continue with the health-behaviour is maintained. Although the processes of initiation and *maintenance* of behaviour are recognised in the TM and other stage models such as the HAPA, there is an implicit assumption that the main cognitive barrier to maintenance is low self-efficacy. So, for example, if a patient is motivated to take their medication and believes realistically that they can carry out the behaviour, then they will continue to do so. Leventhal (1993) has suggested that once self-efficacy and outcome efficacy beliefs are in place, continued behaviour depends on continued motivation. In an attempt to explain the dynamic interaction between cognitions, motivation and behaviour, Leventhal and colleagues have developed a Self-Regulatory Theory as a framework for understanding illness behaviour. This is often referred to as Leventhal's Self-Regulatory Model (SRM).

Leventhal's Self-Regulatory Model Of Illness: From Social Cognition To Self-Regulation

The SRM was derived from early work investigating the impact of fear-arousing communications on preventive health behaviour (see Leventhal *et al.*, 1980). This showed that although a threat message was often necessary to motivate people towards preventive health behaviours such as having a tetanus vaccination or giving up smoking, the threat alone was often insufficient. In order to achieve behavioural change it was necessary to add an action plan to the threat message, e.g. by giving clear instructions for successful action and helping the individual to incorporate this into their daily routine. This cognitive-behavioural approach generated actions which lasted longer than any fear aroused by the threat, which faded within a day or two. Leventhal surmised that the combination of fear and action plan had changed the "cognitive representation" of the threat. This stimulated interest in how people represented health threats and the interaction between representations and behaviour which led to the development of the SRM.

The self-regulatory model: an overview

The fundamental premise of the SRM is a view of the patient as an active problem solver, whose health-related behaviour is an attempt to close the perceived gap between current health status and a future goal state. Threats to health and illness are regarded as a problem and the patient's behaviour is seen as an attempt to solve the problem. Patients respond to illness in a dynamic way based on their interpretation and evaluation of the illness. The choice of a particular coping response (e.g. to take or not to take medication) is influenced by whether it makes sense in the light of their own ideas about the illness and personal experience of symptoms. Thus adherence/non-adherence can be thought of as one of a number of behaviour patterns adopted to cope with the illness as it is perceived. Responses to illness follow three broad stages:

(a) The cognitive representation of the health threat by which the patient identifies the meaning of the health threat. This can be stimulated by internal cues (e.g. symptoms) and or external cues (e.g. information).
(b) The development and implementation of an action plan or coping procedure to deal with the threat.
(c) The appraisal of the outcome of the action plan.

Key features of this model are that the three stages of processing occur in parallel at a cognitive and emotional level and that there is a dynamic interaction between the processes of representation, coping and appraisal. In Figure 3 it can be seen that the interaction proceeds in both directions. For example, the patient's coping and appraisal may arise from a particular and individual representation of the health threat, but, equally the perceived outcome of coping may feed back to influence the representation.

In common with SCMs, the SRM attempts to focus on individual's cognitive representation of the health threat as the key factor determining variations in behaviour. However, the SRM differs from SCMs and stage models in its emphasis on coping appraisal processes and the resultant feedback effect on cognition, emotion and behaviour. Therefore, the interaction between cognition and behaviour is seen as a dynamic process, rather than the result of a single or stage decision. The selection of a coping procedure (taking aspirin) is

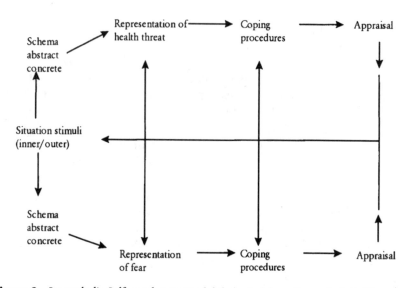

Figure 3   Leventhal's Self-regulatory Model (adapted from Leventhal, 1993).

determined by beliefs about the nature of the illness threat (my headache is stress related and should respond quickly to aspirin). Then this is followed by an appraisal stage in which the patient evaluates the efficacy of their coping strategy (the pain is still there three hours after the aspirin). If the patient appraises a particular coping strategy as being ineffective then this might result in the selection of an alternative coping strategy (I will try a stronger pain killer) or even a change in the representation of the illness (aspirin hasn't worked, this might be something more serious than a head-ache).

The fact that cognitive and emotional processing occur in parallel may be used to explain responses to illness threats which are apparently irrational. For example, a patient may believe that the lump in her breast is likely to be a tumour but delays seeking help because she fears the diagnosis (Phelan, Dobbs and David, 1992). Her behavioural response (to delay seeking help) can be seen as a way of coping with the emotion (fear/distress) generated by the cognitive representation, which may be reinforced by her appraisal that the lump doesn't get bigger and "the less she thinks about it the better she feels".

The SRM emphasises the importance of concrete symptom experi-ence in formulating representations and guiding appraisal of the efficacy of coping. Perceptual experiences are seen to be generally more persuasive than abstract ideas. Pennebaker (1982) provides compelling evidence that illness cognitions and symptom perception are closely linked and that influence is bi-directional. Not only does the experience of symptoms influence the content of illness repre-sentations but arousal of memory based schema initiates a search for confirmatory symptoms (Pennebaker, 1982). The influence of illness representations on symptom perception is further corroborated by recent studies in which people presented with a false diagnosis tended to report symptoms which confirmed their representation (Bishop, 1991).

Personal representations of the illness drives coping and appraisal and the question of how sick individuals conceptualise their illness is central to the SRM. An important difference between the SRM and SCMs is in how relevant beliefs are conceptualised. In both approaches, beliefs are of paramount importance in guiding behaviour. In SCMs, beliefs are characterised as outcome expectan-cies and the values placed on them, or are limited to beliefs about the behaviour. Leventhal and colleagues have devoted much attention to the cognitive representation of illness threats and have identified two important aspects: content (an individuals ideas about the illness) and structure (how these ideas are cognitively organised). They suggest that people form "common-sense" models of disease and illness organised around five components: *identity, cause , consequences, time-line and cure.* Identity consists of concrete symptoms and signs and an abstract label associated with them. Cause relates to ideas about how one gets the disease. Time-line relates to perceptions about the likely course of the condition and how long it will last. Consequences are the expected outcomes in physical, psychological and social terms and cure deals with the persons beliefs about the potential for cure and control (see Leventhal *et al.*, 1992; Leventhal *et al.*, 1997 for a fuller description). The specific content of each component is influenced by the cultural context (Blumhagen, 1980; Farmer, 1988; Farmer and Good, 1991; Landrine and Klonoff, 1992) and by other factors such as past experience and the views of significant others (Leventhal *et al.*, 1992). Although the content of the individual components of illness representations varies between individuals

(Meyer, Leventhal and Gutmann, 1985), the components are stable (Bishop, 1991).

The SRM And Adherence To Treatment

There is empirical support for the utility of the SRM in explaining adherence decisions. Illness representations were related to medication adherence in hypertension (Meyer *et al.*, 1985), and regimen adherence in diabetes (Gonder-Frederick and Cox, 1991). In a recent prospective study, adherence to recommendations to attend rehabilitation classes following a first myocardial infarction was predicted by illness beliefs (identity, consequences, control/cure) elicited during hospital convalescence (Petrie *et al.*, 1996).

Despite a cogently argued rationale for the study of illness cognitions as determinants of treatment adherence (Leventhal *et al.*, 1992; Leventhal and Cameron, 1987), relatively few studies have utilised this approach. A possible reason is that the complexity of the SRM makes it more difficult to operationalise than the SCMs. The recent development of a questionnaire based method for assessing representations of illness (Weinman *et al.*, 1996) makes it easier to operationalise the "representations" construct and may facilitate more widespread use of the SRM in adherence research. (See Petrie and Weinman 1997 for a useful review)

SUMMARY AND CONCLUSIONS

This chapter has described some of the models or concepts which are currently used in health psychology-based adherence research. These models do not commonly provide complete explanations of specific adherence behaviours and no single model seems to be universally valid. Some concepts may be more applicable to particular adherence decisions than to others. SCMs may be more applicable to "single point" decisions about recommendations for maintaining health (e.g. to attend for screening or to wear a condom during sexual intercourse), than for explaining adherence in the context of chronic illness (Connor and Norman, 1996). Stage based models recognise that individuals may be at different stages in their willingness to consider advice. The SRM emphasises that patients make active decisions about whether to follow treatment advice on the basis of whether it makes "common-sense", in the light of their ideas about the nature of the illness and how adherence/non-adherence is perceived to affect it (Leventhal *et al.*, 1992). The SRM emphasises the role of patients' own beliefs about illness. It has recently been suggested that patients ideas about *treatment* also play a key role in guiding adherence decisions (Horne, 1997). The development of measurement scales for assessing cognitive representations of illness (Weinman *et al.*, 1996) and medication (Horne, Weinman and Hankins, 1997) may facilitate the empirical evaluation of these theoretical approaches.

The SCMs, stage models and SRM described in this chapter contribute to our understanding of the psychology of adherence (Conner and Norman, 1996; Petrie and Weinman, 1997). However, we have much to learn about how and when health practitioners should intervene to facilitate adherence to treatment. The capacity of these theoretical approaches to generate effective interventions has yet to be fully evaluated and this remains a key challenge for future adherence research (see Abraham and Hampson, 1996).

ACKNOWLEDGEMENTS

The authors would like to thank Dr Lynn B Myers and Dr Charles Abraham for helpful comments and suggestions. This paper was funded by the Department of Health, Pharmacy Enterprise Scheme award.

REFERENCES

Abraham, C. and Hampson, S.E. (1996) A social cognition approach to health psychology. *Psychology and Health* **11**, 233–241.

Abraham, C. and Sheeran, P. (1997) Congnitive representations and preventative health: a review. In K.J. Petrie and J. Weinman (eds.) *Perceptions of health and illness.* London: Harwood Academic Publishers.

Abraham C., Sheeran. P., Abrams, D. and Speers, R. (1996) Health beliefs and teenage condom use: a prospective study. *Psychology and Health* 11, 641–655.

Ajzen, I. (1985) From intentions to actions: a theory of planned behaviour. In J. Kuhl and J. Beckmann (eds.) *Action-Control: from cognition to behaviour.* Heidelberg: Springer-Verlag.

Ajzen, I. (1988) *Attitudes, personality and behaviour.* Milton Keynes: Open University Press.

Ajzen, I. (1991) The Theory of Planned Behaviour. *Organizational Behavior and Human Decision Processes* **50**, 179–211.

Ajzen, I. and Fishbein, M. (1980) *Understanding attitudes and predicting social behaviour.* Englewood Cliffs, NJ: Prentice Hall.

Alogna, M. (1980) Perception of severity of disease and health locus of control in compliant and non-compliant diabetic patients. *Diabetes Care* **3**, 533–534.

Bagozzi, R.P. (1992) The self-regulation of attitudes, intentions and behaviour. *Social Psychology Quarterly* **55**, 178–204.

Bandura, A. (1977) Self-Efficacy: toward a unifying theory of behavioural change. *Psychological Review* **84**, 191–215.

Bandura, A. (1997) *Self-Efficacy: the exercise of control.* New York: Freeman.

Barker, T (1994) Role of health beliefs in patient compliance with preventive dental advice. *Community Dentistry and Oral Epidemiology* **22**, 327–330.

Barnhoorn, F. and Adriaanse, H. (1992) In search of factors responsible for noncompliance among tuberculosis patients in Wardha District, India. *Social Science and Medicine* **34**, 291–306.

Beck, K.H. (1980) Development and validation of a dental health locus of control scale. *Journal of Preventative Dentistry* **6**, 327–332.

Becker, M.H. and Maiman, L.A. (1975) Sociobehavioural determinants of compliance with health and medical care recommendations. *Medical Care* **13**, 10–24.

Bentler, P.M. and Speckhart, G. (1979) Models of attitude behavior relations. *Psychological Review* **86**, 542–564.

Bishop, G.D. (1991) Understanding the understanding of illness: lay disease representations. In: J.A. Skelton. and R.T. Croyle (eds.) *Mental representation in health and illness.* New York: Springer-Verlag.

Bloom-Cerkoney, K.A. and Hart, L.K. (1980). The relationship between the health belief model and compliance of persons with diabetes mellitus. *Diabetes Care,* **3,** 594–598.

Blumhagen, D. (1980) Hyper-tension: a folk illness with a medical name. *Culture Medicine and Psychiatry* **4,** 197–224.

Bradley, C., Brewin, C.R., Gamsu, D.S. and Moses, J.L. (1984) Development of scales to measure perceived control of diabetes mellitus and diabetes-related health beliefs. *Diabetic Medicine* **1,** 213–218.

Bradley, C., Lewis, K.S., Jennings, A.M. and Ward. (1990) Scales to measure perceived control developed specifically for people with tablet-treated diabetes. *Diabetic Medicine* **7,** 685–694.

Bradley, C. (1994) Measures of perceived control in diabetes. In C. Bradley (ed.) *Handbook of psychology and diabetes.* London: Harwood Academic Publishers.

Brownlee-Duffeck, M., Peterson, L., Simonds, J., Goldstein, D., Kilo, C. and Hoette, S. (1987). The role of health beliefs and regimen adherence and metabolic control of adolescents and adults with diabetes mellitus. *Journal of Consulting and Clinical Psychology* **55,** 139–144.

Bruhn, J.G. (1983) The application of theory in childhood asthma self-help programs. *Journal of Allergy and Clinical Immunology* **72,** 561–77.

Caggiula, A.W. and J.E. Watson, J.E. (1992) Characteristics associated with compliance to cholesterol lowering eating patterns. *Patient Education and Counseling* **19,** 33–41.

Calnan, M. (1984) The health belief model and participation in programmes for the early detection of breast cancer: a comparative analysis. *Social Science and Medicine* **19,** 823–830.

Chan, D.K. and Fishbein, M. (1993) Determinants of college women's intentions to tell their partners to use condoms. *Journal of Applied Social Psychology* **23,** 1455–1470.

Chen, M. and Land, K.C. (1986) Testing the health belief model: LISREL analysis of alternative models of causal relationships between health beliefs and preventative dental behaviour. *Social Psychology Quarterly* **49,** 45–60.

Cochran, S.D. and Gitlin, M.J. (1988) Attitudinal correlates of lithium compliance in bipolar affective disorders. *The Journal of Nervous and Mental Disease* **176,** 457–464.

Conner, M. and Norman, P. (1996) *Predicting health behaviour.* Buckingham: Open University Press.

Conner, M. and Sparks, P. (1996) The theory of planned behaviour and health behaviours. In M. Conner and P. Norman (eds.) *Predicting health behaviour.* Buckingham: Open University Press.

Conner, M., Povey, R., Bell, R. and Norman, P. (1994) GP intervention to produce dietary change. Presented at the British Psychological Society Special Group in Health Psychology Annual Conference, September, Sheffield, UK.

Cummings, K.M., Becker, M.H., Kirscht, J.P. and Levin, N.W. (1981) Intervention strategies to improve compliance with medical regimens by ambulatory haemodialysis patients. *Journal of Behavioural Medicine* **4**, 111–127.

Curry, S.J., Kristal, A.R. and Bowen, D.J. (1992) An application of the stage model of behavior change to dietary fat. *Health Education Research,* **7**, 97–105.

DiClemente, C.C., Prochaska, J.O., Fairhurst, S.K., Velicer, W.F., Velasquez, M.M. and Rossi , J.S. (1991) The process of smoking cessation: an analysis of precontemplation, contemplation and preparation stages of change. *Journal of Consulting and Clinical Psychology* **59**, 295–304.

DiClemente, C.C., Prochaska, J.O. and Gilbertini, M. (1985) Self efficacy and the stages of self-change of smoking. *Cognitive Therapy and Research* **9**, 181–200.

Farmer, P. (1988) Bad blood, spoiled milk: bodily fluids as moral barometers in rural Haiti. *American Ethnologist* **15**, 61–83.

Farmer, P. and Good, B.J. (1991) Illness representations in medical anthropology: a critical review and a case study of the representation of AIDS in Haiti. In J.A. Skelton and R.T. Croyle (eds.) *Mental representations in health and illness.* New York: Springer-Verlag.

Flanders, P.A. and McNamara, J.R. (1984) Prediction of compliance with an over-the-counter acne medication. *Journal of Psychology* **118**, 31–36.

Frazier, P.A., Davis Ali, S.H. and Dahl, K.E. (1994) Correlates of noncompliance among renal transplant recipients. *Clinical Transplantation* **8**, 550–55..

Georgiou, A. and Bradley, C. (1992) The development of a smoking-specific locus of control scale. *Psychology and Health* **6**, 227–246.

Godin, G., Valois, P., Lepage, L. and Desharnais, R. (1992) Predictors of smoking behaviour – an application of Ajzen theory of planned behaviour. *British Journal of Addiction* **87**, 1335–1343.

Godin, G., Valois, P., Jobin, J. and Ross, A. (1991). Prediction of intention to exercise in individuals who have suffered from coronary heart disease. *Journal of Clinical Psychology* **47**, 762–772.

Godin, G., Vezina, L. and LeClerc, O. (1989). Factors influencing the intention of pregnant women to exercise after giving birth. *Public Health Reports* **104**, 188–195.

Gonder-Frederick, L.A. and Cox, D.J. (1991) Symptom perception, symptom beliefs and blood glucose discrimination in the self-treatment of insulin dependent diabetes. In J.A. Skelton and R.T. Croyle (eds.) *Mental representation in health and illness*. New York: Springer-Verlag.

Haefner, D.P. and Kirscht, J.P. (1970) Motivational and behavioural effects of modifying health beliefs. *Public Health Reports* **85**, 478–484.

Harvey, N.S. (1992) Lithium clinic attrition and health locus in attenders compared with a population sample. *Lithium* **3**, 269–273.

Harvey, N.S. and Peet, M. (1991) Lithium maintenance: II. Effects of personality and attitude on health information acquisition and compliance. *British Journal of Psychiatry* **158**, 200–204.

Hazzard, A., Hutchinson, S.J. and Krawiecki, N. (1990). Factors related to adherence to medication regimens in pediatric seizure patients. *Journal of Pediatric Psychology* **15**, 543–555.

Hogan, T.P., Award, A.G. and Eastwood, R. (1983) A self-report scale predictive of drug compliance in schizophrenics: reliability and discriminant validity. *Psychological Medicine* **13**, 177–183.

Horne, R. (1997) Representations of medication and treatment: advances in theory and measurement. In K.J. Petrie and J. Weinman (eds.) *Perceptions of health and illness: current research and applications*. London: Harwood Academic Publishers.

Horne, R and Weinman, J. (1994) Illness cognitions: implications for the treatment of renal disease. In C. Bradley and H. McGee (eds.) *Quality of life and renal care*. London: Harwood Academic Publishers.

Horne, R., Weinman, J. and Hankins, M. (1997) The Beliefs about Medicines Questionnaire (BMQ): a new method for assessing cognitive representations of medication. *Unpublished manuscript.*

Janz, N.K. and Becker, M.H. (1984) The Health Belief Model: a decade later. *Health Education Quarterly* **11,** 1–47.

Johnson, L.R., Magnani, B., Chan, V. and Ferrante, F.M. (1993) Modifiers of patient-controlled analgesia efficacy: I. Locus of Control. *Pain* **39,** 17–22.

Jones, P.K., Jones, S.L. and Katz, J. (1987) Improving compliance for asthma patients visiting the emergency department using a health belief model intervention. *Journal of Asthma* **24,** 199–206.

Kaplan, R.M., Atkins, C.J. and Reinsch, S. (1984) Specific efficacy expectations mediate exercise compliance in patients with COPD. *Health Psychology* **3,** 223–242.

Kelly, G.R., Mamon, J.A. and Scott, J.E. (1987) Utility of the health belief model in examining medication compliance among psychiatric outpatients. *Social Science and Medicine* **25,** 1205–1211.

Kiley, D.J., Lam, C.S. and Pollack, R. (1993) A study of treatment compliance following kidney transplantation. *Transplantation* **55,** 51–56.

Kohlman, C.W., Schuler, M., Petrak, F., Kustner, E., Krohne, H.W. and Beyer, J. (1993) Associations between type of treatment and illness-specific locus of control in type 1 diabetes patients. *Psychology and Health* **8,** 383–391.

Landrine, H. and Klonoff, E.A. (1992) Culture and health-related schema: a review and proposal for inter-disciplinary integration. *Health Psychology* **11,** 267–276.

Levenson, H. (1973a) Multidimensional locus of control in psychiatric patients. *Journal of Consulting and Clinical Psychology* **41,** 397–404.

Levenson, H. (1973b) Activism and powerful others: distinctions within the concept of internal-external control. *Journal of Personality Assessment* **38,** 377–383.

Leventhal, H. (1993) Theories of compliance, and turning necessities intopreferences: Application to adolescent health action. In N. A. Krasnegor, L.H. Epstein, S. Bennett Johnson and S.J. Yaffe, (eds.) *Developmental aspects of health compliance behavior.* Hillsdale, NJ, US: Lawrence Erlbaum Associates.

Leventhal, H., Benjamin, Y., Brownlee, S., Diefenbach, M., Leventhal, E.A., Patrick-Miller, L. and Robitaille, C. (1997) Illness representations: theoretical foundations. In K.J. Petrie and J. Weinman (eds.) *Perceptions of health and illness*. London: Harwood Academic Publishers.

Leventhal, H. and Cameron, L. (1987) Behavioral theories and the problem of compliance. *Patient Education and Counseling* **10**, 117–138.

Leventhal, H., Diefenbach, M. and Leventhal, E.A. (1992) Illness cognition: using common sense to understand treatment adherence and affect cognition interactions. *Cognitive Therapy and Research*. **16**, 143–163.

Leventhal, H., Meyer, D, and Nerenz, D (1980) The common sense representation of illness danger. In S. Rachman (ed.) *Contributions to medical psychology*. Oxford: Pergamon Press.

Marcus, B.H., Selby, V.C., Niaura, R.S. and Rossi, J.S. (1992). Self-efficacy and the stages of exercise behavior change. *Research Quarterly for Exercise and Sport* **63**, 60–66.

McCann, B.S., Bovjberg, V.E., Curry, S.J., Retzlaff, B.M., Walden, C.E. and Knopp, R.H. (1996) Predicting participation in a dietary intervention to lower cholesterol among individuals with hyperlipidemia. *Health Psychology* **15**, 61–64.

McCallum, D.M., Wieb, D.J. and Keith, B.R. (1988) Effects of previous medication experience and health beliefs on intended compliance to an imagined regimen. *Journal of Compliance in Health Care* **3**, 125–134.

Meyer, D., Leventhal, H. and Gutmann, M. (1985) Common-sense models of illness: the example of hypertension. *Health Psychology* **4**, 115–135.

Miller, P., Wikoff, R. and Hiatt, A. (1992) Fishbein's model of reasoned action and compliance behaviour of hypertensive patients. *Nursing Research* **41**, 104–109.

Mullen, P.D., Hersey, J.C. and Iverson, D.C. (1987) Health behaviour models compared. *Social Science and Medicine* **24**, 973–983.

Nelson, E.C., Stason, W.B., Neutra, R.R., Solomon, H.S. and McArdle, P.J. (1978) Impact of patient perceptions on compliance treatment in hypertension. *Medical Care* **16**, 893–906.

Naea De Valle, M. and Norman, P. (1992) Causal attributions, health locus of control beliefs and lifestyle changes among pre-operative coronary patients. *Psychology and Health* **7**, 201–211.

Norman, P. and Bennett, P. (1996) Health Locus of Control. In M. Conner and P. Norman (eds.) *Predicting health behaviour.* Buckingham: Open University Press.

Norman, P. and Conner, M. (1996) The role of social cognition models in predicting health behaviours: future directions. In M. Conner and P. Norman (eds.) *Predicting health behaviour.* Buckingham: Open University Press.

Norman, P. and Smith, L. (1995). The theory of planned behaviour and exercise: an investigation into the role of prior behaviour, behavioral intentions and attitude variability. *European Journal of Social Psychology* **25,** 403–501.

Pan, P. and Tantam D. (1989) Clinical characteristics, health beliefs and compliance with maintenance treatment: a comparison between regular and irregular attenders at a depot clinic. *Acta Psychiatrica Scandinavica* **79,** 564–570.

Pennebaker, J. (1982) *The psychology of physical symptoms.* New York: Springer Verlag.

Petrie, K.J. and Weinman. J. (eds.) (1997) *Perceptions of health and illness: current research and applications.* London: Harwood Academic Publishers.

Petrie, K.J., Weinman, J., Sharpe, N. and Buckley, J. (1996) Predicting return to work and functioning following myocardial infarction: the role of the patient's view of their illness. *British Medical Journal* **312,** 1191–1194.

Phelan, M., Dobbs, J. and David, A.S. (1992) 'I thought it would go away': patient denial in breast cancer. *Journal of the Royal Society of Medicine* **85,** 206–207.

Prochaska , J.O. and DiClemente, C.C. (1983) Stages and processes of self-change of smoking: toward an integrative model of change. *Journal of Consulting and Clinical Psychology* **51,** 390–395.

Reynaert, C., Janne, P., Delire, V., Pirard, M.., Randour, P., Collard, E., Installe, E., Coche, E. and Cassiers, L. (1995) To control or be controlled? From health locus of control to morphine control during patient-controlled analgesia. *Psychotherapy and Psychosomatics* **64,** 74–81.

Ried, L.D. and Christensen, D.B. (1988) A psychosocial perspective in the explanation of patients' drug-taking behavior. *Social Science and Medicine* **27,** 277–285.

Ried, L.D., Oleen, M.A., Martinson, O.B. and Pluhar, R. (1985) Explaining intention to comply with antihypertensive regimens:

the utility of health beliefs and the theory of reasoned action. *Journal of Social and Administrative Pharmacy* **3**, 42–52.

Rosenstock, I. (1974) The health belief model and preventative behaviour. *Health Education Monographs* **2**, 354–386.

Rotter, J.B. (1966) Generalised expectancies for internal versus external control of reinforcement. *Psychological Monographs* **80**, (Whole no. 609) 1–28.

Rotter, J.B. (1954) *Social learning and clinical psychology*. Englewood Cliffs, NJ: Prentice-Hall.

Schwarzer, R. (1992) Self-efficacy in the adoption and maintenance of health behaviors: theoretical approaches and a new model. In R. Schwarzer (ed.) *Self-efficacy: thought control of action*. London: Hemisphere.

Schwarzer, R. and Fuchs, R. (1996) Self-efficacy and health behaviours. In M. Conner and P. Norman (eds.) *Predicting health behaviour*. Buckingham: Open University Press.

Sheeran, P. and Abraham, C. (1996) The health belief model. In M. Conner and P. Norman (eds.) *Predicting Health Behaviour*. Buckingham: Open University Press.

Stroebe, W. and Stroebe, M.S. (1995) *Social psychology and health*. Pacific Grove, CA, US: Brooks/Cole Publishing Co.

Sutton, S.S. and Eiser, J.R. (1990) The decision to wear a seat belt: the role of cognitive factors, fear and prior behaviour. *Psychology and Health* **4**, 111–123.

Suris-Rangel, A.C., DiClemente, C.C. and Dunn, J.R. (1988) Stages and processes in weight control for Mexican American women. New York: 22nd Annual AABT Convention.

Taylor, D.W. (1979) A test of the health belief model in hypertension. In R.B. Haynes, D.L. Sackett and D.W. Taylor (eds.) *Compliance in health care*. Baltimore: John Hopkins University Press.

Tennen, H., Affleck, G. and Gershman, K. (1986) Self-blame among parents of infants with perinatal complications : the role of self-protective motives. *Journal of Personality and Social Psychology* **50**, 690–696.

Urban, N., White, E. Anderson, G.L., Curry, S. and Kristal, A.R. (1992) Correlates of maintenance of a low-fat diet among women in the Women's Health Trial. *Preventive Medicine* **21**, 279–291.

Velicer, W.F., Prochaska, J.O., Rossi J.S. and Snow, M.G. (1992) Assessing outcome in smoking cessation studies. *Psychological Bulletin*, **111**, 23–41.

Wallston. K.A., Smith, R.P., King, J.E. and Smith, M.S. (1991) Desire for control and choice of antiemetic treatment for cancer chemotherapy. *Western Journal of Nursing Research* **13**, 12–29.

Wallston, K.A., Wallston, B.S. and DeVellis, R. (1978) Development of the multidimensional health locus of control (MHLC) scales. *Health Education Monographs* **6**, 160–170.

Wallston, K.A., Wallston, B.S. Kaplan, G. and Maides, S. (1976) Development and validation of the health locus of control (HLC) scale. *Journal of Consulting and Clinical Psychology* **44** 580–585.

Wallston, K.A., Stein, M.J. and Smith, C.A.. (1994) Form C of the MHLC scales: a condition-specific measure of locus of control *Journal of Personality Assessment* 63, 534–553.

Weiner, B. (1979) A theory of motivation for some classroom experience. *Journal of Educational Psychology* **6**, 160–170.

Weinman, J., Petrie, K.J., Moss-Morris, R. and Horne, R. (1996) The Illness Perception Questionnaire: a new method for assessing cognitive representations of illness. *Psychology and Health* **11**, 431–445.

Weinstein, N.D. (1988) The precaution adoption process. *Health Psychology* **7**, 355–386.

West, K.P., Durant, R.H. and Pendergrast, R. (1993). An experimental test of adolescents' compliance with dental appointments. *Journal of Adolescent Health*, 14, 384–389.

Wilson B.M. (1995) Promoting compliance: the patient-provider partnership. *Advances in Renal Replacement Therapy* **2**, 199–206.

Wright, S.J., Brownbridge, G., Fielding, D. and Stratton, P. (1990) Family attributions and adjustment to dialysis in adolescent end-stage renal failure. *Psychology and Health* **5**, 77–88.

Zimmerman, R.S. and Vernberg, D. (1994) Models of preventive health behaviour: comparison, critique and meta-analysis. *Advances in Medical Sociology* **4**, 45–67.

3

Doctor-Patient Communication and Adherence to Treatment

Lorraine M. Noble

The purpose of this chapter is to provide a framework for the issue of patient adherence to treatment in the context of the doctor-patient relationship and to show how communication between the doctor and the patient can have a profound impact on this. It will begin with a discussion of the concept of "adherence to treatment", in which it will be shown that the conceptualisations of both adherence and the doctor-patient relationship are inextricably intertwined in their assumptions and the way they have shaped the literature. The role of doctor-patient communication in influencing adherence will then be considered, specifically focusing on three key domains: (a) patients' beliefs about illness and treatment, (b) information exchange between the doctor and the patient, and (c) the impact of the nature of the doctor-patient relationship. This discussion should be taken in the context of the wider literature which has demonstrated that doctor-patient communication significantly influences a variety of outcomes, including not only adherence but also patients' knowledge, satisfaction, physical functioning and health status (e.g. Ley, 1977; Green, 1978; Hall *et al.*, 1988; Wooley *et al.*, 1978; Wartman *et al.*, 1983).

THE CONCEPT OF ADHERENCE TO TREATMENT

Much of the literature has been characterised by the assumption that "adherence" or "compliance" means that the patient should simply follow the recommendations made by the doctor. Haynes (1979) defined "patient compliance" as "the extent to which a person's behaviour (in terms of taking medications, following diets, or executing lifestyle changes) coincides with medical or health advice." This definition has been echoed by others (e.g. Hopp and Gerken, 1983) but is often an implicit and unquestioned assumption in many studies in this field. Whilst apparently straightforward, this conceptualisation of adherence contains many assumptions within it, all of which *can* be called into question.

It assumes that the treatment being recommended is without doubt the best course of action for the particular patient. Several lines of research have found otherwise. A number of studies have found that doctors themselves often fail to adhere to professional guidelines about recommended treatment regimes. The term "professional non-compliance" was coined by Philip Ley, who found that 51% to 100% of patients did not receive appropriate medication or advice (Ley, 1981). More recently, Yeo *et al.* (1994) found that general practitioners (GPs) adhered poorly to recommendations for prescribing benzodiazepines (tranquillizers), even following a well-constructed educational intervention. Despite the doctors' intentions to alter their behaviour, they greatly underestimated how much they actually prescribed benzodiazepines and were unable to complete the agreed task to review certain prescriptions. Yeo *et al.* concluded "we do not always do what we mean to do [.. or ...] what we think we do." Similarly, McMillan *et al.* (1991) found poor adherence to guidelines for the management of neonatal hyperbilirubinemia (jaundice in newly born babies): 26 out of 45 doctors never prescribed according to the guidelines, and the remainder only prescribed according to the guidelines for a proportion of infants in their care.

In addition to the doctor's choice of treatment, patients may not receive the most appropriate treatment due to inaccuracies in the recording of information and poor communication among health professionals. Hulka *et al.* (1976) and Fletcher *et al.* (1979) both found that doctors were unaware of about a fifth of prescribed medications being taken by patients, some of which included combinations with potentially dangerous interactions. Ross (1991), comparing GPs', district nurses' and patients' perceptions of medication regimes, found that for 57 patients, in only 5% was there complete agreement in the number and type of medications. In addition, 44% of patients were taking prescribed medications which had not been recorded by either the GP or the nurse. This raises a point made by Ley (1981), who suggested that a patient cannot be said to be "non-compliant" if the records of the treatment regime are inaccurate.

Becker (1985) emphasised that the positive relationship between adherence and health outcome, although often assumed, is not absolute. At times, patients who adhere to the recommended treatment do not recover, and those who do not adhere, or who adhere partially to the regime, do recover. There are a variety of reasons for this, including incorrect diagnosis of the problem, inappropriate treatment recommendations, and spontaneous remission due to the activities of the host's natural defences (Hessen-Klemens and Lapinska, 1984; Fletcher, 1989). Even when the patient's condition has been correctly diagnosed and the appropriate medication has been prescribed in accordance with guidelines for recommended dosages, the effects of the treatment are not guaranteed. This is because recommended dosages are based on published reports of the average dose required for groups of people under ideal conditions. However, individual patients can vary in their absorption and metabolism of the medication. For some patients, the recommended dose may be too much or too little. Consequently, some patients who take their medication intermittently will actually receive the correct dose and others who take the medication as recommended will not receive enough.

A further problem with the assumption that the patient should simply "follow the doctor's advice" is that it presumes a certain relationship between the doctor and the patient, in which the patient is a passive and obedient recipient (Trostle, 1988). Kjellern *et al.* (1995) argued that this conceptualisation is based on a model of power and control rather than one of co-operation to achieve a mutual goal, i.e. an improvement in the person's health. Indeed the terminology used illustrates the nature of the relationship that is assumed: Stimson (1974) found that terms such as "disobedience", "non-compliance", "resisting", "rejecting", "deviant", "unco-operative" and "defaulting" were all commonly used. Currently "compliance" is still the most popular term used in the medical literature, although many writers now advocate the more neutral term "adherence".

A consequence of this model of the doctor-patient relationship is that any problems with adherence are assumed to be due to the patient. Early studies attempted to identify the "typical refuser of medication" (Richards, 1964), the "error-prone patient" (Schwartz *et al.*, 1962), or the "unco-operative type" (Porter, 1969). However, considerable research efforts have failed to identify any stable personality traits or socio-demographic characteristics that predict which patients will or will not "comply" (Ley, 1979; Lane, 1983; Leventhal and Cameron 1987; Gabbard-Alley 1995). Indeed, doctors' own adherence to medical treatment is no better than that of patients in general (Blackwell, 1973; Blackwell *et al.*, 1978; Shangold, 1979).

The final problem with the traditional conceptualisation of adherence is the assumption that the patient will unquestioningly follow any advice that is given. The evidence is that patients come to the doctor with a more complex agenda and are more active in their own health care than this conceptualisation suggests. Regimes tend to be modified or distorted rather than completely accepted or abandoned. In describing this, Kjellern *et al.* (1995) suggested that adherence should be viewed as a matter of "more or less" rather than "yes or no". Whilst some of the modifications that patients make to their regimes are unintentional as a result of not being able to understand or recall the advice (Ley, 1977), patients also actively alter the recommended course of treatment, depending on their beliefs about the adequacy of the proposed regime (Stimson, 1974; Hayes-Bautista, 1976; Zola, 1980; Hessen-Klemen and Lapinska, 1984). This can result in a number of outcomes: partial adherence to the recommendations, partial adherence supplemented by other patient-generated remedies, and even over-adherence, in which the patient increases the frequency or intensity of the prescribed treatment.

The conceptualisation of adherence is important, as it underpins any attempt to address the problem of non-adherence. Certainly the wealth of evidence has demonstrated that it is a more complex issue than that of "the doctor instructs and the patient follows". However, the traditional view of adherence, which is still very prevalent in the literature also has implications for the nature of the doctor patient relationship and the communication that arises from this.

ADHERENCE AND THE DOCTOR-PATIENT RELATIONSHIP

The problem of non-adherence has wider implications for the doctor-patient relationship than simply that the patient does not obtain the benefits of treatment. There is evidence that non-adherence is seen as a contentious issue in interactions between doctors and patients, and that both parties feel threatened by this (Hessen-Klemens, 1987; Ross and Phipps, 1986). Doctors feels threatened because their experience and medical authority are being questioned and because they are often baffled by patients' failure to follow the appropriate course of action despite their own best efforts. Patients feels threatened because they feel inadequately prepared for what is expected of them in following the recommendations and they are aware that any admission of "non-compliance" may count against them in terms of withdrawal of medical care.

Hessen-Klemens (1987) suggested that non-adherence is seen as a frustrating event by doctors, who react by the use of "ego-defensive" strategies. In a study of 109 audiotaped consultations, Hessen-Klemens found 30 events in which there was evidence that the patient was not adhering to the recommendations as prescribed. The most common strategies used by the doctors were "medical threat" (threatening the patient with the dire consequences that would result if the patient failed to take the advice), "carrying the doctor's point in an indulgent atmosphere" (the doctor allowed the patient to express their objections but these were not taken into account in formulating the treatment plan), and "authoritarian tactics" (the doctor stressed their own superior position or the patient's obligation to comply). Other research has produced similar findings. Interviewing patients about their doctors' strategies to their non-adherence, Hayes-Bautista (1976) identified two types of approach: "convincing" (attempting to change the patients' mind) and "countering" (attempting to minimise the patients' interference with the treatment). A further study (Appelbaum and Roth, 1983), using direct observation of inpatients who had refused treatment, found that the strategies used were mainly forced treatment or forceful persuasion (i.e. telling patients that they had no choice). Also used were "coax and wheedle" tactics, giving more information, or simply denying that refusal had occurred. In all three studies, doctors only rarely attempted to elicit from the patient the reasons why they were not adhering.

A more recent study (Essex *et al.*, 1990) attempted to improve the care of patients with long-term mental illness by introducing a scheme in which patients held a copy of their own records. Patients who were receiving care from at least two sources (including a GP and a psychiatric nurse or a psychiatrist), were asked to bring their record to all of their appointments. The record included information about the patient's diagnosis, current treatment, the roles of the various professionals and services available to the patient. The scheme was designed to improve communication between patients and all the professionals involved in their care, and to ensure that all parties had access to accurate and up-to-date information, particularly about medication changes. The system was extremely popular with patients, 72% of whom took their records to 50% or more of appointments. However, the investigators, who included a consultant psychiatrist, were unable to persuade any of the 25 psychiatrists they had approached about potential involvement in this scheme to participate: the psychiatrists regarded the scheme with great misgivings and were unhappy about patients having access to their own records. The investigators concluded that the psychiatrists felt that this was a challenge to their authority, despite the clear benefits of the scheme to patient care. Ross and Phipps (1986) commented that such power struggles can only lead to a deterioration in the situation, with the patient becoming even less likely to follow the doctor's advice. This may lead to a complete breakdown in the working relationship, which may be terminated by either the doctor or the patient, although in practice this is seldom an option for the patient.

These phenomena can be explained in terms of the traditional conceptualisation of the doctor-patient relationship, which very much goes hand in hand with the traditional view of "compliance to treatment". In both, the doctor is perceived as the expert who is in charge of the patient's care and who knows best. Consequently, any problems are seen as being located within the patient. A number of studies have illustrated this, by attempting to produce typologies of patients who cause problems for their doctors (Groves, 1978; Gerrard and Riddell, 1988; O'Dowd, 1988). Groves (1978) described four types of "hateful patients" ("dependent clingers", "entitled demanders", "manipulative help rejecters" and "self-destructive deniers"). Gerrard and Riddell (1988) provided an anecdotal description of ten categories of "difficult patients," including those who "demand help persistently but are expert at blocking it", or who "make the doctor pay for real and imagined grievances and are most animated when they are successful", or even those who are "wicked, manipulative, and playing games". In a similar vein, O'Dowd (1988) described problems associated with being consulted by "heartsink" patients, who "exasperate, defeat and overwhelm their doctors by their behaviour." Rather tellingly, O'Dowd was unable to identify any common characteristics which linked the patients: "[they are] a disparate group of individuals whose only common thread seems to be the distress they cause their doctor and the practice."

This view of patient culpability for problems is by no means an obsolete concept. In a study considering types of consultations which doctors find difficult, Levinson *et al.* (1993) identified seven broad categories in doctors' descriptions: lack of trust or agreement, lack of understanding, feeling distressed, too many problems, lack of adherence, demanding or controlling patient, and special problems (e.g. drug or alcohol dependence, chronic pain). Levinson *et al.* found that doctors attributed the cause most frequently to the patient (50%), followed by difficulties with communication (20%) and factors concerned with the practice setting (10%). Articles which advance the "patient-blaming" approach have been published in the most widely read and prestigious medical journals: both the O'Dowd and the Gerrard and Riddell papers were published in the British Medical Journal, and a further paper (Wright, 1993) considering the issue of non-adherence was published in the Lancet. Wright's paper began with one of Hilaire Belloc's *cautionary tales* "Matilda told such dreadful lies..." and placed most emphasis on behavioural techniques to "gain compliance", such as a pill bottle that sounded a tone when the dose was due and would only stop when the bottle was opened.

The consequence of defining both the doctor-patient relationship and adherence in this way is that the issue of non-adherence becomes a forbidden subject, which both parties are uncomfortable about discussing. Doctors are poor at identifying non-adherence and consistently over-estimate their patients' rates of adherence, and in fact in many studies their estimates have been found to be no better than chance (Becker, 1985). Doctors even have difficulty in identifying the consequences of adherence, i.e. improvements in their patients' health status. Hessen-Klemens and Lapinska (1984) found that doctors' evaluations of their patients' health were significantly influenced by a number of factors which are unreliably associated with health status, such as the patient being complimentary towards the doctor. Often doctors rely on casual reports from patients, but over-reporting of adherence is high, even as much as 100% (Kasl, 1975; Gordis *et al.*, 1969). Whilst the unreliability of self-reports of adherence has led some investigators to conclude that patients are irresponsible and not to be trusted (e.g. Wright, 1993), closer examination suggests that patients are behaving in such a way as to attempt to preserve a relationship with the doctor and avoid confrontation (Fletcher,1989).

MODERN APPROACHES TO ADHERENCE AND THE ROLE OF DOCTOR-PATIENT COMMUNICATION

Meichenbaum and Turk (1987) suggested the concept of adherence, rather than "compliance", implies "a more active, voluntary collaborative involvement...in a mutually acceptable course of behaviour to produce a desired preventative or therapeutic result." Their recommendations included "establishing clinical relationships in which patients are active participants, and where patients' explanatory models of their illness, worries and concerns about their illness and expectations about treatment are explored." In effect, this approach conceptualises both the doctor and the patient as experts in their own domains (Cameron and Gregor, 1987). The doctor's expertise is in making medical diagnoses and providing appropriate treatment. The patient's expertise is in being able to identify changes in their health and knowing how a given treatment can be implemented in the context of their own lifestyle. This requires a reconceptualisation of the doctor-patient relationship, from one in which the aim is simply to "increase compliance" to one which actively accommodates patients' responses to medical care (Donovan and Blake, 1992). Zola (1980) described this change from one of "medication compliance" to "therapeutic alliance".

This is analogous to a recent reconceptualisation of "informed consent" (Hope, 1996). Hope criticised the prevailing notion of informed consent as something to be extracted from a fairly passive patient. The current model is that the doctor decides and proposes the course of action, which the patient is permitted only to accept or veto. Hope argued that this power of veto is thought to ensure that the patient's autonomy has been respected, which is not in fact the case, as the patient has had little input into the process until the end point. He showed how many of the difficulties doctors have in practice in their attempts to seek consent arise directly from this flawed model of consent, and outlined an alternative model to overcome these difficulties, in which the patient is engaged in the decision-making process at a much earlier stage.

Patients' Beliefs

The beliefs that patients have about illness and treatment are often very different to those of their doctors. There is evidence that these beliefs have a major impact on patients' acceptance of prescribed treatments, yet this is an aspect seldom explored during normal consultations. Early studies of lay beliefs found that patients make attributions about the cause of their illness and hold certain notions about the nature of the illness itself. For example, cancer was found to be perceived as an invading enemy of cells which rendered the patient passive and helpless, and was attributed to a variety of causes, including previous venereal disease, the effects of an old injury, inheritance or contagion (Bellak, 1952; Abrams and Finesinger, 1953).

The potential impact of patients' beliefs about illness on adherence was highlighted in a series of studies of 800 consultations from a paediatric emergency clinic (Korsch et al., 1968; Francis et al., 1969). It was found that a large proportion of parents attending the clinic blamed themselves for their child's illness, often worrying that the cause had been a preventable, environmental hazard (such as the child "getting a chill" or something that the child had eaten). Many parents had hoped that the doctor would provide information about the reason for the illness, but this was seldom forthcoming, and parents' beliefs about this issue were rarely explored during the consultation. The unmet expectation for information about the cause of the child's illness was significantly related to parents' failure to adhere to medical advice. Patients also have beliefs about treatment itself. Stimson (1974) studied patients' beliefs about medication and found a number of misconceptions that were related to patients' non-adherence to prescribed treatments. These included beliefs that medication should be taken only when the person feels ill and stopped when they feel better, that the body needs a rest from medicines from time to time, and that people can become dependent on medication or immune to the effect of a medication with prolonged use. None of these beliefs had been discussed with the doctor. Since the early work considering lay beliefs of illness, a number of formal models of patients' beliefs have been developed, many of which have been found to be linked to adherence. Four models are particularly relevant to the issue of how doctor-patient communication relates to adherence. These models are more fully described by Horne and Weinman in Chapter 2.

Health belief model (e.g. Becker and Maiman, 1975; 1980; Becker, 1985). This model states that a person's motivation to follow medical advice is related to four factors: the person's level of interest in (and concern about) health matters, their perception of how susceptible they are to an illness, their perception of the severity of the illness and its consequences, and the balance of costs and benefits in engaging in the behaviour. The concept of self-efficacy (the person's perception of how capable they feel in dealing with the situation) was later incorporated into this model (Rosenstock *et al.,* 1988). Studies attempting to link health beliefs and adherence have found positive relationships (Becker, 1985) although there have been mixed findings (Bruhn, 1983). However, there is evidence that identifying and addressing patients' health beliefs during a consultation is effective in improving adherence. Inui *et al.* (1976) conducted an intervention study which involved training a group of doctors in a hypertension clinic. The doctors were given a tutorial (1–2 hours in length) explaining why patients might not adhere to treatment and suggesting strategies based on the health belief model. The intervention led to an increased proportion of time spent by the doctors on patient education, leading to more accurate patient knowledge and beliefs about hypertension and its treatment, higher rates of adherence to treatment and improved blood pressure control.

Locus of control (Rotter, 1966). Part of Rotter's Social Learning Theory, the concept of "locus of control" refers to the extent to which the person feels that they have control over what happens in a situation (internal locus) or that the situation is being controlled by other factors (external locus). Often in the literature there is confusion about whether this construct refers to a person's beliefs about a given situation or whether people can be classified along a stable personality dimension of "internals" and "externals". The problem with the latter conceptualisation is the simplistic view that "internals" are more active in their own treatment and in many respects make "better" patients (e.g. Hopp and Gerken, 1983). Whilst findings concerning the relationship between locus of control and adherence have been mixed (Bruhn, 1983; Wilson, 1995), there is evidence that adherence is more likely if the patient's locus of control matches the requirements of the situation (e.g. Lowery and DuCette, 1976). Wilson (1995) suggested that the doctor's approach to the patient should differ depending on the patient's presentation of locus of control. For example, if a person demonstrates an internal locus, the doctor should draw attention to parts of the treatment that are affected by the patient's behaviour and give the patient the opportunity to suggest solutions or at least choose between alternatives.

The Transtheoretical Model or Stages of Change Model (e.g. Prochaska and DiClemente, 1983). Although this is a less widely-discussed model, it provides an additional perspective which is often neglected. Prochaska and DiClemente suggested that there are a number of distinct stages that a person progresses through when making changes to their health-related behaviour. At the "precontemplative" stage, the person is not even considering change and may not even believe that there is a problem to be addressed. The person may then progress to "contemplation" (thinking about a behaviour change), to "decision" (making definite plans), and to "action" (carrying out behaviour change). Once the behaviours are in place, the person is in the "maintenance" stage, although there may be "relapse" which takes the person back to an earlier point in the cycle. If the person is successful in the maintenance stage and the behaviours have the desired effect, the person may then "exit" from the cycle completely. Prochaska and DiClemente described the process by which the health professional can identify a person's stage and encourage them to move towards the next stage. They termed this "motivational interviewing". This framework has been successfully applied to a variety of situations, including smoking (DiClemente *et al.*, 1991; Velicer *et al.*, 1992, Gritz *et al.*, 1992), dietary modification and weight control (Suris-Rangel *et al.*, 1988; Curry *et al.*, 1992) and health screening (Prochaska *et al.*, 1994). The importance of this model is that it does not presume that a person attending a doctor necessarily has decided that they have a problem that they wish to be treated, a common assumption in the adherence literature. The model proposes that the approach that a doctor should use must be tailored to the patient's stage. For example, it would be ineffective to discuss in detail how a patient can change their eating habits for the purpose of losing weight, if the person is happy with their current weight or is still considering the potential consequences to their lifestyle of going on a diet.

Self-regulation model (e.g. Leventhal and Cameron, 1987). This conceptualises a patient as an "active problem-solver" who attempts to bridge a perceived gap between their current and ideal state. This involves three main components: the patient's representation of the health threat (its causes and the likely consequences), their action plan for dealing with the threat, and their appraisal of how effective their coping efforts have been. Leventhal and Cameron suggested that failures of communication between the doctor and the patient in any of these three areas can lead to non-adherence, although in practice the latter two components are most likely to be neglected. They described research which found that in tape-recorded consultations with hypertensive patients, doctors talked almost exclusively about the nature of the illness and its consequences, rarely provided information on how to implement the intervention (a diet) and how to cope with problems, and almost never gave information on how patients could appraise their own coping efforts (e.g. how much weight would be lost each week if the diet was successful).

Information Exchange

Eliciting information. Much of the research considering communication and adherence has focused on how doctors provide information about treatment, but there is evidence that the likelihood of the patient adhering to recommendations can be determined at a much earlier stage. Even from the outset, the manner in which the doctor elicits information from the patient at the beginning of the consultation can determine the eventual outcome. Firstly, in terms of the quality of the information obtained by the doctor about the nature of the problem. A number of studies have found that doctors tend to over-control the interview, which impedes the collection of accurate and complete information (Beckman and Frankel, 1984; Burack and Carpenter, 1983; Platt and McMath, 1979). Beckman and Frankel (1984) discovered that patients were interrupted on average 18 seconds after beginning their description of the problem, mostly after the expression of a single stated concern. They found that only 23% of the 73 patients actually completed their statements and only one patient who had been interrupted continued with the statement. Interruption appeared to stop the spontaneous flow of information from the patient, which was not regained during the remainder of the ·interview. A later study (Beckman *et al.*, 1985) found that the time patients took to complete their opening description was usually less than one minute, but that doctors tended to interrupt between 5 and 50 seconds into this. It would be expected that this form of interviewing would lead to an impoverished description of the patient's problem, and indeed this is the case. In a study by Roter and Hall (1987) doctors interviewed a simulated patient who had been briefed in a role of a 60 year old man with chronic obstructive pulmonary disease. On the whole, doctors elicited less than 50% of the medical information available. The type of questions asked emerged as ʿone of the most important variables in accounting for the variation, with open questions accounting for more than four times the variation in patient disclosure than closed questions. The consequence of over-controlling the interview and failing to elicit all of the relevant information is that patients feel, often with some justification, that the diagnosis and treatment are likely to be inappropriate and therefore not worth following (Stimson, 1974).

Further studies have found that doctors often focus almost exclusively on the biomedical aspects of the patient's history (such as the presenting symptoms), and lack both confidence and skill in addressing other areas (Ley, 1982a). There is evidence that a number of outcome variables improve if doctors address patients' concerns and worries (Wooley *et al.*, 1978; DiMatteo and Hays, 1980; Starfield *et al.*, 1981; Romm *et al.*, 1976), but these are rarely identified and psychosocial issues are seldom discussed (Korsch *et al.*, 1968; Starfield *et al.*, 1981; Sotosky *et al.*, 1992; Daltroy *et al.*, 1991). Doctors have been found to give poor estimates of patients' health status and tend to underestimate the extent to which patients' activities are limited by their condition, both of which are associated with higher levels of patient dissatisfaction (Wartman *et al.*, 1983).

There is evidence that if doctors discuss the issue of adherence with patients then it is more likely to occur. In a meta-analysis, Hall *et al.* (1988) found a positive correlation between doctors asking questions about adherence and actual levels of adherence. However, the manner in which the topic is raised is important. Fletcher (1989) and Sanson-Fisher *et al.* (1989) both suggested that doctors should make it acceptable for patients to discuss non-adherence, for example, by prefacing a question about medication with a comment that they themselves sometimes forget to take medication or that other patients have had difficulties with the regime in the past. In practice, doctors have been found to use both successful and unsuccessful strategies. Steele *et al.* (1990), in an observational study of 75 consultations in a hypertensive clinic, found two types of strategy used by doctors to elicit information about adherence. One approach was "indirect", often characterised by vague questions or questions in which adherence was assumed, e.g. when a patient was asked simply to report on any changes resulting from taking the medication. The second approach was termed "information intensive" and involved the doctor asking quite specific questions about how the patient was taking the medication and what changes had occurred. Steele *et al.* found that doctors using the indirect style were able to predict their patients' adherence no better than chance, whereas 20% of the doctors using the "information-intensive" style were 80% successful in predicting adherence. Steele *et al.* also noted that doctors using the indirect style ran the risk of inadvertently reinforcing non-adherence, by commenting on an improvement in the patient's condition that the patient knew was not due to taking the prescribed treatment.

Zola (1980) made the point that too often non-adherence is only addressed as an issue when it has already occurred, by which time it can be too late. He suggested that prevention was better than cure, describing with astonishment the approach of a group of doctors treating essential hypertension whom he found were unanimous in their decision not to tell their patients that the first course of treatment recommended was unlikely to work. Unsurprisingly, the levels of non-adherence in this patient population were very high.

Giving information. The aspect of medical care with which patients express most dissatisfaction is the information given to them by their doctors (McKinlay, 1972). Doctors themselves demonstrate poor skills in educating patients and feel unprepared for this part of their role (Russell *et al.*, 1985; Kenney *et al.*, 1988; Mittelmark *et al.*, 1988; Lewis *et al.*, 1991; Palchik *et al.*, 1991). The most common problem is that doctors consistently underestimate the amount of information that patients want (Daltroy, 1993). Doctors tend to over-estimate the amount of time they spend on patient education and concentrate most on providing information and instructions, with little time spent on checking how the information is being received and what the patient understands and wishes to know (McClellan, 1986).

The premise that patients should be given full information about their condition and treatment has not been universally upheld. Ley (1982a) summarised research considering areas in which full communication with the patient has traditionally been considered "potentially harmful". These areas included severe or terminal illness (information is not given on the grounds that the patient will be happier not knowing), less serious illness and investigative procedures (information is not given as it is believed that the patient may become anxious or depressed), and medication (information is not given as it is believed that it would increase the incidence of side-effects or decrease adherence). Ley concluded that there was no evidence of "harmful effects" resulting from giving patients information in any of these areas, in fact quite the reverse. The two areas which have aroused the most debate are the issues of breaking bad news and giving information about medication. However the research in both areas is unequivocal. Studies have consistently shown that the majority of patients want to know if a diagnosis of cancer or terminal illness has been made (Ley, 1977; 1982b). Regarding the provision of information about medication side-effects, there is no evidence that side-effects will be increased or that adherence will be reduced (Myers and Calvert, 1973; 1976; 1978; Morris and Kanouse, 1982; Mazucca, 1982; Devine and Cook, 1983; Quaid *et al.*, 1990). Even so, omissions and even distortions in the information given to patients are still common (Rimer *et al.*, 1984; Scherwitz *et al.*, 1985; Katz *et al.*, 1992).

Research has consistently demonstrated that patients' understanding of their condition and treatment is positively related to adherence (Burgoon *et al.*, 1987) and that adherence, satisfaction, recall and understanding are all related to the amount and type of information given (Hall *et al.*, 1988). But patients often lack even the most basic information about their treatments. Svarstad (1976), in a study of patients prescribed medication at a neighbourhood health centre, discovered that 50% did not know how long they were to continue on the medication, 25% did not know the correct dosage, and 15% could not report the frequency with which they were to take the medication. This knowledge was related to adherence: 70% of patients who understood the recommendations adhered, whereas only 15% of those who made one or more mistakes in recalling the recommendations adhered. When the clarity of the instructions given during the consultation was rated from the audiotapes, of those who received clear instructions 60% understood and 50% adhered, whereas of those receiving confusing instructions, 40% understood and 30% adhered. Similarly, Daltroy *et al.* (1991) found that four months after a prescription had been made, patients adhered to 58% of prescriptions whose purpose they understood and 29% of prescriptions whose purpose they did not understand. Again, clarity of instructions was important: Daltroy *et al.* (1992) found that when a rheumatologist made a clear statement about the purpose of a non-steroidal anti-inflammatory drug, 79% of patients were adhering four months later. When such a statement was not made, 33% of patients adhered.

A considerable body of research has been established concerning patients' understanding and recall of treatment recommendations. Patients frequently do not understand what they have been told (Ley, 1977; 1982a) and this can be due to a number of factors. Many patients do not have elementary "medical" knowledge (such as the positions of various organs in the body) on which doctors' explanations are often based. In addition, patients may have misconceptions which militate against understanding and which can lead to the rejection of advice as unhelpful or positively detrimental (Stimson, 1974; Stoeckle and Barsky, 1980). The language used by doctors can be another problem, particularly in the use of medical jargon. For example, Korsch *et al.* (1968) found a number of phrases which led to some confusion among the parents attending the paediatric clinic: e.g. "lumber puncture" was thought to mean that the child's lungs would be drained and "incubation period" was taken to be the amount of time the child should stay in bed. In addition, written information is also frequently above the level which would be understood by the majority of the population. Ley (1982a) reviewed a number of studies which applied readability formulae to leaflets intended for different patient groups (readability is a measure of how easy written information is to understand). Ley found that only a fifth of the leaflets (17/85) would be understood by 75% or more of the population.

Ley (1982a) provided a clear summary of the literature on factors influencing recall of information. Failure to recall information is high, even immediately following the consultation. Diagnostic statements appear to be recalled better than instructions, although this may be due to this information being presented earlier in the consultation and because it is perceived to be more important by the patient. In most studies, anxiety has been found to have a Yerkes-Dodson relationship with recall, i.e. a mild to moderate level is optimal, whereas a very high level of anxiety or very little concern both reduce recall. Ley (1977) suggested a number of recommendations to improve patients' recall of information, based on interventions which had been shown to be successful. These were: (1) provide patients with instructions and advice at the start of the information to be presented; (2) stress the importance of the instructions and advice; (3) use short words and sentences; (4) give the patient the framework of the information to be provided and signal the beginning of each new segment before providing the detail; (5) repeat important information, and (6) make advice as specific, detailed and concrete as possible. Wilson (1995) suggested that patients also need guidance on problem-solving. For example, if a patient has been prescribed a special diet, the advice should be sufficiently concrete to enable the person to follow a detailed plan, but abstract enough to allow for contingencies (e.g. how to choose an appropriate substitute from the relevant food group if a particular food is unavailable).

Calibration of the information given appears to be one of the most difficult tasks for doctors: how to tailor the language and pace of the information to the level the patient will understand and how to balance the content of the information between what the patient wants to know and what the doctor feels the patient needs to know. Maynard (1989) collected qualitative data which illustrated different styles of information-giving demonstrated by doctors giving the diagnosis that a child had developmental disabilities. Maynard contrasted two styles: "interactional" and "non-interactional". In the "non-interactional" style, the doctor assumed the starting point and provided information according to a doctor-defined pace and language. Such information would frequently be rejected by the recipient because of the terminology (e.g. use of the word "retarded") or because the explanation did not match with the parent's conceptualisation of the situation. In the "interactional" style, the doctor took time before giving the diagnosis to ask the parent about their view of the situation and current concerns, and then linked the information being provided with the parent's account. Daltroy (1993) described a model which included a sequence of steps that a doctor can use to ensure that the information given meets the needs of both the patient and the doctor: (1) the patient is encouraged to express all their concerns; (2) the patient's concerns are discussed; (3) the doctor and the patient share models of disease and symptoms; (4) the doctor and the patient share goals for treatment; (5) treatment goals are agreed and priorities set; (6) the doctor and the patient share models of treatment; (7) potential barriers to adherence are identified; (8) plans are made to overcome anticipated barriers to adherence and (9) the doctor provides written information on the disease and the treatment regime. Sanson-Fisher *et al.* (1989) also emphasised the importance of feedback, both from doctor to patient and vice versa. The doctor must constantly check throughout the interview that the patient understands and is in agreement with the plan being discussed. This involves more than simply asking "do you understand?" It should involve checking that the patient can recall salient details of the regime or can demonstrate a procedure, and is able to mention any areas about which they feel unsure. The patient needs to know that what they have understood from the discussion is the correct way to proceed, and when the course of treatment is underway, that their condition is responding as expected.

Relationship Factors

The consultation between the doctor and the patient involves more than the impartial exchange of information in a neutral environment. The patient is faced with an uncertain threat to their health, which they must place in the hands of professionals who are often complete strangers. In addition, their sense of vulnerability is heightened by being in a strange environment, sometimes in a state of undress, and often meeting the doctor in a setting which can either be overheard or overlooked by others (Zola, 1980). There is a substantial body of evidence that a patient needs to feel secure in the care being given in order to obtain the most benefit and that this requires the establishment of a good working relationship. This evidence comes from two strands of research:the first considering the effects of the affective quality of the doctor-patient relationship, and the second considering the role of patient participation in the consultation.

The affective quality of the doctor-patient relationship. Early studies exploring the link between the quality of the doctor-patient interaction and adherence found clear evidence of a positive relationship. Davis (1968; 1971) studying patterns of interaction present in 223 consultations, found that adherence was poorer when there was unresolved tension in the consultation, when the doctor failed to provide feedback in response to the patient's questions, and when a passive doctor was consulted by an active patient. In a series of studies of 800 consultations from a paediatric clinic (Korsch *et al.*, 1968; Francis *et al.*, 1969; Freemon *et al.*, 1971), higher adherence was found to be related to the doctor being perceived by as being "friendly" rather than "business-like" and with a greater proportion of the doctors' statements indicating positive rather than negative affect.

More recent studies have confirmed the presence of a relationship between the nature of emotional exchange and adherence (DiMatteo *et al.*, 1993). Hessen-Klemens and Lapinska (1984) found that recall and adherence improved when the doctor was emotionally supportive (by providing encouragement and reassurance) and when the patient was treated as an equal partner in the exchange. Similarly Hall *et al.* (1988) found that adherence was greater among patients whose doctors expressed encouragement, reassurance and support, and was lower when doctors expressed anger, anxiety or other negative emotions. In addition to the effects of doctors expressing affect, it appears that the ability to identify patients' emotions is also important. DiMatteo *et al.* (1986) found that doctors' sensitivity to non-verbal communication was related to their patients' adherence in terms of keeping appointments. In a review of the literature, Squier (1990) concluded that there is strong evidence that the affective quality of the doctor-patient relationship is a key determinant of both patient satisfaction and adherence to treatment. In particular, warmth, caring, positive regard, lack of tension, and non-verbal expressiveness appear to be the most important elements in establishing and maintaining a good working relationship (DiMatteo, 1979; Friedman. 1979).

Traditionally, it was thought that fear was a useful tool that could be used by the medical profession in motivating patients to improve their adherence, and over the years this issue has aroused some lively debate (Ley, 1977). It has become apparent that the relationship is considerably more complex than simply that of increasing the level of fear to increase the amount of adherence. Recent work has confirmed that fear arousal as a technique should be used with caution, as it can easily lead to avoidance and cause the situation to deteriorate (Becker, 1985). It is most effective under a specific set of circumstances: that is, when a person has initially been little concerned about the illness, there is a defined course of action which is effective against the illness and when the action can be quickly and easily undertaken by the recipient of the fear-arousing message. The deliberate use of fear arousal under other circumstances, for example, when there is no clear course of action or the condition is not amenable to treatment, would be pointless if not unethical.

Patient participation. An observational study by Svarstad (1974) identified a number of strategies frequently used by doctors to control and limit patient-initiated communications. These included the intentional use of technical jargon, looking at the clock, interrupting the patient, ignoring the patient's communication, "mumbling" to indicate that the doctor was thinking and should not be disturbed, and walking out of the room without indicating to the patient that the interview was coming to a close. Svarstad found that the use of these strategies was extremely efficient in limiting patient-initiated communications. Unfortunately, doctors using such strategies do so at a cost, and the cost is to adherence. Rost (1989) considered the impact of patient participation with adherence to medication prescribed during that consultation. Four types of "patient participation" were considered: patients answering doctors' questions; patients volunteering information; patients interrupting their doctors and patients asking questions of their doctors. Rost found that patients' adherence was significantly related to the opportunity to be able to offer information voluntarily and to answer questions that they had been asked. Whether patients interrupted their doctors made no difference and few patients asked their doctor any questions. Other studies have confirmed the link between participation and adherence. In their meta-analysis, Hall *et al.* (1988) found a positive relationship between enlisting patient participation and adherence. Partnership building was also positively related to patients' understanding and ability to recall information they had been given by the doctor, and satisfaction with their medical care.

A number of researchers have considered the effects of increasing patient participation. Roter (1977) conducted an intervention to train patients how to ask their doctor questions. This was effective in that patients became more active and were more likely to attend for future appointments, but the trained patients experienced more dissatisfaction with their treatment and were rated as showing more anger and anxiety in the consultations than control patients. It appeared that the change from the traditional passive role was not an easy one. However, further studies have found that training patients to be more active has more beneficial than detrimental consequences. Kaplan *et al.* (1989) trained patients to ask more questions during the consultation and to be more active in making decisions about their own treatment. The intervention was effective in enabling patients to seek information from their doctors, and led to improved physiological markers of functioning and increased health status of trained patients compared to controls. Daltroy *et al.* (1991) conducted an intervention over the telephone to train patients to be more active in their communication with their rheumatologist. The intervention led to a decreased number of cancellations and failure to attend, and increased patients' self-reported ability to communicate with their doctor.

Increased patient participation means not only that there will be more discussion about treatment, but that this will entail negotiation and compromise. Clearly in some conditions, the treatment options are more flexible than in others. Wilson (1995) suggested that patients are willing to negotiate and seek some workable alternative when barriers to adherence are identified. Contrary to expectations, this does not diminish the patient's faith in the suggested course of action, rather, the feeling of ownership is more likely to enhance the patient's willingness to follow the regime. In situations where a complex or difficult regime is unavoidable, Sanson-Fisher *et al.* (1989) suggested that the course of treatment be built up slowly wherever possible. In extreme circumstances, re-negotiation of medical goals may be required. Zola (1980) suggested that "if a four times a day prescription is medically best but socially intolerable, then a one-a-day form should not be second choice, but the best choice."

CONCLUSION

The model of "adherence to treatment" is necessarily more complex than the traditional model of "compliance". It is no longer feasible to assume that patients will unquestioningly follow any instructions given to them by doctors. Patients expect to take a more active role in their own care, they want to be able to evaluate for themselves whether the treatment being suggested is the best available, and they want to feel secure that they are receiving good medical care from a doctor they can trust rather than a series of routine procedures given impersonally. The consequence of this is that adherence cannot be taken for granted; it is not the "default setting". In fact it is probably more helpful to construe adherence as a behaviour which results only when a particular set of circumstances arises. These will include: that the patient wishes to undertake treatment; is satisfied that the treatment being offered is the most appropriate course of action; can fully understand and is able to undertake the behaviours required; is not impeded in any way during the course of the behaviour and is able to monitor progress towards the end goal.

This change in the concept of adherence necessarily means that the process of communication will be more complex. This can seem daunting, particularly to the majority of practicing doctors who are not familiar with the research findings and who are unlikely to have had more than the most cursory training in communication with patients. Change is further hampered by the routines and assumptions currently in place which doctors use to organise their everyday work, which often undermine the possibility of moving towards a patient-centred approach, but are rarely questioned with regard to the implicit values they contain (Barnard, 1985).

The modern conception of adherence is in essence a contract between the doctor and the patient, with responsibilities on both sides. The more explicit and well-defined the contract, the more likely it is that it will be adhered to. Preparation is paramount. The issue of difficulties with adherence should be pre-empted by providing the opportunity for the appropriate information to be exchanged in the context of a supportive relationship. Where difficulties do arise, the doctor must first identify the source of the problem before implementing strategies in an attempt to address them. Jenkins (1979) suggested that "as with any complex physical diagnosis or difficult problem-solving procedure, it takes time and effort to diagnose a problem in health-related behaviour. Some physicians may not be able to make this investment; others will judge the future benefits to warrant the effort."

The good news is that we now know that non-adherence is not the inexplicable and baffling phenomenon that it was originally considered to be. Both adherence and non-adherence are behaviours that can be reliably predicted and one of the key determinants in this is the nature of the communication between the patient and the doctor.

REFERENCES

Abrams, R.D. and Finesinger, J.E. (1953) Guilt reactions in patients with cancer. *Cancer* **6**, 474–482.

Appelbaum, P. and Roth, L. (1983) Patients who refuse treatment in medical hospitals. *Journal of the American Medical Association* **250**, 1296–1301.

Barnard, D. (1985) Unsung questions of medical ethics. *Social Science and Medicine* **21**, 243–249.

Becker, M.H. (1985) Patient adherence to prescribed therapies. *Medical Care* **23**, 539–555.

Becker, M.H. and Maiman, L.A. (1975) Sociobehavioral determinants of compliance with health and medical care recommendations. *Medical Care* **13**, 10–24.

Becker, M.H. and Maiman, L.A. (1980) Strategies for enhancing patient compliance. *Journal of Community Health* **6**, 113–135.

Beckman, H.B. and Frankel, R.M. (1984) The effect of physician behavior on the collection of data. *Annals of Internal Medicine* **101**, 692–696.

Beckman, H.B., Frankel, R.M. and Darnley, J. (1985) Soliciting the patients' complete agenda: a relationship to the distribution of concerns. *Clinical Research* **33**, 714A.

Bellak, L. (1952) *Psychology of physical illness*. New York: Grune and Stratton.

Ben-Sira, Z. (1976) The function of the professional's affective behavior in client satisfaction: a revised approach to social interaction theory. *Journal of Health and Social Behavior* **17**, 3–11.

Blackwell, B. (1973) Drug therapy: patient compliance. *New England Journal of Medicine* **289**, 249–253.

Blackwell, B., Griffin, B., Magill, M. and Bencse, R. (1978) Teaching medical students about treatment compliance. *Journal of Medical Education* **53**, 672–675.

Bruhn, J.G. (1983) The application of theory in childhood asthma self-help programs. *Journal of Allergy and Clinical Immunology* **72**, 561–577

Burack, R.C. and Carpenter, R.R. (1983) The predictive value of the presenting complaint. *Journal of Family Practice* **16**, 749–754.

Burgoon, J.K., Pfau, M., Parrott, R., Birk, T., Coker, R. and Burgoon, M. (1987) Relational communication, satisfaction, compliance-gaining strategies and compliance in communication between physicians and patients. *Communication Monographs* **54**, 307–324.

Cameron, K. and Gregor, F. (1987) Chronic illness and compliance. *Journal of Advanced Nursing* **12**, 671–676.

Curry, S.J., Kristal, A.R. and Bowen, D.J. (1992) An application of the stage model of behavior change to dietary fat. *Health Education Research* **7**, 97–105.

Daltroy, L.H. (1993) Doctor-patient communication in rheumatological disorders. *Ballire's Clinical Rheumatology* **7**, 221–239.

Daltroy, L.H., Katz, J.N. and Liang, M.H. (1992) Doctor-patient communication and adherence to arthritis treatments. *Arthritis Care and Research* **5**, S19.

Daltroy, L.H., Katz, J.N., Morlino, C.I. and Liang, M.H. (1991) Improving doctor-patient communication. *Arthritis Care and Research* **4**, S19.

Davis, M.S. (1968) Variations in patients' compliance with doctors' advice: an empirical analysis of patterns of communication. *American Journal of Public Health* **58**, 274–288.

Davis, M.S. (1971) Variations in patients' compliance with doctors' advice: medical practice and doctor-patient interaction. *Psychiatric Medicine* **2**, 31.

Devine, E.C. and Cook, T.D. (1983) A meta-analytic analysis of effects of psychoeducational interventions on length of post-surgical hospital stay. *Nursing Research* **32**, 267–273.

DiClemente, C.C., Prochaska, J.O., Fairhurst, S.K., Velicer, W.F., Velasquez, M.M. and Rossi, J.S. (1991) The process of smoking cessation: an analysis of precontemplation, contemplation and preparation stages of change. *Journal of Consulting and Clinical Psychology* **59**, 295–304.

DiMatteo, M.R. (1979) A social-psychological analysis of physician-patient rapport: toward a science of the art of medicine. *Journal of Social Issues* **35**, 12–33.

DiMatteo, M.R. and DiNicola, D.D. (1982) *Achieving patient compliance: the psychology of the medical practitioner's role.* New York: Pergamon Press.

DiMatteo, M.R. and Hays, R. (1980) The significance of patients' perceptions of physician conduct: a study of patient satisfaction in a family practice center. *Journal of Community Health* **6**, 18–34.

DiMatteo, M.R., Hays, R., Prince, L.M. (1986) Relationship of physicians' non-verbal communication skills to patient satisfaction, appointment non-compliance, and physician workload. *Health Psychology* **5**, 581–594.

DiMatteo, M.R., Sherbourne, C.D., Hays, R.D., Ordway, L., Kravitz, R.L., McGlynn, E.A., Kaplan, S. and Rogers, W.H. (1993) Physician's characteristics influence patients' adherence to medical treatment: results from the medical outcomes study. *Health Psychology* **12**, 93–102.

Donovan, J.L. and Blake, D.R. (1992) Patient non-compliance: deviance or reasoned decision-making? *Social Science and Medicine* **34**, 507–13.

Essex, B., Roig, R. and Renshaw, J. (1990) Pilot study of records of shared care for people with mental illnesses. *British Medical Journal* **300**, 1442–1446.

Fletcher, C. (1980) Listening and talking to patients. I. The problem. II. The clinical interview. III. The exposition. IV. Some special problems. *British Medical Journal* **281**, 845, 931, 994, 1056.

Fletcher, R.H. (1989) Patient compliance with therapeutic advice: a modern view. *The Mount Sinai Journal of Medicine* **56**, 453–458.

Fletcher, S.W., Fletcher, R.H., Thomas, D.C. and Hamann, C. (1979) Patients' understanding of prescribed drugs. *Journal of Community Health* **4**, 183–89.

Freemon, B., Negrete, V.F., Davis, M. and Korsch, B.M. (1971) Gaps in doctor-patient communication: doctor-patient interaction analysis. *Paediatric Research* 298–311.

Friedman, H.S. (1979) Non-verbal communication between patients and medical practitioners. *Journal of Social Issues* **35**, 82–99.

Francis, V., Korsch, B.M. and Morris, M.J. (1969) Gaps in doctor-patient communication: patients' response to medical advice. *New England Journal of Medicine* **280**, 535–540.

Gordis, L., Markowitz, M., and Lilienfeld, A.M. (1969) Why patients don't follow medical advice: a study of children on long-term anti-streptococcal prophylaxis. *Journal of Paediatrics* **75**, 957–968.

Green, L.W. (1978) Determining the impact and effectiveness of health education as it relates to federal policy. *Health Education Monographs (suppl. 1)* **6**, 28–66.

Gritz, E.R. and Bastani, R. (1993) Cancer prevention – behavior changes: the short and the long of it. *Preventive Medicine* **22**, 676–688.

Gritz, E.R., Berman, B.A., Bastani, R. and Wu, M. (1992) A randomised trial of a self-help smoking cessation intervention in a nonvolunteer female population: testing the limits of the public health model. *Health Psychology* **11**, 280–289.

Gabbard-Alley, A.S. (1995) Health communication and gender: a review and critique. *Health Communication* **7**, 35–54.

Gerrard, T.J. and Riddell, J.D. (1988) Difficult patients: black holes and secrets. *British Medical Journal* **297**, 530–32.

Groves, J.E. (1978) Taking care of the hateful patient. *The New England Journal of Medicine* **298**, 883–887.

Hall, J.A., Roter, D.L. and Katz, N.R. (1988) Correlates of provider behavior: a meta-analysis. *Medical Care* **26**, 657–675.

Hayes-Bautista, D.E. (1976) Modifying the treatment: patient compliance, patient control and medical care. *Social Science and Medicine* **10**, 233–238.

Haynes, R.B. (1979) Determinants of compliance: the disease and the mechanism of treatment. In R. B. Haynes, D.W. Taylor D.W. and D.L. Sackett (eds.) *Compliance in Health Care.* Baltimore: Johns Hopkins University Press .

Hessen-Klemens, I. (1987) Patients' non-compliance and how doctors manage this. *Social Science and Medicine* **24**, 409–416.

Hessen-Klemens, I. and Lapinska, E. (1984) Doctor-patient interaction, patients' health behavior and effects of treatment. *Social Science and Medicine* **19**, 9–18.

Hope, T. (1996) Don't 'consent' patients, help them to decide. *Health Care Analysis* **4**, 73–76.

Hopp, J.W. and Gerken, C.M. (1983) Making an educational diagnosis to improve patient education: the pulmonary rehabilitation team. *Respiratory Care* **28**, 1456–1461.

Hulka, B.S., Cassel, J.C., Kupper, L.L. and Burdette, J.A. (1976) Communication, compliance, concordance between physicians and patients with prescribed medications. *American Journal of Public Health* **66**, 847–853.

Inui, T.S. and Carter, W.B. (1985) Problems and prospects for health services research on provider-patient communication. *Medical Care* **23**, 521–538.

Inui, T.S., Yourtee, E.L. and Williamson, J.W. (1976) Improved outcomes in hypertension after physician tutorials: a controlled trial. *Annals of Internal Medicine* **84**, 646–651.

Jenkins, C.D. (1979) An approach to the diagnosis and treatment of problems in health-related behaviour. *International Journal of Health Education (Suppl. 2)* **22**, 1–24.

Kaplan, S.H., Greenfield, S. and Ware, J.E. Jr (1989) Impact of the doctor-patient relationship on the outcomes of chronic disease. In M. Stewart and D. Roter (eds.) *Communicating with medical patients* Newbury Park: Sage.

Kasl, S.V. (1975) Social-psychological characteristics associated with behaviors which reduce cardiovascular risk. In A.J. Enelow and J.B. Henderson (eds.) *Applying behavioral science to cardiovascular risk* . Dallas, Texas: American Heart Association.

Katz, J.N., Daltroy, L.H., Brennan, T.A. and Liang, M.H. (1992) Informed consent and the prescription of non-steroidal anti-inflammatory drugs. *Arthritis and Rheumatism* **35**, 1257–1263.

Kenney, R.D., Lyles, M.E., Turner, R.C., White, S.T., Gonsalez, J.J., Irons, T.G., Sanchez, C.J., Rogers, C.S., Campbell, E.E. and Villagra, V.G. (1988) Smoking cessation counseling by resident physicians in internal medicine, family practice and pediatrics. *Archives of Internal Medicine* **148**, 2469–2473.

Kjellern, K.I., Ahlner, J. and Slj, R. (1995) Taking hypertensive medication – controlling or co-operating with patients? *International Journal of Cardiology* **47**, 257–268.

Korsch, B.M., Gozzi, E.K. and Francis, V. (1968) Gaps in doctor-patient communication: Doctor-patient interaction and patient satisfaction. *Pediatrics* **42**, 855–871.

Lane, S.D. (1983) Compliance, satisfaction and physician-patient communication. In R. Bostrom (ed.) *Communication yearbook 7*. Beverley Hills, CA: Sage .

Leventhal, H. and Cameron, L. (1987) Behavioral theories and the problem of compliance. *Patient Education and Counseling* **10**, 117–138.

Levinson, W., Stiles, W.B., Inui, T.S. and Engle, R. (1993) Physician frustration in communicating with patients. *Medical Care* **31**, 285–295.

Lewis, C.E., Clancy, C., Leake, B. and Schwartz, J.S. (1991) The counseling practices of internists. *Annals of Internal Medicine* **114**, 54–58.

Ley, P. (1977) Psychological studies of doctor-patient communication. In S. Rachman (ed.) *Contributions to medical psychology. volume 1*. Oxford: Pegamon Press.

Ley, P. (1979) The psychology of compliance. In D.J. Oborne, M.M. Gruneberg and J.R. Eiser (eds.) *Research in Psychology and Medicine. volume 2* London: Academic Press .

Ley, P. (1981) Professional non-compliance: a neglected problem. *British Journal of Clinical Psychology* **20**, 151–154.

Ley, P. (1982a) Satisfaction, compliance and communication. *British Journal of Clinical Psychology* **21**, 241–254.

Ley, P. (1982b) Giving information to patients. In J.R. Eiser (ed.) *Social psychology and behavioral science*. New York: John Wiley and Sons .

Lowery, B.J. and DuCette, J.P. (1976) Disease-related learning and disease control in diabetics as a function of locus of control. *Nursing Research* **25**, 358–362.

Maynard, D. (1989) Notes on the delivery and reception of diagnostic news regarding mental disabilities. In D. Helm, T. Anderson, A. Meehan and A. Rawls (eds.) *The interactional order: new directions in the study of the social order*. New York: Irvington .

Mazucca, S.A. (1982) Does patient education in chronic disease have therapeutic value? *Journal of Chronic Diseases* **35**, 521–529.

McClellan, W. (1986) The physician and patient education: a review. *Patient Education and Counseling* **8**, 151–163.

McKinlay, J.B. (1972) Some approaches and problems in the study of the use of services: an overview. *Journal of Health and Social Behavior* **13**, 115–152.

McMillan, D.D., Lockyer, J.M., Magnan, L., Akierman, A. and Parboosingh, J.T. (1991) Effect of educational programme and interview on adoption of guidelines for the management of neonatal hyperbilirubinemia. *Canadian Medical Association Journal* **144**, 707–712.

Meichenbaum, D. and Turk D.C. (1987) *Facilitating treatment adherence: a practitioner's guidebook* . New York: Plenum Press .

Mittelmark, M.B., Leupker, R.V., Grimm, R. Jr., Kottke, T.E. and Blackburn H. (1988) The role of physicians in a community-wide programme for prevention of cardiovascular diseases: the Minnesota Heart Health Program. *Public Health Reports* **103**, 360–365.

Morris, L.A. and Kanouse, D.E. (1982) Informing patients about drug side-effects. *Journal of Behavioral Medicine* **5**, 363–373.

Myers, E.D. and Calvert, E.J. (1973) Effects of forwarning on the occurrence of side-effects and discontinuance of medication in patients on amitryptiline. *British Journal of Psychiatry* **122**, 461–464.

Myers, E.D. and Calvert, E.J. (1976) Effects of forwarning on the occurrence of side-effects and discontinuance of medication in patients on dothiepin. *Journal of International Medical Research* **4**, 237–240.

Myers, E.D. and Calvert, E.J. (1978) Knowledge of side-effects and perseverence with medication. *British Journal of Psychiatry* **132**, 526–527.

O'Dowd, T.C. (1988) Five years of heartsink patients in general practice. *British Medical Journal* **297**, 528–530.

Palchik ,N.S., Laing, T.J., Connell, K.J., Daltroy, L.H., Friedman, C.P., Hull, A.L. and Mazzuca S.A. (1991) Research priorities for professional education. *Arthritis and Rheumatism* **34**, 234–240.

Platt, F.W. and McMath, J.C. (1979) Clinical hypocompetence: the interview. *Annals of Internal Medicine* **91**, 898–902.

Porter, A.M.W. (1969) Drug defaulting in a general practice. *British Medical Journal* **1**, 218–222.

Prochaska, J.O. and DiClemente, C.C. (1983) Stages and processes of self-change of smoking: toward an integrative model of change. *Journal of Consulting and Clinical Psychology* **51**, 390–395.

Prochaska, J.O., Velicer, W.F., Rossi, J.S., Goldstein, M.G., Marcus, B., Rakowski, W., Fiore, C., Harlow, L.L., Redding, C.A., Rosenbloom, D. and Rossi S.R. (1994). Stages of change and decisional balance for twelve problem behaviors. *Health Psychology* **13**, 39–46.

Quaid, K.A., Faden, R. R., Vining, E.P. and Freeman J.M. (1990) Informed consent for a prescription drug: impact of disclosed information on patient understanding and medical outcomes. *Patient Education and Counseling* **15**, 249–259.

Richards, A.D. (1964) Attitude and drug acceptance. *British Journal of Psychiatry* **110**, 46.

Rimer, B., Jones, W.L., Keintz, M.K., Catalono, R.B. and Engstrom P.F. (1984) Informed consent: a crucial step in cancer patient education. *Health Education Quarterly (Suppl.)* **19**, 30–42.

Romm, F.J., Hulka, B.S. and Mayo F. (1976) Correlates of outcome in patients with congestive heart failure. *Medical Care* **14**, 765–776.

Rosenstock, I.M., Strecher, V.J. and Becker M.H. (1988) Social learning theory and the health belief model. *Health Education Quarterly* **15**, 178–193.

Ross, F.M. (1991) Patient compliance: whose responsibility? *Social Science and Medicine* **32**, 89–94.

Ross, J.L. and Phipps, E. (1986) Physician-patient power struggles: their role in non-compliance. *Family Medicine* **18**, 99–101.

Rost, K. (1989) The influence of patient participation on satisfaction and compliance. *The Diabetes Educator* **15**, 139–143.

Rotter, J.B. (1966) Generalised expectancies for internal vs. external control of reinforcement. *Psychological Monographs* **80**, 1–28.

Roter, D. (1977) Patient participation in the patient-provider interaction: the effects of patient question asking on the quality of interaction, satisfaction and compliance. *Health Education Monographs* **5**, 281–315.

Roter, D. and Frankel, R. (1992) Quantitative and qualitative approaches to the evaluation of the medical dialogue. *Social Science and Medicine* **34**, 1097–1103.

Roter, D. and Hall, J.A. (1987) Physician interviewing styles and medical information gained from patients. *Journal of General Internal Medicine* **2**, 325–329.

Russell, M.L., Insull, W. Jr. and Probstfield J.L. (1985) Examination of medical professions for counseling on medication adherence. *American Journal of Medicine* **78**, 277–382.

Sanson-Fisher, R.W., Campbell, E.M., Redman, S. and Hennrikus D.J. (1989) Patient-provider interactions and patient outcomes. *The Diabetes Educator* **15**, 134–138.

Scherwitz, L., Hennrikus, D., Yusim, S., Lester, J. and Valbona C. (1985) Physician communication to patients regarding medication. *Patient Education and Counseling* **7**, 121–136.

Schwartz, D., Wang, M., Zeitz, L. and Goss M.E.W. (1962) Medication errors made by elderly and chronically ill patients. *American Journal of Public Health* **52**, 2018.

Shangold, M.M. (1979) The health care of physicians: do as I say not as I do. *Journal of Medical Education* **54**, 668.

Sotosky, J.R., McGrory, C.H., Metzger, D.S. and DeHoratius R.J. (1992) Arthritis problem indicator: preliminary report on a new tool for use in the primary care setting. *Arthritis Care and Research* **5**, 157–162.

Squier, R.W. (1990) A model of empathic understanding and adherence to treatment regimens in practitioner-patient relationships. *Social Science and Medicine* **30**, 325–339.

Starfield, B., Wray, C., Hess, K., Gross, R., Birke, P. and D'Lugoff B.C. (1981) The influence of patient-practitioner agreement on outcome of care. *American Journal of Public Health* **71**, 127–131.

Steele, D.J., Jackson, T.C. and Gutmann, M.C. (1990) Have you been taking your pills? The adherence monitoring sequence in the medical interview. *Journal of Family Practice* **30**, 294–299.

Stimson, G.V. (1974) Obeying doctor's orders: a view from the other side. *Social Science and Medicine* **8**, 97–104.

Stoeckle, J.D. and Barsky, A.J. (1980) Attributions: uses of social science knowledge in the 'doctoring' of primary care. In I. Eisenberg and A. Kleinman (eds.) *The relevance of social science for medicine.* Dordrecht: D. Reidel Publishing Company.

Suris-Rangel, A.C., DiClemente, C.C. and Dunn J.R. (1988) *Stages and processes in weight control for Mexican American women.* New York: 22nd Annual AABT Convention.

Svarstad, B. (1974) *The patient-physician encounter: an observational study of communication and outcome.* Unpublished PhD thesis: University of Wisconsin.

Svarstad, B. (1976) Physician-patient communication and patient conformity with medical advice. In M. Mechanic (ed.) *The growth of bureaucratic medicine: an inquiry into the dynamics of patient behavior and the organisation of medical care.* New York: Wiley.

Trostle, J.A. (1988) Medical compliance as an ideology. *Social Science and Medicine* **27**, 1299–1308.

Velicer, W.F., Prochaska, J.O., Rossi, J.S. and Snow M.G. (1992) Assessing outcome in smoking cessation studies. *Psychological Bulletin* **111**, 23–41.

Wartman, S.A., Morlock, L.L., Malitz, F.E. and Palm E. (1983) The impact of divergent evaluations by physicians and patients of patients' complaints. *Public Health Reports* **98**, 1414–1415.

Wilson, B.M. (1995) Promoting compliance: the patient-provider partnership. *Advances in Renal Replacement Therapy* **2**, 199–206.

Wooley, F.R., Kane, R.L., Hughes, C.C. and Wright D.D. (1978) The effects of doctor-patient communication on satisfaction and outcome of care. *Social Science and Medicine* **12**, 123–128.

Wright, E.C. (1993) Non-compliance – or how many aunts has Matilda? *The Lancet* **342**, 909–913.

Yeo, G.T., de-Burgh, S.P., Letton, T., Shaw, J., Donnelly, N., Swinburn, M.E., Phillips, S., Bridges-Webb, C. and Mant, A. (1994) Educational visiting and hypnosedative prescribing in general practice. *Family Practice* **11**, 57–61.

Zola, I.K. (1980) Structural constraints in the doctor-patient relationship: the case of non-compliance. In I. Eisenberg and A. Kleinman (eds.) *The relevance of social science for medicine.* Dordrecht: D. Reidel Publishing Company.

4

The Influence of Written Information on Patient Knowledge and Adherence to Treatment

D.K. Raynor

Most treatment regimes require the patient to be given a certain amount of information if they are to be able to adhere to the treatment. However, it is apparent that there are two key reasons why there is no direct link between provision of information and adherence:

- the provision of information does not necessarily result in the transfer of knowledge;
- the transfer of knowledge does not necessarily lead to a change in behaviour or attitude.

These two factors underpin any discussion on information and adherence.

Increasing acceptance by health professionals (HPs) of the relative ineffectiveness in effectiveness of their verbal interventions appears to be one reason why the written form has become an important method for delivering information to patients (Mays, 1994). Original work such as that of Ley (1973), showed that, after five minutes, patients had forgotten around half of the verbal instructions given to them. More recently, patients were shown to remember about a third of verbal information given by pharmacists after 24 hours (Wilson *et al.*, 1992). Furthermore, HPs often have insufficient time to give all the necessary information verbally (Raynor, 1992a).

Another reason for the greater use of written information may be the increasing sophistication of some types of treatment, which often means that greater understanding and input is required of the patient. The shift towards written information appears to be particularly marked in the field of drug therapy. It is this area of treatment which I will use to demonstrate the principles governing the relationship between written information, knowledge and adherence.

HOW CAN INFORMATION INFLUENCE ADHERENCE?

Information has the potential to positively influence adherence in a number of ways:

- Patients who want to adhere but need more information to allow them to do so;
- Patients who have fears and misconceptions about their treatment which may be countered by providing information;
- Patients dissatisfied with their care (in general or specifically relating to the amount and quality of the information given). Equally, information might have a negative effect on adherence, through the provision of facts which cause a patient to decide not to adhere.

Positive influence can be direct or indirect (see Table 1). Direct influence comes through giving basic information on "how to" i.e. enabling information. For medication, this may simply be the number of tablets to take and when to take them. If a non-standard form of treatment is used (e.g. an inhaler or suppository), enabling information on administration is particularly important. The influence here is on unintentional non-adherence i.e. where patients want to adhere, but lack certain information to allow them to do so (Raynor, 1992a).

Indirect influence on adherence comes through three main avenues, which are largely related to intentional non-adherence, where patients make a conscious decision not to adhere (Raynor, 1992a). The first is the correction of misunderstanding. For example, many patients believe that alcohol cannot be taken while taking any antibiotics (Penwarden and Raynor, 1996). In fact, this applies to only a small minority of antibiotics. If information is provided stating that alcohol can be taken, this may cause a patient to change a decision not to take an antibiotic. The second avenue relates to a change in attitude to treatment e.g. countering patients' erroneous views about the addictive potential of corticosteroid therapy. Also relevant here is information which emphasises to the patient the benefits they will gain from the treatment. However, simple information provision alone is unlikely to bring about an immediate change in long-standing beliefs and attitudes which are firmly held.

The third avenue relates to a general effect on satisfaction with treatment, one of the characteristics of the patient-health service interaction associated with adherence (Ley, 1988). The quality of doctor-patient communication is a key factor in adherence (DiMatteo and DiNicola, 1982) and this effect is likely to be mirrored for other HPs.

Table 1 Methods by which information can positively influence adherence

Category	Type of Information	Example of Information
Direct	Basic enabling information	When to take medicines during the day
	Detailed enabling information on use of non-standard treatments	How to use an asthma inhaler
Indirect	Information which corrects misunderstanding	The ability to drink alcohol while taking certain medications
	Information which alters attitude to treatment	The lack of addictive potential of steroids The benefits of treatment
	Information which makes the patient more satisfied with their care	A well designed leaflet relevant to the patient's needs⸱

Information can have a negative influence on adherence (see Table 2) through provision of information on topics such as side-effects, efficacy or contra-indications. Gibbs, Waters and George (1989a) found that a leaflet on non-steroidal anti-inflammatory drugs (NSAIDs: the mainstay of drug treatment for rheumatoid arthritis) caused a small number of patients to stop taking these tablets. They had been prescribed the drug for relatively minor symptoms, which they perceived as too minor to risk the side-effects described. This type of behaviour has been described as "intelligent non-adherence", where patients decide not to adhere for appropriate reasons (Weintraub, 1981). However, describing the relative risk of adverse effects is difficult (Anon. 1996), and leaflets generally resort to words like "rarely" or "infrequently". This may make an informed decision difficult to make.

Information can also have a negative effect when too much information is provided. Weinman (1990) described two types of "coping style": patients who cope by becoming involved in their treatment and who welcome detailed information and patients who cope by avoiding the issues associated with their treatment and who do not desire detailed information. Negative results may also arise when patients receive conflicting information from a number of different sources e.g. a patient with diabetes may receive information on their treatment from a doctor, nurse, dietician and pharmacist. Any contradiction is likely to lead to a negative effect. Conversely, if each piece of information reinforces and complements the others, the result is likely to be an effective overall message.

Table 2 Methods by which information can negatively influence adherence

Category	Type of Information	Example of Information
Direct	Information on risks of treatment	The side-effects of drugs
Indirect	Excessive amounts of information leading to dissatisfaction	Long or multiple leaflets which are not relevant to the patient
	Conflicting information from different sources	Conflicting verbal and/or written information from several professionals

Donovan, Blake and Fleming (1989) remind us that "the patient is not a blank sheet". Patients have a complex set of lay beliefs and "knowledge", drawn from their own experiences, the media, friends and family (Stockwell-Morris and Schultz, 1993). The influence of family and friends' beliefs is particularly important, as their influence is one of the few patient-related aspects accepted as being firmly linked with adherence (Haynes, 1976). Attitudes towards the benefits of following medical advice are therefore developed in the light of these non-professional sources of information. Information from a professional source will always be filtered through this existing background information. The powerful influence of such sources of information on adherence to treatment should not be underestimated.

The effect of information is complex because treatment knowledge is made up of independent components, and good knowledge of one component does not guarantee the same knowledge of other aspects (Ascione, Kirscht and Shimp, 1986). In respect of medication, patients are generally most knowledgeable about the dose schedule and purpose of the medicine, with knowledge about side-effects being generally poor (Pullar *et al.*, 1989; Eagleton, Walker and Barber, 1993; Sullivan and George, 1996).

The evidence that patients want more information about their treatment has been described as overwhelming (Weinman, 1990). However, there is some evidence that the elderly are less receptive to more information (Livingstone, 1995). The International Medical Benefit Risk Foundation (IMBRF) (1993) suggested the minimum information patients should be given about medication was : name and dose, purpose and benefits, how to take, special precautions and adverse events. This is roughly comparable with what patients themselves say they would like (Sutton, Smart and Herring, 1989). However, a study cited by Myers (1995) found some marked differences in the patients' and doctors' views in this respect. In particular, doctors were reluctant to give information on side-effects and lifestyle changes, which were amongst the patients' priorities.

WHAT ARE THE MAIN CATEGORIES OF WRITTEN INFORMATION?

Leaflets and booklets relevant to certain disease states (from manufacturers, patients' organisations and the NHS) have been described elsewhere (Allen and Sweeney, 1985, Axon *et al.*, 1989) and the place of leaflets in general has been usefully reviewed by McIver (1993). It has been suggested that the public tends to ignore much printed information on health which is general in nature (Meredith, Emberton and Wood, 1995), although this has been challenged (Dixon, 1995). Perhaps, it depends on the relevance and quality of the information. Leaflets relating to a patient's specific medicines were said to be read by just under three-quarters of patients (Ley, 1988).

The label remains the single most important source of information about medicines for a patient. Verbal information is largely forgotten and leaflets may be ignored or thrown away (Raynor and Silletto, 1982). However size clearly limits the potential of the label as an information source. The inclusion of "additional labels" which added to the basic dose and frequency instructions became mandatory in the UK in 1987. These provide limited information on storage and handling, timing of doses and potential side-effects.

The influence of labelling on adherence was studied in the early 1980s (Adult Literacy Support Services Fund, 1981; Raynor and Silletto, 1982). Many wordings on labels were shown to be misunderstood e.g. "every 8 hours" was interpreted as two doses per day by 52% of patients and 39% thought that: "Caution: avoid alcohol while taking this preparation" meant that a little alcohol could be taken. The influence of such misunderstanding on patients' ability to adhere is clear. Later, Barber and Raynor (1989) found that plain English versions of traditional wordings were generally more memorable, understandable and acceptable. However, the study also highlighted the problem of expressing complex ideas (e.g. drug-induced photosensitivity) in two or three short lines.

WHAT IS THE EFFECT OF PATIENT INFORMATION LEAFLETS ON KNOWLEDGE AND ADHERENCE?

The inadequacies of providing information verbally or on a label leads logically to the provision of information in leaflet form (generally known as Patient Information Leaflets: PILs). Many studies have examined the effect of such leaflets on patient knowledge and, to a lesser extent, adherence.

USA Studies

Until the 1980s, most studies came from the USA. Five papers in the 1970s on antibiotics all reported increased adherence in patients given written information (Colcher and Bass, 1972; Madden, 1973; Sharpe and Mikeal, 1974; Linkewich *et al.*, 1974; Lima *et al.*, 1976). However, the written intervention was generally accompanied by other interventions, notably verbal information. A one page information leaflet on medication used in long-term therapy had no significant effect on adherence (Clinite and Kabat, 1976). A study of an information sheet on diuretics compared distribution by the doctor or the pharmacist (DeTullio *et al.*, 1986). Patients preferred to receive the sheet from their doctor, but their satisfaction with the information given did not differ between the two groups. Patients in both groups had significantly increased overall knowledge compared with a control group. Johnson *et al.*, (1986) tested a one page information sheet which described the medicine's purpose, dose regime and common side-effects. The improvement in knowledge was small (although statistically significant).

Early studies of leaflets for oral contraceptives in the USA (Fleckenstein *et al.*, 1976; Morris, Mazis and Gordon, 1977) suggested that such leaflets were received, read and understood. A series of studies on leaflets on other drugs confirmed these findings. Overall, 72% of patients said they had read the leaflet. The leaflets were kept by about half the patients and were more likely to be read by patients receiving the medicine for the first time. Most patients found the leaflets helpful in understanding their medicine and this was confirmed by objective testing. However, although 80% of patients said the leaflet helped their understanding, it appeared to have minimal effect on attitudes and behaviour and it made patients neither more likely not less likely to adhere (Anon., 1981). In a later study of the oral contraceptive leaflet, 61% of a sample of recipients had read all of the leaflet and 10% had read none of the leaflet. On average, patients could correctly answer just under half of the questions asked of them about the information contained in the leaflet. Twenty-one percent said it was difficult to understand (Sands, Robinson and Orlando, 1984).

Culbertson *et al.*, (1988) tested the effect of a modified version of leaflets produced by the major US provider of medical information for patients, the US Pharmacopoeia, when given with brief verbal information. Fifty seven percent of the study group responded. Of the respondents, 45% said the information was responsible for changing the way they took their medicines.

UK Studies

Early work in the UK centred on leaflets for patients being discharged from hospital. In one study, patients were given information on diagnosis and medication either verbally or through a short leaflet. At follow-up, all the points of information were better recalled by the leaflet group (Ellis *et al.*, 1979). A later study of an antibiotic leaflet showed a significant increase in both knowledge and adherence. These leaflets were well designed, used simple language, and a "question and answer" format (Dodds, 1986).

Three studies by Kay used a series of well-designed pieces of written information for medication, including a question and answer format, and simple language. Two of the studies showed significantly increased patients' knowledge when followed-up by telephone (Kay, Moss and Rees, 1987; Punchak and Kay, 1988). The third leaflet was tested on inpatients, who were questioned before receiving the information and then 3 or more days later. Results indicated significantly superior recall of many of the points of information (Kay and Bailie, 1987).

Hawkey and Hawkey (1989) studied 12 leaflets on gastro-intestinal disease (commended by the Plain English Campaign) on over 1000 patients. A postal questionnaire had a response rate of 65%. Knowledge was significantly better in the leaflet group, although up to 30% of patients found the information worrying. The leaflets were reported to be either an equally good or better source of information than the doctor, and most patients found the leaflets easy to read.

Brief leaflets (A6 in size) for cardiology drugs were prepared with advice from the Plain English Campaign and given to patients along with verbal information. Compared with verbal information alone, the leaflets resulted in significantly greater recall, especially about missed doses and side-effects (followed-up by postal questionnaire). Patients given written information were more satisfied with their information provision and drug treatment (Baker *et al.*, 1991). However, in the above studies, where patients were followed-up by post or telephone, it is possible that they could have read their responses directly from the leaflets.

Southampton Leaflets

The most widely studied leaflets in the UK are those developed by George and his co-workers in Southampton. They were first described in 1983 (George, Waters and Nicholas) and were generic in style, i.e. they contained information relating to a group of drugs, rather than a specific drug. Leaflets for penicillins and NSAIDs were tested in a controlled study of nearly 200 general practice patients. Almost all of the patients thought that the leaflets were "very clear" or "clear," and two-thirds thought the leaflets were helpful, although 20–31% said they were unnecessary. There was a small increase in knowledge in the patients who received the leaflets and there was a non-significant trend for an increase in satisfaction with treatment. Adherence was significantly increased only for penicillins. Two second-generation leaflets were then prepared (one-sided and two-sided) with input from a graphic artist and an educational psychologist. Both leaflets contained an essentially similar side of fairly detailed information (the total content of the one-sided leaflet). The two-sided leaflet contained brief summarised information on the other side. Generally the leaflets followed the principles of plain English in terms of content and design.

Gibbs, Waters and George (1987) compared the two-sided leaflets for NSAIDs and Penicillins, with the one-sided version. The two-sided design was preferred by 85% of patients. Patients were given three minutes to read the leaflet, after which 48% could name the main side-effects (two-sided) compared with 29% (one-sided). Following this study, 174 patients who were actually prescribed a drug were supplied with a leaflet. There were no significant differences in resulting patient knowledge between the two styles. However, satisfaction was significantly better with the two-sided leaflet. There was no effect on adherence.

In two further controlled studies the two-sided style of leaflet was used for six different groups of drugs. There was a small increase in patient knowledge in the leaflet group compared with control. There was no significant effect on adherence, but satisfaction with the information given was significantly higher in patients who received the leaflets (Gibbs *et al.*, 1989a; 1989b). A subsequent postal questionnaire indicated significant differences in knowledge between control and leaflet group. The most marked benefit was for information about drug side-effects. Satisfaction was significantly better in the leaflet group (Gibbs, Waters and George, 1990). These two-sided leaflets were eventually adopted by the Association of British Pharmaceutical Industry (ABPI) as the basis for their guidelines on the production of PILs (ABPI, 1988).

WRITTEN OR VERBAL INFORMATION?

Studies investigating verbal communication alone have shown a variable effect on knowledge of, and adherence to, medication; it can increase knowledge, but it is less likely to improve adherence

(Raynor, 1992a). Some researchers including Mazzuca (1982) and Haynes *et al.* (1987) are consequently sceptical about the effect of providing verbal information and education. One of the difficulties in assessing such studies is the wide variations in the nature of the verbal intervention (length of time taken, degree of interaction, use of summarising, checking for recall, etc.). In many cases the nature of the intervention is not described in detail and simply described as "counselling".

It has been suggested that written information reinforced by verbal information is the most effective means of transmitting information to patients (Kessler, 1991; IMBRF, 1993). There is some evidence to support this, although it is not conclusive (Raynor, 1991). The combination of verbal and written information was shown to be clearly superior to the individual interventions, particularly with respect to knowledge, in some studies. Woroniecki *et al.* (1982) looked at long-term recall, after 8 weeks, in patients given verbal information plus written information or verbal information alone. Knowledge was increased by 31% in the former group, compared with a 20% increase in the latter group, a significant difference. McBean and Blackburn (1982) also found a statistically significant increase in knowledge in patients given both written and verbal information, but not with verbal information alone. There was a non-significant trend for adherence to increase. Similarly, Gauld (1981) found that patients recalled information about their condition significantly more completely when they were given verbal reinforcement of written information, than with verbal information alone, although there was no significant increase in adherence. Baker *et al.* (1991) also found that the combination maximised recall of information.

Two of the most comprehensive reviews of information and its effect on adherence concluded that a combination of written and verbal information produces the highest level of knowledge and adherence (Morris and Halperin, 1979; Ley, 1988). Other authors have concurred (Cochrane, 1992; Rheinstein, McGinnis and Nightingale, 1995) and it seems clear that written instructions without a verbal explanation will not fully educate a patient (Smith, 1983).

The combination of verbal and written information can maximise the potential improvement in knowledge and adherence for a number of reasons.

- .Repetition and reinforcement will result from the pharmacist or doctor going through the leaflet briefly with the patient and summarising the contents. The patient then reads the same information at home. Such reinforcement increases patients' uptake and recall of information (Ley, 1979).
- Verbal reinforcement shows the patient that the professional feels that the written information is important and relevant to the patient (Raynor, 1992a).
- Patients appear to prefer the combination of the two methods (Harvey *et al.*, 1991; Dodds and King, 1989). Doak, Doak and Root (1985) suggest that giving the verbal information first, telling the patient that the written information is important, and preferably taking the patient through it is better than simply handing the written information over.

PATIENT INFORMATION LEAFLET INITIATIVES IN THE USA AND UK

In the USA in the 1970s, pressure from consumer and professional bodies led to proposals for the compulsory supply of leaflets inside medicine packs. However, objections led to the development of a voluntary system, with the American Medical Association, US Pharmacopoeia, American Society of Hospital Pharmacists amongst others all preparing PILs, for supply to patients by doctors and pharmacists. However, in the mid 1990s, it was felt that substantial numbers of patients were still not getting sufficient written information with their medicines. Initiatives were then set up to ensure that by the year 2000, at least 75% of patients would receive a useful and easy-to-understand leaflet conforming to certain standards. These leaflets will be mandatory for selected drugs with particular risks (Rheinstein *et al.*, 1995).

In some European countries, PILs have been available for some time, notably in the Netherlands, France and Germany, although the content and method of distribution varies. In Sweden, generic leaflets covering over 70 drug groups are provided by pharmacists. Similarly, in Sweden there is a medicines information compendium available for patients (Baudrihaye, 1991).

In the UK, there were similar arguments about PILs as in the USA (Anon., 1978) and it has similarly proved difficult to reach a consensus. Until the late 1980s, PILs were provided with only a small number of medicines. An industry working party subsequently recommended that PILs should be prepared by manufacturers and supplied sealed in medicine packs (ABPI, 1987). Some felt that these new leaflets might resemble previous poor quality industry-produced leaflets and preferred that unbiased HPs should produce them, as in the USA (Anon., 1987). It was also suggested that manufacturers might include too much information to protect themselves against litigation (George, 1987).

A subsequent document: "Patient information: advice on the drafting of leaflets" (ABPI, 1988) alleviated many of the fears, by recommending that leaflets should be succinct, intelligible and have a uniform design. The advice was also largely consistent with good practice in terms of text design and layout. The two-sided style of leaflet developed by George and his team in Southampton was adopted i.e. a summary on one side and detailed information on the other. These new style leaflets began to appear in 1989.

Subsequently, a European Community directive was published (EC Directive 92/27/EEC), which requires that all medicines supplied to patients should be accompanied by a comprehensive information leaflet (known as a "patient user leaflet"). The amount of information which has to be included is much more than the Southampton leaflets. It must include dose instructions and all contra-indications and precautions mentioned in the written information supplied to HPs (known as the Data Sheet). However, all information should be written "in a manner which is understandable to the patient" (Drug and Therapeutics Bulletin, 1995).

When the Directive was launched, the Council of the European Community, said that they hoped that "improved information will improve patient compliance" (Donnelly, 1991). The Directive was subsequently implemented in the UK through the development of a patient pack dispensing system (medicine pack plus PIL). Similarly, this launch promoted the benefits relating to adherence. These claims were made despite lack of evidence for such an effect. The inclusion of leaflets within medicines packs, although a reliable method of making sure the patient actually receives the written information, is clearly no guarantee that they will read it, or change their behaviour as a result.

If patients do read leaflets supplied inside medicine packs, it could be argued that even the limited effects on knowledge and adherence suggested by controlled studies cannot be assured. This is because of the differences between a package insert and the style of leaflet generally tested in the studies described above. On the whole, including the Southampton studies, leaflets tested have been personally handed out by doctors or pharmacists. The effect of written information is likely to depend on the method of distribution (Morris and Halperin, 1979). The leaflets studied have also generally been an unfolded piece of good quality paper or card. This is in marked contrast to the thin, multiply folded package inserts, found sealed within a medicine pack. Equally, most of the evidence is based on a leaflet for one of a patient's medicines. Again there will be a different situation when all medicines come with such a leaflet. Consequently, great care needs to be taken in extrapolating the results of most studies to leaflets provided as package inserts on a universal basis.

A major advantage of a single universal PIL for each drug is the opportunity it gives for HPs to base their verbal information on a common source. Repetition is an effective method of increasing recall of information (Ley, 1979). A universal PIL will help to ensure that the information given to patients by all professionals is consistent, hence maximising the repetition effect.

INDIVIDUALISED WRITTEN INFORMATION

Written information which is individualised or personalised for a patient can have an effect on adherence which is over and above that possible with standardised information. This may be achieved in two ways.

- Through increased satisfaction: patients like personalised information and may be more likely to read it and accept it (Sellu, 1987).
- Through incorporation of a behavioural component: it is possible to tailor a treatment to a patients daily routine (Raynor, 1992a).

Medicine reminder charts incorporate both such elements and are particularly useful for patients on multiple medication. Such charts consist of a simple grid showing a sample day's regimen (see Figure 1). The medicines names are included on the horizontal axis and on the vertical axis are four daily events to which the patient can relate (usually meal times and bedtime). Each daily dose is marked in the

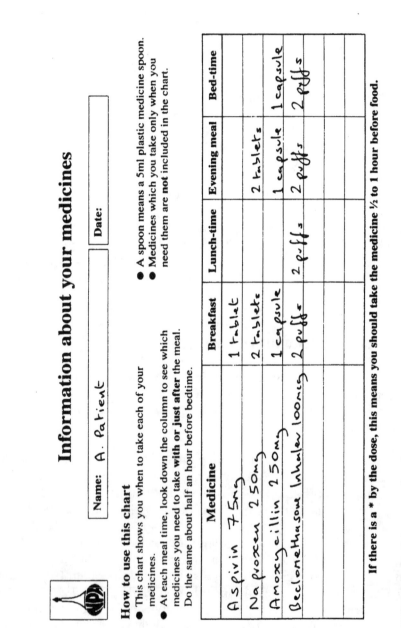

Information about your medicines

Name: A. Patient	Date:

How to use this chart

● This chart shows you when to take each of your medicines.
● At each meal time, look down the column to see which medicines you need to take with or just after the meal. Do the same about half an hour before bedtime.

● A spoon means a 5ml plastic medicine spoon.
● Medicines which you take only when you need them are not included in the chart.

Medicine	Breakfast	Lunch-time	Evening meal	Bed-time
Aspirin 75mg	1 tablet			
Naproxen 250mg	2 tablets		2 tablets	
Amoxycillin 250mg	1 capsule		1 capsule	1 capsule
Beclomethasone Inhaler 100mcg	2 puffs	2 puffs	2 puffs	2 puffs

If there is a * by the dose, this means you should take the medicine ½ to 1 hour before food.

FIGURE 1   Medicine reminder chart

appropriate box. The chart allows the patient to relate the doses of each medicine to each other, as well as to a time of day which is part of their routine. These daily events then act as cues for medicine taking. At each event (e.g. at breakfast), the patient can look down the column and see which medicines they need to take. (For a discussion of event-based tasks, see Ellis, Chapter 5).

Two major trials of reminder charts have been carried out in the UK. In Nottingham, an information booklet was devised which incorporated a reminder chart. Patients discharged from hospital with the chart had significantly better knowledge of drug name, dose frequency and purpose (Sandler *et al.*, 1989a). Adherence was not measured, but satisfaction was improved (Sandler *et al.*, 1989b).

In Leeds, a computer-generated chart produced automatically by the dispensary labelling computer was developed in the early 1990s. The design and wording was devised in co-operation with the Plain English Campaign. The timing and naming of the daily events were researched in the local community prior to being chosen (Raynor, 1991). The chart significantly improved adherence in patients on discharge from hospital., Full knowledge of the patient's regime was found in 83% of patients given the chart, compared with 47% of the control group. Eighty five percent of patients given the chart took more than 85% of their doses, compared with 61% of those not given the chart (Raynor, Booth and Blenkinsopp, 1993). Since then, two manually completed charts have been produced, based on this design (Figure 1).

Medicine reminder charts can be used by pharmacists as an aide-memoire to help them to go through medicines with a patient. After this, they can ask the patient to use the chart to show how they will take their medicines. This feedback allows evaluation of the patient's learning, and emphasises the usefulness and importance of the chart for the patient when at home. The cueing effect of reminder charts can be maximised by individualising the named events for each patient according to their particular daily routine (Raynor, in press).

THE LINK BETWEEN WRITTEN INFORMATION, TRANSFER OF KNOWLEDGE AND ADHERENCE

Looking at all the factors associated with non-adherence, lack of knowledge appears to be more amenable to change than most

(Lipton *et al.*, 1995). However, as articulated by Gibbs (1995), people appear to find it difficult to believe that providing information will not automatically have a positive effect on adherence. The reason for the lack of a strong link relates to the complex path from the provision of information to a change in behaviour.

In some of the studies reviewed, the written information studied was published, and the results could be interpreted in the light of the quality of the information. In others the text (but not the design) was included or even just a vague description. Valid assessments of trials of written information can only be made if the quality of the written information can be analysed. In addition, in many studies it is difficult to isolate the effect of the written information, as it was combined with other interventions.

Mazucca (1982) conducted a meta-analysis of 30 papers on patient education in chronic disease. He found that increasing patient knowledge alone is rarely successful in improving adherence. A review of over 20 studies also reported no strong evidence of a link between knowledge and non-adherence (Anon., 1992). In one group of patients, those with a good level of knowledge were the poorer adherers (Al-Deagi, McElnay and Scott, 1995). In another, an individualised programme of medication education and individualisation resulted in increased adherence in the study patients, but this was independent of any change in their medication knowledge (Horne, Coombes and Weinman, 1995)

The largest gap in patients knowledge about medicines is the lack of awareness and understanding of side-effects (IMBRF, 1993). It was previously believed that patients will wrongly claim to have specific side-effects if they are warned about them. This has not been borne out in practice. In general, it appears that information given on side-effects tends to increase the number of patients who correctly link an effect with the medicine, rather than resulting in spurious claims (Morris and Kanouse, 1982; George *et al.*, 1983).

Adherence in long-term therapy is not thought to be increased by written information unless combined with additional social support and motivational based interventions which are tailored to patients needs i.e. a combination of educational and behavioural strategies (Morris and Halperin 1979; Stockwell-Morris and Schultz 1992). In Mazzuca's meta-analysis (1982) of patient education studies in chronic disease, he also concluded that most effective programmes involved a behavioural, regime-orientated, aspect. He felt that patients need less knowledge about their disease and more about integrating their treatment regime with their lifestyle. This is borne out by the positive effect of medicine reminder charts on adherence, where the patient's regime is related to their daily routine.

Written information generally has a positive effect on knowledge, if it is well written and has appropriate design and layout (Raynor, 1992a). Ley and Morris (1984) reviewed 32 studies of written information, only one of which resulted in no knowledge gain. Non-individualised information is unlikely to improve adherence on its own and the only consistent improvement in adherence via written information is for short course antibiotics. This effect may relate to the specific issue of completing the course (Morris and Halperin, 1979), although it is possible that such information only has a short-term effect (possibly through satisfaction).

PREPARING EFFECTIVE WRITTEN INFORMATION

The potential influence of a piece of written information on knowledge and adherence could be said to be associated with three essential elements:

- how it is delivered to the patient;
- the design and layout;
- the content.
  All three are important, yet prominence is usually given to content. This is unfortunate, as the quality of the content is irrelevant if the information is not actually read. Inappropriate delivery and poor design both play a key role in determining the latter.

There are a number of accepted principles relating to preparing effective written information which have been distilled below from key texts. These should be referred to for further detail:

- Writing plain English (Plain English Campaign, 1984).
- Teaching patients with low literacy skills (Doak *et al.*, 1985).
- Writing patient information: a pharmacists guide (Raynor, 1992b).
- See It Right (Royal National Institute for the Blind, 1993)

Method of Delivery

How information is delivered is important, because getting the information to the patient is an essential first step. In addition, it may also affect the patient's perception of the relevance and importance of the information. There is an inherent contradiction here, as the methods which are more likely to guarantee delivery to the patient (e.g. within a pack of medicine) may be those least likely to invest importance and relevance. The maximum effect is to be expected from the professional personally handing over the information and, if possible, going through it, highlighting important points (Mayeaux *et al.*, 1996). However, the performance of HPs in ensuring delivery of written information to patients can be poor (Gibbs, 1995).

Design and Layout

The design and layout affects whether a patient pays attention to a piece of information. If it looks relevant, useful and easy to read, it seems more likely that the target reader will read the information. Relevance can be helped by clear titles and headings to which the reader can relate e.g. question headings such as: "What is this medicine for?" Patients learn when information is important to them personally (Doak *et al.*, 1985). The inclusion of a patients' name can also be a powerful indicator of relevance. If the information is too long, many patients will not read it (Morris and Kanouse, 1980), but this has to be balanced against the right of patients to receive all relevant information. The best approach may be to include all relevant information but present it well. Illustrations can be used to reinforce or explain specific parts of the text. However, they may just be a distraction if used in isolation.

Information will look easy to read, and be easier to read, if it is well organised. This is aided by use of the following:

- clear headings; question headings are particularly effective,
- plenty of white space; too much text on a page will put off the reader,

- bullet points; bulleted lists are also better remembered and under-stood than paragraphs:
- lower case in bold type for emphasis, text in capitals is less easy to read,
- familiar type face and large print size; a minimum print size of 12 point is suggested by the Royal National Institute for the Blind (RNIB, 1993; Raynor, 1992b).

Content

The style of writing needs to be clear, direct, personal and conversational (Dolinsky *et al.*, 1983). Writing as you speak is one of the key recommendations of the Plain English Campaign (1984). It is self-evident that easy to read information maximises the number of people who can understand the information. There appears to be little evidence that the more well-educated are put off or less satisfied with clear, simple information. However, it is apparent that PILs for medicines in the USA and UK are generally written at levels well above the average national reading age of 10 -14 years (Basara and Juergens, 1994; Vahabi and Ferris, 1995).

The understandability of text can be maximised by the use of:

- Simple words
- Translated jargon
- Short sentences
- Active verbs
- Specific instructions, and
- Positive phrasing (Raynor, 1992b)

Piloting of Written Information

Considerable time elapsed between the initial development of written information for patients and consideration of how easy it is to read (usually described as "readability"; Smith, 1992). However, an inappropriate emphasis was then given to readability formulae. These give an estimate of the reading age needed for a particular piece of information. They are based on word and sentence length (or word difficulty) and take no account of layout, typeface, motivation of the reader or previous knowledge. It is salutary to note that any passage would receive the same reading score, whether it was written forwards or backwards! They can be a useful guide, but should not be relied upon. Patients opinion of readability does not necessarily agree with formula score (Morris, Myers and Thilman, 1980). If such a formula is used, the FOG test can be simply applied, as described by Albert and Chadwick (1992). This test is a broad measure of the proportion of long sentences and long words in a document.

Leaflet writers need to write for audience acceptance, rather than a favourable reading score. There is no substitute for piloting material on a sample of the intended audience (Vahabi and Ferris, 1995). In 1991, none of the drug companies producing PILs had tested them on patients (Dodds, 1993). Later, Bradley *et al.* (1995) found that most companies producing PILs for over-the-counter medicines had no formal testing procedure, with just a quarter having a volunteer panel.

WHO DOES WRITTEN INFORMATION EXCLUDE?

Written information has the potential to exclude significant minorities of the population:

- blind and partially sighted people;
- people with reading difficulties;
- non-English speakers.

  The numbers who are excluded in the first two categories can be minimised by taking into account some of the recommendations described above for clear and simple information. In particular, large print is useful for the partially sighted and use of plain English helps those with reading difficulties. However, this will clearly be insufficient for people with no sight and those who are illiterate (Raynor and Yerrasimou, in press).

Patient information and advice continues to rely almost exclusively on written material, despite problems with literacy (IMBRF, 1993). More imaginative methods are needed, including the use of audio and video tapes as ways of transmitting information. The use of written information in foreign languages most commonly used in the ethnic minority populations in the UK is increasingly being used. However there is evidence that a large number are illiterate in their own language (Tufnell *et al.*, 1994).

ADHERENCE AND WRITTEN INFORMATION: THE WAY FORWARD

The provision of information for patients is likely to continue to play a key role in the joint management of treatment by HPs and patients. Adherence to treatment, however, will never be guaranteed by the provision of information alone, written or otherwise. The factors which influence adherence are so many and so varied that addressing one aspect alone cannot be expected to make a significant difference (Gibbs, 1995).

In simple terms, the facilitation of adherence can be considered to have two main strands:

- education;
- motivation (Roter and Hall, 1994).

A patient who understands their treatment regime will not follow it without sufficient motivation. Conversely, a patient who is motivated to follow their regime cannot do so, if they have insufficient information. So, either element alone is likely to be insufficient to assure adherence. Information can improve patient knowledge, but this may only lead to improved adherence if it is in a framework where issues relating to motivation are also addressed.

Well-written and designed written information can contribute to patient education. However, evidence that combined face-to-face and written information may maximise this effect suggests that written information should not replace verbal intervention. The provision of good written information can also improve satisfaction (Gibbs *et al.*, 1989a; 1989b) and satisfaction is positively associated with adherence (Ley, 1988).

Written information has a number of distinct advantages over verbal information. The patient can refer to it on subsequent occasions and can read as much or as little as they wish, assuming the information is well organised. The written information is also available to partners, family and carers, influential providers of information to the patient (Gibbs, 1995). Written information can also help to overcome professional non-adherence (Ley, 1988). If a doctor prescribes a medicine for a non-licensed indication or dose, they will have to explain to the patient why their instructions differ from the information provided on the leaflet.

As written information alone will generally not improve adherence, there is an argument against devoting resources to such information provision. However, this line of argument is not sustainable in the light of another powerful agenda: patient empowerment. It is now generally accepted that patients have a fundamental right to comprehensive information about their treatment, including medicines, (Morris and Halperin, 1979; Anon., 1978). In the 1990s this has been strongly promoted by the UK by the Department of Health in the "Patients Charter," with patients being encouraged to take more responsibility for their health.

Computer-generated written information is likely to be the start of the impact of new technology (Raynor *et al.*, 1993). In the future, leaflets are likely to be complemented and possibly superseded by interactive computer-based information. This will allow a greater level of individualisation of information – providing bespoke information which is tailored to an individual patient's requirements. However, it will take some time before the elderly population are confident to use such computer-based methods. The telephone is also likely to become more important as a medium for communication on health. In the meantime, the use of written information can improve knowledge, and create the potential for improved adherence. For maximum effect, the emphasis should be on a combination of interventions, including written information which is accessible, easy-to-read and relevant to the patient.

REFERENCES

Adult Literacy Support Services Fund. (1981) *Understanding labels: problems for poor readers.* London: BSS.
Albert, T. and Chadwick, S. (1992) How readable are practice leaflets? *British Medical Journal* **305**, 1266–1268.

Al-Deagi, F.A., McElnay J.C. and Scott, M.G. (1995) Factors leading to non-compliance in elderly patients. *Pharmaceutical Journal* **255**, R8.

Allen, K.F. and Sweeney, S.J. (1985) The availability and design of patient information leaflets. *Pharmaceutical Journal* **235**, 181–3.

Anon. (1978) Patient package inserts. *British Medical Journal* **2**, 586.

Anon. (1981) Rand corporation issues PPI study findings. *American Pharmacy* **NS21**, 588.

Anon. (1987) Telling patients about their medicines. *Lancet* **ii**, 1064.

Anon. (1992) Compliance and knowledge not linked after all? *Pharmaceutical Journal* **248**, 186.

Anon. (1996) The drug information gap. *Health Which?* **October**, 167–170.

Ascione, F.J. and Shimp, L.A. (1984) The effectiveness of four education strategies in the elderly. *Drug Intelligence and Clinical Pharmacy* **18**, 926–931.

Ascione, F.J., Kirscht, J.P. and Shimp, L.A. (1986) An assessment of different components of patient medication knowledge. *Medical Care* **24**, 1018–1028.

Association of British Pharmaceutical Industry. (1987) *Information to patients on medicines.* London: ABPI.

Association of British Pharmaceutical Industry. (1988) *Patient information: advice on the drafting of leaflets.* London: ABPI.

Axon, R.A., Lane, G.R., Whittome, J. and Clarke, C. (1989) Patient information sources. *British Journal of Pharmaceutical Practice* **11**, 314–319.

Baudrihaye, N. (1991) Assessment of current situation in Europe and way forward. In R.D. Mann (ed) *Patient information in medicine.* Carnforth UK: Parthenon.

Baker, D., Roberts, D.E., Newcombe, R.G. and Fox, K.A.A. (1991) Evaluation of drug information for cardiology patients. *British Journal of Clinical Pharmacology* **31**, 525–531.

Barber, N.D. and Raynor, D.K. (1989) Understanding medicine labels: the effect of plain English. *Pharmaceutical Journal* **242**, R13–17.

Basara, L.R. and Juergens J.P. (1994) Patient package insert readability and design. *American Pharmacy* **NS34**, 48–53.

Bradley, B., McClusker, E., Scott, E. and Li Wan Po, A. (1995) Patient information leaflets on over-the-counter (OTC) medicines: the manufacturer's perspective. *Journal of Clinical Pharmacology and Therapeutics* **20**, 37–40.

Clinite, J.C. and Kabat, H.F. (1976) Improving patient compliance. *Journal of the American Pharmaceutical Association* **16**, 74–76.

Cochrane, B.M. (1992) Information for patients. *International Journal of Pharmacy Practice* **1**, 121–122.

Colcher, I.S. and Bass, J.W. (1972) Penicillin treatment of streptococcal pharyngitis: a comparison of schedules and the role of specific counselling. *Journal of the American Medical Association* **222**, 657–659.

Culbertson, V.L., Arthur, T.G., Rhodes, P.J. and Rhodes, R.S. (1988) Consumer preferences for verbal and written medication information. *Drug Intelligence and Clinical Pharmacy* **22**, 390–396.

DeTullio, P.L., Eraker, S.A., Jepson, C, Becker, M.H., Fujimoto, E., Diaz, C.L., Loveland, R.B. and Strecher, V.J. (1986) Patient medication instruction and provider interactions. *Health Education Quarterly* **13**, 51–60.

DiMatteo, M.R. and DiNicola, D.D. (1982) *Achieving patient compliance: the psychology of medical practitioners' role.* New York: Pergammon Press.

Dixon, M. (1995) Assertions about patient information are not supported. *British Medical Journal* **311**, 946.

Doak, C.G., Doak, L.G. and Root, J.H. (1985) *Teaching patients with low literacy skills.* Philadelphia: Lippincott.

Dodds, L.J. (1986) Effect of information leaflets on compliance with antibiotic therapy. *Pharmaceutical Journal* **236**, 48–52.

Dodds, L.J. and King, R.W. (1989) Factors affecting attitudes to the provision of information with prescribed drugs. *Pharmaceutical Journal* **242**, R7–12.

Dodds, L.J. (1993) Industry-produced patient information leaflets: are hospital pharmacies making used of them? *Pharmaceutical Journal* **250**, 311–314.

Dolinsky, D., Gross, S.M., Deutsch, T, Demestihas, E. and Dolinsky, R. (1983) Application of psychological principles to the design of written patient information. *American Journal of Hospital Pharmacy* **40**, 266–271.

Donnelly, M.C. (1991) Background to patient information in the European Community. In R.D. Mann (ed) *Patient information in medicine.* Carnforth UK: Parthenon.

Donovan, J.L., Blake, D.R. and Fleming, W.G. (1989) The patient is not a blank sheet. *British Journal of Rheumatology* **28**, 58–61.

Drug and Therapeutics Bulletin (1995) Patient pack prescribing and the provision of patient information leaflets **33**, 86–88.

Eagleton, J.M., Walker, F.S. and Barber, N.D. (1993) An investigation into patient compliance with hospital discharge medication in a local population. *International Journal of Pharmacy Practice* **2**, 107–110.

Ellis, D.A., Hopkin, J.M., Leitch, A.G. and Crofton, J. (1979) "Doctors orders": controlled trial of supplementary, written information for patients. *British Medical Journal* **1**, 456.

Fleckenstein, L., Joubert, P., Lawrence, R., Patsner, B., Mazullo, J.M. and Lasagne, L. (1976) Oral contraceptive patient information. *Journal of the American Medical Association* **235**, 1331–1336.

Gauld, V.A. (1981) Written advice, compliance and recall. *Journal of the Royal College of General Practitioners* **31**, 553–556.

George, C.F., Waters, W.E. and Nicholas, J.A. (1983) Prescription information leaflets, a pilot study in general practice. *British Medical Journal* **287**, 1193–1196.

George, C.F. (1987) Telling patients about their medicines. *British Medical Journal* **294**, 1566–1567.

Gibbs, S., Waters, W.E. and George, C.F. (1987) The design of prescription information leaflets and feasibility of their use in general practice. *Pharmaceutical Medicine* **2**, 23–33.

Gibbs, S., Waters, W.E. and George, C.F. (1989a) The benefits of prescription information leaflets (1). *British Journal of Clinical Pharmacology* **27**, 723–739.

Gibbs, S., Waters, W.E. and George, C.F. (1989b) The benefits of prescription information leaflets (2). *British Journal of Clinical Pharmacology* **28**, 345–351.

Gibbs, S., Waters, W.E. and George, C.F. (1990) Communicating information to patients about medicine. *Journal of the Royal Society of Medicine* **83**, 292–297.

Gibbs, S. (1995) Medicines and the role of patient information leaflets. In J. Griffin (ed) *Health Education and the Consumer.* London: Office of Health Economics.

Harvey, J.L. and Plumridge, R.J. (1991) Comparative attitudes to verbal and written medication information among hospital outpatients. *Drug Intelligence and Clinical Pharmacy* **25**, 925–928.

Hawkey, G.M. and Hawkey, C.J. (1989) Effect of information leaflets on knowledge in patients with gastro-intestinal diseases. *Gut* **30**, 1641–1646.

Haynes, R.B. (1976) A critical review of the determinants of patient compliance. In D.L. Sackett and R.B. Haynes (eds) *Compliance with therapeutic regimens*, Baltimore: Johns Hopkins University Press.

Haynes, R.B., Wang, E and Da Mota Gomes, M. (1987) A critical review of interventions to improve compliance. *Patient Education and Counselling* **10**, 155–166.

Horne, R., Coombes, J. and Weinman, J. (1995) Impact of a hospital-based programme of pharmaceutical care on elderly patients' adherence. *Pharmaceutical Journal* **255**, R10.

International Medical Benefit Risk Foundation (1993) *Improving patient information and education on medicines*. Geneva: IMBRF.

Johnson, M.W., Mitch, W.E., Sherwood, J., Lopes, L., Schmidt, A. and Hartley, H. (1986) The impact of a drug information sheet on the understanding and attitudes of patients about drugs. *Journal of the American Medical Association* **256**, 2722–2723.

Kay, E.A., Moss, I.G. and Rees, J.A. (1987) Patient information on anti-malarial therapy for rheumatoid arthritis. *Pharmaceutical Journal* **239**, 19–20.

Kay, E.A. and Bailie, G.R. (1987) Educating patients about sub-lingual glyceryl trinitrate. *Pharmaceutical Journal* **239**, R3.

Kessler, D.A. (1991) Communicating with patients about their medications. *New England Journal of Medicine* **325**, 1650–1652.

Ley, P. (1973) Communication in the clinical setting. *British Journal of Orthodontics* **1**, 173–177.

Ley, P. (1979) Memory for medical information. *British Journal of Social and Clinical Psychology* **18**, 245–255.

Ley, P. (1988) *Communicating with the patient*. London: Croom Helm.

Ley, P. and Morris, L.A. (1984) Psychological aspects of written information for patients. In S. Rachman (ed) *Contributions to medical psychology*. Volume 3. Oxford: Pergammon Press.

Lima, J., Nazarian, L, Charney, E and Lahti, C. (1976) Compliance with short-term anti-microbial therapy. *Pediatrics* **57**, 383–386.

Linkewich, J.A., Catalano, R.B. and Flack, H.L. (1974) The effect of packaging and instruction on out-patient compliance with medication regimes. *Drug Intelligence and Clinical Pharmacy* **8**, 10–15.

Lipton, H.L., Byrns, P.J., Soumerai, S.B. and Chrischilles, E.A. (1995) Pharmacists as agents of change for rational drug therapy. *Inter-*

national Journal of Technology Assessment in Healthcare **11**, 485–508.

Livingstone, C. (1995) The views of elderly people on information from community pharmacists about prescribed medicines. *Pharmaceutical Journal* **255**, R7.

Madden, E.E. (1973) Evaluation of outpatient pharmacy patient counselling. *Journal of the American Pharmaceutical Association* **NS13**, 437–443.

Mayeaux, E.J., Murphy, P.W., Arnold, C, Davis, T.C., Jackson, R.H and Sentell, T.(1996) Improving patient education for patients with low literacy skills. *American Family Physician* **53**, 205–211.

Mays, N.O. (1994) *Health Services Research in Pharmacy.* University of Manchester: Pharmacy Practice Research Resource Centre.

Mazzuca, S.A. (1982) Does patient education in chronic disease have therapeutic value? *Journal of Chronic Disease* **35**, 521–529.

McBean, B.J. and Blackburn, J.L. (1982) An evaluation of four methods of pharmacist-conducted patient education. *Canadian Pharmaceutical Journal* **115**, 1167–1172.

McIver, S. (1993) *Obtaining the views of users of health services about quality of information.* London: Kings Fund.

Meredith, P., Emberton, M. and Wood ,C. (1995) New directions in information for patients. *British Medical Journal* **311**, 3–4.

Morris, L.A., Mazis, M. and Gordon, E. (1977) A survey of the effects of oral contraceptive patient information. *Journal of the American Medical Association* **238**, 2504–2508.

Morris, L.A., Myers, A and Thilman, D.G. (1980) Application of the readability concept to patient-orientated drug information. *American Journal of Hospital Pharmacy* **37**, 1504–1509.

Morris, L.A. and Halperin, J.A. (1979) Effects of written drug information on patient knowledge and compliance, a literature review. *American Journal of Public Health* **69**, 47–52.

Morris, L.A. and Kanouse, D.E. (1982) Informing patients about drug side-effects. *Journal of Behavioural Medicine* **5**, 363–374.

Morris, L.A. and Kanouse, D.E. (1980) Consumer reactions to differing amounts of written drug information. *Drug Intelligence and Clinical Pharmacy* **14**, 531–535.

Myers, L.B. (1995) Taking a healthy interest in psychology. *Pharmaceutical Journal* **253**, 783.

Penwarden, J. and Raynor, D.K. (1996) Can I drink alcohol with this medicine? *Pharmacy in Practice* **6**, 111.

Plain English Campaign. (1984) *Writing plain English*. Stockport UK: Plain English Campaign.

Pullar, T., Roach, P, Mellor, E.J., McNeece, J., Judd, A., Feely, M and Cooke, J. (1989) Patients knowledge concerning their medications on discharge from hospital. *Journal of Clinical Pharmacology and Therapeutics* **14**, 57–59.

Punchak, S.S. and Kay, E.A. (1988) Educating arthritic patients about their drugs. *Pharmaceutical Journal* **241**, 247–249.

Raynor, D.K. and Silletto, M. (1982) Patient non-comprehension of labelled instructions. *Pharmaceutical Journal* **229**, 648–649.

Raynor, D.K. (1991) *Patient information and its influence on medication compliance*. Unpublished PhD Thesis. University of Bradford.

Raynor, D.K. (1992a) Patient compliance, the pharmacist's role. *International Journal of Pharmacy Practice* **1**, 126–135.

Raynor, D.K. (1992b) Writing patient information – a pharmacist's guide. *Pharmaceutical Journal* **249**, 180–182.

Raynor, D.K., Booth, T.G. and Blenkinsopp, A. (1993) Effects of computer generated reminder charts on patients' compliance with drug regimens. *British Medical Journal* **306**, 1158–1161.

Raynor, D.K. *In press* Medicine reminder charts, maximising benefits for pharmacists and patients. *Pharmaceutical Journal.*

Raynor, D.K. and Yerrasimou, N. *In press* Medicine information-leaving behind blind people? *British Medical Journal.*

Rheinstein, P.H., McGinnis, T.J. and Nightingale, S.L. (1995) The patient information and education initiative. *American Family Physician* **52**, 2377–2382.

Roter, D.L. and Hall, J.A. (1994) Strategies for enhancing patient adherence to medical recommendations. *Journal of the American Medical Association* **271**, 80.

Royal National Institute for the Blind. (1993) *See it right*. London: RNIB.

Sandler, D.A., Mitchell, J.R.A., Fellows, A. and Garner, S.T. (1989a) Is an information booklet for patients at a teaching hospital useful and helpful? *British Medical Journal* **298**, 870–874.

Sandler, D.A., Heaton, C., Garner, S.T. and Mitchell, J.R.A.(1989b) Patients' and GP's satisfaction with information given on discharge from hospital. *British Medical Journal* **299**, 1511–1513.

Sands, C.D., Robinson, J.D. and Orlando, J.B. (1984) The oral contraceptive PPI, its effect on patient knowledge. *Drug Intelligence and Clinical Pharmacy* **18**, 730–735.

Sellu, D.P. (1987) Computer-generated information leaflets for surgical patients. *British Journal of Clinical Practice* **41**, 612–617.

Sharpe, T.S. and Mikeal, R.L. (1974) Patient compliance with antibiotic regimens. *American Journal of Hospital Pharmacy* **31**, 479–484.

Smith, D.L. (1983) The information needs of the patient. *Pharmacy International* **4**, 168–172.

Smith, T. (1992) Information for patients. *British Medical Journal* **305**, 1242.

Stockwell-Morris, L. and Schultz, R.M. (1992) Patient compliance – an overview. *Journal of Clinical Pharmacology and Therapeutics* **17**, 283–295.

Stockwell-Morris, L. and Schultz, R.M. (1993) Medication compliance, the patient's perspective. *Clinical Therapeutics* **15**, 593–606.

Sullivan, M.J. and George, C.F. (1996) Medicine taking in Southampton, a second look. *British Journal of Clinical Pharmacology* **42**, 567–571.

Sutton, A., Smart, J.D. and Herring, C.N. (1989) Patient information leaflets – the patients' perspective. *Pharmaceutical Journal* **243**, R43.

Tufnell, D.J., Nuttall, K., Raistrick, J. and Jackson, T.L. (1994) Use of translated written material to communicate with non-English speaking patients. *British Medical Journal* **309**, 992.

Vahabi, V. and Ferris, L. (1995) Improving written patient education materials, a review of the evidence. *Health Education Journal* **54**, 99–106.

Weinman, J. (1990) Providing written information for patients, psychological considerations. *Journal of the Royal Society of Medicine* **83**, 303–305.

Weintraub, M. (1981) Intelligent non-compliance with special emphasis on the elderly. *Contemporary Pharmacy Practice* **4**, 8–11.

Wilson, M., Robinson, E.J., Blenkinsopp, A. and Panton, R. (1992) Customers recall of information given in community pharmacies. *International Journal of Pharmacy Practice* **1**, 52–59.

Woroniecki, C.L., McKercher, P.L., Flagler, D.G., Berchou, R and Cook J.A. (1982) Effect of pharmacist counselling on drug information recall. *American Journal of Hospital Pharmacy* **39**, 1907–1910.

5

Prospective Memory and Medicine Taking

Judi Ellis

As the range of topics addressed in this book reveals, adherence to treatment is a question of interest to a number of disciplines and is clearly influenced by many different factors. The primary aim of this chapter is to focus on one aspect of "treatment", namely medicine taking, and to examine the role of memory processes in this activity. In particular, I examine the importance of memory for delayed intentions (prospective remembering) for successful medicine taking. As I hope to make apparent, this is an aspect of remembering that emphasises the close relations between memory, attention and planning and, in an everyday environment, one that is frequently influenced by personal and social factors. Thus, its successful operation is affected by many of the factors and contextual variables examined in other chapters.

When a course of medicine is prescribed and presented to a patient the health professional concerned assumes, unless there is clear evidence to the contrary, that the patient has formed an intention to take this medicine in the manner that the prescriber has outlined. It is then the patient's responsibility to recall this intention at the appropriate times and to act accordingly. Importantly, this recall has to occur some time after the original instructions have been conveyed. Moreover, recall is rarely directly prompted (e.g. by a reminder from someone else) and often must occur while the patient is engaged on other, often unrelated activities. Prospective memory researchers focus on investigating the different variables that influence the probability of recall.

PROSPECTIVE MEMORY: THE BASIC TASK

The core of a prospective memory task is an intention to act in a particular way at some specified moment in the future. The crux of the problem that we experience in realising our intentions is that in many instances we cannot act on them immediately; these delayed intentions are the focus of concern in prospective memory research (Brandimonte, Einstein and McDaniel, 1996).

When an intention is formed, one has to encode the *content* of that intention: the action (*what* to do); the retrieval criteria (*when* to do it) and the intent (*that* there is something you wish to do at some point). This content must be retained over a period of delay or retention interval (of minutes, hours, days etc.), then recalled and enacted when a situation that satisfies the retrieval criteria occurs. Clearly, there is also some need for evaluating whether the intention has been fully or partially satisfied and to retain a record of this event. The latter potentially allows us to recall whether the intention has or has not been satisfied and therefore can prevent us from repeatedly carrying out an intention that we have previously realised or failing to realise an unsatisfied one (for further details, see Ellis, 1996).

From the above (truncated) description of a prospective memory task, it is clear that many different factors could influence the probability of recalling any one intention. Probably the simplest way of examining these variables is to classify them, initially, as ones that occur at either encoding, retention, or retrieval although it has to be borne in mind that the effects of a variable at one "stage" are often dependent on or influence the effects of a variable at another stage. For example, intentions encoded with an under-specified retrieval criteria ("phone Mary this *afternoon* ") are more vulnerable to failure than ones with a more precise criteria ("phone Mary at the *afternoon coffee break* ") (Ellis, 1988). This is in part because although the former may come to mind more often (Ellis and Nimmo-Smith, 1993), these recall occasions are frequently inconvenient (e.g. you are not near a telephone or you are in a meeting) (Ellis, Shallice and Cooper, 1996). A review of other influential variables is presented in the following sections of this chapter. For the moment, however, it is important to consider in more detail the place of prospective remembering in the context of adherence to medicines.

MEDICINE TAKING: THE PRESENCE AND ABSENCE OF A PROSPECTIVE COMPONENT

Consider an instruction to take a course of tablets twice a day for a period of 10 days. The translation of this instruction into an intention will be strongly influenced by a patient's beliefs about the benefits of following this advice and the consequences of failing to take it. If the tablets are designed to provide a cure for an ailment these beliefs will, in turn, be affected by the nature of that ailment, for example, whether or not it (i) causes serious or mild discomfort and/or (ii) may disappear "naturally" or persist without treatment. A complaint that causes considerable discomfort and that will persist without treatment has high personal consequences and benefits. On the other hand, one that is likely to gradually disappear and that causes mild discomfort is relatively low on these features (cf. Park and Kidder, 1996).

Attributions of personal importance are strongly related to perceived benefits and consequences (e.g. Ellis, 1988) and, as we shall see, personal importance plays an influential role in prospective remembering. One reason for this is that it may affect the status of an intention i.e. the intent aspect which may be encoded as a "wish" rather than as a "will". Something that is merely a vague desire (wish) is not a firm intention to act (cf. Kuhl, 1983; 1986) and therefore prospective remembering is *not* relevant if an instruction is encoded in this manner. Personal importance also affects the intentional strength of an intention; benefits and consequences are derived for the main part from the relations between an intention and other longer term goals, aims and personal themes (cf. Ortony, Clore and Collins, 1988), such as the effects of one's illness on work efficiency. Intentional strength may cause changes in the threshold or activation level of an encoded intention, thus rendering it more accessible to recall when its retrieval criteria occur (see Ellis, 1996; Goschke and Kuhl, 1996).

Encoding of an instruction also depends on the patient's understanding and interpretation of those instructions. Clearly these are strongly influenced by the complexity of the instructions, the clarity of their delivery (by the health professional) and on whether they are given in a purely verbal form with no written record. While these issues are examined elsewhere (see Noble, Chapter 3 and Raynor, Chapter 4) it is important to note their relevance in the current context. Failure to carry out, or the incorrect enactment of, an intention that is a direct consequence of failure to encode it accurately (through errors of presentation) is not typically regarded as a failure of prospective remembering, although it may be misinterpreted as such (Kvavilashvili and Ellis, 1996). However, faulty encoding that is primarily a consequence of individual differences in memory specific to a delayed intention is clearly relevant both to health practitioners and prospective memory researchers.

Encoding, as mentioned previously, is also relevant for future retrieval even when an intention has been "correctly" (as instructed in this context) retained. The retrieval criterion or criteria is particularly important here. Consider the earlier instruction to take a specific tablet twice a day for 10 days. The retrieval criteria (twice a day, repeated 10 times) are clearly underspecified and provide poor cues for future recall. The recoding of these into "after breakfast and after dinner" would provide useful additional cues or anchoring events (Ellis *et al.*, 1996; Maylor, 1990) since it would provide a link between routine daily activities and the "non-routine" intention. Also, the deliberate use of an external reminder (external memory aids) may assist the identification of a recall criteria (e.g. a timer) but may be of only marginal use if there is no external record of what to do at this time (Harris, 1980).

The enrichment of retrieval criteria is generally a result of planning processes applied by an individual either when an intention is formed and/or if it is recollected during a retention interval. It is possible, however, that individuals might vary in the frequency and efficacy with which they apply these processes with concomitant effects on the likelihood of future recall. Planning processes, therefore, especially applied to retrieval criteria are clearly relevant to prospective remembering.

Recollections of one's intention during a delay period (between instructions and the first occasion for taking medicine or between medicine occasions) are also thought to play an important role in prospective remembering (e.g. Harris and Wilkins, 1982). In the context of medicine taking, recollections during these delay periods may be more likely to occur if the intention is important or if one has an ailment which causes obvious physical discomfort. Recollections have been suggested to act by refreshing an encoded intention and/ or to lead to planning and re-coding. One's activity during a delay period is likely to be important for both the occurrence of and the nature of a recollection. For example, an attentionally demanding or absorbing activity appears to reduce the likelihood of such recollections and may affect the type of processing that occurs on these occasions (Ellis and Nimmo-Smith, 1993). The nature of one's activity at the moment when a situation occurs that should be perceived as a retrieval criterion is also important and influences the likelihood of recognising the retrieval criterion (e.g. Ellis, Milne and McGann, 1996).

Finally, evaluative processes that occur following an occasion for recalling a delayed intention are clearly pertinent when that intention has to be realised more than once e.g. "every day for 10 days". Memory for what you have and have not done could be crucial in this context with failures leading to either an overdose (failure to recall that one has taken a tablet that morning) or an ineffective course of treatment (failure to recall that one hasn't taken the tablet). In some circumstances, of course, there are (or one could create) external records of success but these can be either prohibitively expensive or only partially effective (e.g. counting the number of remaining tablets; Park and Kidder, 1996). Evaluative processes, when an intention (to take a tablet twice a day) has to be repeatedly recalled (for 10 days), may influence prospective remembering from one recall occasion to the next.

In conclusion, assuming an intention has been formed and the instructions for the content of this intention have been correctly conveyed and understood, patients' prospective remembering skills and the variables that foster effective remembering are relevant to the study of medicine taking. Whether or not they are typically *major* factors in non-adherence behaviours is a question that I will return to after a brief review of relevant research on prospective remembering.

PROSPECTIVE REMEMBERING IN YOUNG ADULTS

Early research tended to take the form of field studies in which people were asked, during the course of their everyday lives, to mail cards or telephone the researcher at prescribed times (e.g. Meacham and Leiman, 1975). The problems that these investigations raise, in terms of experimental control over extraneous or confounding variables, has led to the current focus on laboratory simulations which, by and large, replicate and expand on the findings from earlier studies. However, some field research still takes place that directly examines medicine taking behaviours.

The primary laboratory paradigm (Einstein and McDaniel, 1990; Ellis, Williams and Baddeley, 1990; Harris and Wilkins, 1982) is to embed the criterion for realising a delayed intention in a concurrent, relatively demanding activity. This criterion (e.g. a specific word or event) typically occurs several times (3–8 presentations) during this task. This repeated intention design is superficially equivalent to taking a specific type of tablet at breakfast for several days. Other studies use a modification in which the same action is required in response to more than one criterion, where each can appear on either one or more occasions (multiple-criteria intention design; cf. taking the tablet on four occasions during the day). A delay, filled with unrelated tasks, is interposed between instructions for the delayed intention(s) and the start of the "concurrent" or background task.

A few studies, however, have examined performance when a particular intention is presented once only. One such experiment revealed the facilitative effects on performance of relative import- ance and suggests that unimportant intentions may be particularly vulnerable when the delay period is filled by an interesting and absorbing activity (Kvavilashvili,1987). Using a repeated criterion design, Brandimonte and Passolunghi (1994) have confirmed the relevance of one's activity during this period and present findings that suggest forgetting (failure to retain one's intention) occurs pri- marily in the first few minutes after encoding (i.e. no effects of extending the delay period from 15–30 minutes, e.g. Einstein and McDaniel,1990).

The above findings have been replicated in both laboratory and field studies and indicate the importance of encoding processes, particularly when the intention is relatively unimportant (low per- ceived personal consequences and/or benefits) (for examples see Harris, 1984). They also suggest that one's activity during a delay period (e.g. between tablet times) may affect recall. One possibility is that these activities may distract one from noticing a retrieval situ- ation (e.g. Einstein and McDaniel,1996; Ellis, 1996). There is certainly some evidence that we are less likely to spontaneously recollect naturally occurring intentions, prior to the time for performance, while occupied by an activity that is attentionally demanding (Ellis and Nimmo-Smith, 1993). Several studies indicate the positive relation between such recollections and the likelihood of performing an intention (e.g. Harris and Wilkins, 1984; Kvavilashvili, 1987). While the prescriber clearly cannot dictate the patient's daily activities, he/she can identify both the type of ailment (in terms of its severity) and the character of the patient's lifestyle and perhaps suggest appropriate strategies that could increase the salience of the retrieval context. However, we should note that recollections may be induced by symptoms that are obvious (to the patient) early on in the treatment period; the role of "spontaneous" recollections may be more important at a later stage when such symptoms have dissipated, and in cases of medicine taking when few obvious symptoms are present at any stage.

Most recent research in prospective remembering has focused on factors that are thought to directly influence the probability of recognising a retrieval context when a situation that matches it occurs. Both laboratory and field studies have confirmed the benefits of adopting an external memory aid such as a timer, post-it stickers or placing a relevant object in a prominent and/or unusual place (e.g. Meacham and Leiman, 1975; Einstein and McDaniel, 1990). It has been assumed, moreover, that the primary benefits of such explicit strategies are to facilitate recollections of the intention during a delay period and/or immediately prior to the moment for recall (e.g. Harris and Wilkins, 1982).

A recent study by Vortac, Edwards and Manning (1995) suggests that memory aids are reliably beneficial only when they prompt recollection close to the moment for action. Thus, any effective deliberate retrieval strategy, such as an external memory aid, should be directed at timely retrieval (the *when* aspect of an intention) as well as providing some indication of the action to be recalled and performed (the *what* aspect; cf. Harris, 1980). Research by Azrin and Powell (1969) indicates the benefits of such aids for adherence behaviours. They employed an apparatus that emitted a tone at the time(s) for medication and which could be turned off only by turning a knob – the pill could then be dispensed. Azrin and Powell reported a marked increase in adherence when this apparatus was employed (see also, Leirer *et al.,* 1989; Tanke and Leirer, 1993).

The likelihood of a successful recall can be influenced also by changes to different aspects of the retrieval criterion itself. For example, increasing the distinctiveness of the criterion with respect to the context in which it occurs has clear beneficial effects (Brandimonte and Passolunghi, 1994; Einstein and McDaniel, 1990; McDaniel and Einstein, 1993). Similarly, a retrieval criterion that is a specific instance of a class of events is generally more easily recognised than one that merely denotes the class from which such an event is drawn (Einstein *et al.*, 1995; Ellis and Milne, in press).

The above findings indicate that one way of enhancing the probability of recognising a situation as one associated with a delayed intention (and thereby improving prospective remembering) is to make it more prominent in the context in which it occurs. For example, a medicine bottle put out the night before with a cereal packet is likely to attract attention since it is conceptually distinctive from breakfast items. This feature would not work if one already has at this time to take another long-term type of medication, contained in a similar bottle. However, physical distinctiveness could be employed here by, for example, putting a coloured label on the new medicine bottle. Specificity of the context, on the other hand, is achieved by encoding it (or re-coding at a recollection) as "breakfast" rather than with "a meal", or even "eating cereal" instead of "breakfast". This, incidentally, illustrates the close relation between encoding and retrieval operations and the value of planning (when appropriate) at encoding. Planning processes directed towards the "when" aspect of recall require us to predict, based on knowledge of our daily schedule or routine, where we will be, what we will be doing, other people who are usually present etc. at different times of the day. This knowledge allows us to encode a more specific and/or distinctive retrieval criterion within this (anticipated) context (Ellis, 1996; Ellis, Shallice and Cooper, 1996).

A recent distinction in the prospective memory literature concerns the basic character of a retrieval criterion; whether it is time-based or event-based (Einstein and McDaniel, 1990). The former would be an instruction to take medication at a particular time or during a time period while an event-based equivalent would be to do this at a meal or at a particular meal. It has been suggested that recognition of event-based criteria is less attentional demanding and supported by the external cue that the event provides for recognition (e.g. Einstein and McDaniel, 1996). It should be noted that most of the studies reviewed here employed event-based criteria. However, in their everyday lives people often recode a time-based criterion into an event-based one (choosing an event that typically occurs at that time or in that time period, cf. planning discussion above). Moreover, they often increase the effectiveness of this recoding by selecting a routine daily event (Maylor, 1990). Interestingly, this strategy may be difficult to adopt if a medication has to be taken several times a day as it might prove difficult to find evenly spaced routine events and this, as Park and Kidder (1996) have suggested, may explain the recent finding of poor adherence with a high (4 times a day) daily dosage (Kruse *et al.*, 1991).

As I mentioned earlier, different types of prospective memory tasks have been employed in laboratory studies. Both repeated-criteria and multiple-criteria designs have interesting implications for adherence research, although it should be noted that all have been studied with much shorter time intervals between presentation of a criterion than is typically the case in medicine taking tasks. Consider first a repeated-criterion task, such as taking a particular type of tablet twice a day for 10 days. Recent research in the laboratory suggests that prospective remembering improves from the first to the last few presentations of the criterion (Burkes, 1994). Thus, it could be assumed that the types of strategies mentioned earlier would be most effective early on in a medicine taking period. However, this may depend on the nature of the initial ailment. As noted earlier, if it produces obvious symptoms these are likely to provide either a constant or an intermittent reminder of the need to take medication. Later on, however, if these abate, the types of strategies described earlier may become increasingly important if effective treatment requires completion of a prescribed course (e.g. many antibiotics). On the other hand, if a course of medication is prescribed as a preventative measure then these strategies are likely to be most important during the early stages of medication. Later on, the act of taking them should have been absorbed into normal everyday activity (cf. Ellis *et al.*,1996; Lewis, Ellis and Milne, 1996). Multiple-criteria designs also indicate improved performance, from the first to the second presentation (Ellis and Milne, in press); (cf. taking a tablet on three different occasions during the day for several days).

The distinction between repeated and multiple criteria designs may be relevant when one considers the potential need for evaluative processes and the retention of a record of one's actions. As Park and Kidder (1996) note, multiple acts of medication may become confused with one another and it may be difficult to recall whether or not a tablet has been taken on a particular occasion. For example, if one encodes the instruction "three times a day" as "at (3) meal-times" then remembering that a tablet has been taken with a (the first) meal, on a particular day, may cause one to (mis-) remember taking one with the current meal. The likelihood of mis-remembering an event is thought to be lower if there is clear external evidence that an event has or has not occurred (Koriat, Ben-Zur and Druch, 1990). This has received some support from recent studies of adherence behaviours; providing people with a device that provides accurate time and date information about the last use of a medicine increases adherence behaviour (Nides *et al.*, 1993; McKenney, Munroe and Wright, 1992). As Park and Kidder observe, these studies indicate that memory confusions concerning the occurrence of pill-taking may be a substantial factor in adherence failures.

PROSPECTIVE REMEMBERING IN OLDER ADULTS

A considerable number of studies on prospective remembering have been concerned primarily with the effects of increased age on performance. With regard to other tests of memory, older people (60 years+) have been shown repeatedly to have poorer memory than younger people on most tasks (e.g. free recall of word lists, prose passages etc.). These tasks also include the comprehension and memory for medical information given in a laboratory setting (Morrell, Park and Poon, 1989) when poor recall was observed even when people were allowed unlimited time for reading and learning the instructions. Relatively few studies, however, have demonstrated a similar pattern in prospective remembering tasks; indeed, some field studies have shown the opposite effect of higher performance in older people (e.g. Maylor, 1993; Patten and Meit, 1993; West, 1988).

Current evidence (reviewed in Maylor, 1996) suggests that elderly people (70+) do not perform as well as younger ones (both young-old, 60–70 years and young, under 50 years) on laboratory based prospective memory tasks. These differences are particularly apparent when the task is relatively complex in terms of remembering to do the same action in response to several different retrieval criteria (i.e. multiple-criteria tasks). They are also marked when the task is a (repeated-criterion) time-based one (Einstein *et al.*, 1995), which, in the laboratory, cannot be converted into an event-based task. However, studies by Einstein and his colleagues have frequently failed to observe a decrement associated with age on repeated-criterion event-based tasks (e.g. Einstein and McDaniel, 1990; Einstein *et al.*, 1995; McDaniel and Einstein, 1993). One explanation of this anomaly, as Maylor (1996) points out, is that in contrast to other researchers, Einstein and his colleagues structure the concurrent, background task specifically to reduce the cognitive demands of this activity. (Older people are given fewer items to learn and recall, for example, than their younger counterparts in an ongoing word list task). This practice might conceivably mask the disadvantage of depleted attentional processing resources typically observed in many older people.

The above discussion indicates that older patients, in particular, may need to be encouraged to employ a number of different strategies to assist prospective remembering; for example, converting a time-based task into an event-based one and, in multiple-criteria tasks, to encode retrieval criteria more specifically or to make them more distinctive events when they occur. However, field studies, as described earlier, typically do not reveal such marked deficits with ageing. It is commonly thought that this is because experience has taught older people to use compensatory strategies which they can, of course, employ in everyday life but not in the laboratory.

Studies of adherence behaviours provide strong evidence for the claim that "failures" here may be largely attributable to faulty encoding of the content of an intention or errors in recall of whether one has actually performed an action. Two types of error can occur in the latter situation. We may incorrectly "remember" that we have already taken a tablet and thus omit to take one (omission) or we might incorrectly "remember" that we haven't take one and so taken an extra dose (addition). Thus, Park *et al.* (1992) observed that older adults' (aged 71+) adherence was improved by the use of two devices: one that assisted memory for a past action (having taken or not taken a tablet) and one that assisted memory for the original instructions. Similarly, Morrell, Park and Poon (1990) report that older adults (aged 71+), who showed lower levels of adherence than "younger" persons (aged 60–70), benefited from the use of various devices designed to support comprehension of and memory for the medication instructions.

In summary, it would seem that in a real world task such as medicine taking prospective memory, performance in the elderly is primarily a problem of recalling the content of the intention or of recalling past performance or non-performance correctly. However, while it is clear that neither an incorrect addition nor an incorrect omission should be regarded as failures of prospective remembering, these two errors are not equally easy to determine, even with an accurate recording device. Although with the latter it will be apparent that an incorrect addition has occurred, an apparently incorrect omission in reality may be either: (a) failure in prospective remembering (intention not recalled) or (b) a true incorrect omission. Thus, some care should be taken in interpreting such data.

PROSPECTIVE REMEMBERING IN CHILDREN

Unfortunately, only a handful of studies have been conducted on children's prospective memory abilities. Anecdotal evidence suggests that younger children are less skilled on these tasks than older ones. The interesting questions therefore are (i) is there experimental evidence for this supposed difference and (ii) is any difference specific to the cognitive skills required for prospective remembering or a consequence of children's social or other cognitive skill development ? At present we are largely limited to examining only the first of these questions; the latter must await the outcome of more detailed and extensive research.

Thus far, studies indicate a trend for 7–8 year old children to be more successful than 6–7 year old ones but this difference apparently disappears when the task is more motivating for children (Meacham and Columbo, 1980; Meacham and Dumitru, 1976). Moreover, age effects in older children (10 and 14 year olds) may vary with the environmental context of the study, the gender stereotypic nature of the task and the gender of the child. Using a time-based task in which they examined ability to recall this task in terms of clock watching behaviours, Ceci and Bronfenbrenner (1985) observed differences only when the task was conducted in the laboratory. Moreover, these effects were most marked for boys carrying out a stereotypic "male" task; with girls the comparable trend was not statistically reliable. Finally, a study of much younger children (2–4 years) failed to reveal any age differences but demonstrated that performance is reliant on the level of interest (cf. personal importance) of a task (Somerville, Welman and Cultice, 1983).

Clearly, it would be foolish to make any strong claims about children's prospective memory abilities, and thus their possible adherence behaviours, on the basis of findings from a handful of studies examining performance on a variety of tasks and studying different age groups. However, these studies do verify findings from research with adults with regard to the benefits of providing cues that aid recall when the retrieval criterion occurs, with some indication that such cues may be particularly beneficial for young children. As Beal (1988) points out, younger (less than 7–8) children often fail to prepare appropriate internal (planning) or external (e.g. related object) cues because they appear to " assume they will remember automatically in the future"; they appear to be overconfident that when a set of retrieval criteria appear the task will "spring to mind".

A recent set of laboratory experiments offers some new avenues for research that appear to have direct relevance for attempts to improve children's adherence behaviours. Passolunghi, Brandimonte and Cornoldi's (1995) findings suggest that age effects may depend on the modality in which the prospective remembering task is encoded. Thus, while younger children (7–8 years) are advantaged by visual encoding of a retrieval criterion, older children (10–11 year olds) are advantaged by motoric practice of the action to be performed when the criterion occurs. Age effects were particularly apparent, also, when verbal encodings were encouraged. Since, as the authors note, instructions for a delayed intention task are typically conveyed in a verbal form their results suggest that younger children may be disadvantaged.

Health practitioners, and others, reading the above may think that young children's inherent prospective remembering skills are largely irrelevant for everyday adherence behaviours since one might expect an adult to oversee a child's medication programme. However, in many if not the majority of instances children have to take or continue a course of medication while at school or in child care. In the UK, at least, most authorities are reluctant to take responsibility for the administration of medication; frequently, therefore, the child takes primary responsibility for the accurate recall of medicine taking behaviours. Thus, children's adherence behaviour and their prospective remembering skills may be a very important area of research.

SUMMARY AND CONCLUSIONS

The most vulnerable intentions are those that are not perceived to be of high importance, by the patient (cf. Kvavilashvili, 1987; Meacham and Leiman, 1975). While it is probable that most instructions for medication that are translated into an intention, by the patient, are attributed with relatively high importance it must be recognised that this variable can change over the course of treatment. Although a prescriber may have little control over this aspect of encoding, the other factors that have been considered in this review suggest a number of measures that could be introduced at the initial prescribing episode. These factors can act directly to assist retrieval or indirectly facilitate retrieval through enriched encoding processing. For example, it is clear that a critical factor in prospective remembering is the recognition that a particular situation matches the retrieval criterion for an intention. Recognition can be aided by the use of a deliberate aid to cue recall on this occasion or by planning processes that are directed at increasing the distinctiveness or specificity of this criterion. Recoding a time-based instruction into an event-based format, especially if these events are associated with routine activities, also appears to be a beneficial strategy, particularly for elderly persons. When medicine has to be taken several times a day, moreover, it would be worthwhile to discuss the possible events that might coincide with the prescribed times for medication; again, this may be particularly useful for elderly patients and for young children. Finally, the nature of the ailment needs to be taken into account when advice on the above strategies is provided.

With reference to particular groups of patients, this review has highlighted the problems that elderly people appear to experience in (a) encoding and retaining instructions and (b) recalling whether or not they have complied with them on any one occasion. Particular measures to reduce these difficulties seem advisable. Children also may have problems at encoding (although future research may highlight other areas of difficulty). Younger children (7–8 and under), for example, may be disadvantaged by verbal instructions and may benefit from the inclusion of illustrative examples of possible retrieval occasions. For a discussion of adherence in children see Bryon, Chapter 7, and for a discussion of adherence in the elderly see McElnay and McCallion, Chapter 9.

As the studies and theories reviewed here have revealed, prospective remembering is quite clearly an important component in medicine taking in particular and adherence in general. However, are failures of prospective remembering a major contributor to poor adherence ? This is a difficult question to answer as it is not always clear whether or not other explanations of non-adherence have been excluded from a particular study. Research on the effectiveness of techniques designed to facilitate recall and/or to improve memory for past recall occasions do, on the whole, show clear improvement in adherence behaviours. The studies referred to in this chapter suggest that these techniques may most benefit younger children and elderly patients. However, these studies also indicate the importance of actions and processing that occur at encoding – when instructions are given to the patient. In some instances efficient planning at this time may reduce the likelihood of recall failures in the future and such processes may mask the importance of prospective remembering in adherence behaviours. It will almost certainly be the case, however, that the importance of prospective processes will vary with the nature of the condition underlying treatment and an individual's beliefs about that condition and about treatment. As Park and Kidder (1996) comment, "(t)he act of remembering to take a medication at the appointed time represents only the final point in a complex chain of cognitive and psychosocial behaviors that begins when an individual is prescribed a medication".

REFERENCES

Azrin, N.H. and Powell, J. (1969) Behavioral engineering: the use of response priming to improve prescribed self-medication. *Journal of Applied Behavior Analysis* **2**, 39–42.

Beal, C.R. (1988) The development of prospective memory skills. In M.M.Gruneberg, P.E. Morris and R.N.Sykes (eds) *Practical aspects of memory: current research and issues.* Chichester: Wiley.

Brandimonte, M., Einstein, G.O. and McDaniel, M.A. (eds.) (1996) *Prospective memory: theory and applications.* Mahwah, NJ: Lawrence Erlbaum.

Brandimonte, M.A. and Passolunghi, M.C. (1994) The effect of cue-familiarity, cue-distinctiveness and retention interval on prospective memory. *Quarterly Journal of Psychology* **47**, 565–588.

Burkes, M.E. (1994) The effect of local context on prospective memory performance in a semantic processing task. Presented at the Practical Aspects of Memory Conference, August, College Park, MD. USA.

Ceci, S.J. and Bronfenbrenner, U. (1985) "Don't foget to take the cup-cakes out of the oven": prospective memory, strategic time-monitoring and context. *Child Development* **56**, 152–164.

Einstein, G.O. and McDaniel, M.A. (1990) Normal aging and prospective memory. *Journal of Experimental Psychology: Learning, Memory and Cognition* **16**, 717–726.

Einstein, G.O. and McDaniel, M.A. (1996) Retrieval processes in prospective memory: theoretical approaches and some new empirical findings. In M. Brandimonte, G.O. Einstein and M.A.McDaniel (eds) *Prospective memory: theory and applications.* Mahwah, NJ: Lawrence Erlbaum.

Einstein, G.O., Holland, L.J., McDaniel, M.A. and Guynn, M.J. (1992) Age-related deficits in prospective memory: the influence of task complexity. *Psychology and Aging* **7**, 471–478.

Einstein, G.O., McDaniel, M.A., Richardson, S.L.,Guynn, M.J. and Cunfer, A.R. (1995) Aging and prospective memory: examining the influences of self-initiated retrieval. *Journal of Experimental Psychology: Learning, Memory and Cognition* **21**, 996–1007.

Ellis, J.A. (1988) Memory for future intentions: investigating pulses and steps. In M.M.Gruneberg, P.E. Morris and R.N. Sykes (eds) *Practical aspects of memory: current research and issues.* Chichester: Wiley.

Ellis, J.A. (1996) Prospective memory or the realisation of delayed intentions: a conceptual framework for research. In M. Brandimonte, G.O. Einstein and M.A. McDaniel (eds) *Prospective memory: theory and applications.* Mahwah, NJ: Lawrence Erlbaum.

Ellis, J.A. and Milne, A. *in press* The effects of retrieval cue specificity on delayed intention realisation. *Quarterly Journal of Experimental Psychology.*

Ellis, J.A., Milne, A. and McGann, D. (1996) *Conceptual and perceptual processes in a prospective remembering.* Presented at the 37th Annual Meeting of the Psychonomic Society, November, Chicago, USA.

Ellis, J.A. and Nimmo-Smith, I. (1993) Memory for naturally-occurring intentions: A study of cognitive and affective factors. *Memory* **1,** 107–126.

Ellis, J.A., Shallice,T and Cooper, R. (1996) Memory for, and the realisation of, future intentions. *Manuscript under review.*

Ellis, J.A., Williams, J.M.G. and Baddeley, A.D.(1990) *Retrospective and prospective remembering: common and distinct processes.* Presented at the meeting of the Experimental Psychology Society, April, Manchester, UK.

Goschke, T. and Kuhl, J. (1996) Remembering what to do: explicit and implicit memory for intentions. In M. Brandimonte, G.O. Einstein and M.A. McDaniel (eds) *Prospective memory: theory and applications.* Mahwah, NJ: Lawrence Erlbaum.

Harris, J.E. (1980) Memory aids people use: two interview studies. *Memory and Cognition* **8,** 31–38.

Harris, J.E. (1984) Remembering to do things: a forgotten topic. In J.E. Harris and P.E. Morris (eds) *Everyday memory, actions and absent-mindedness.* London: Academic Press.

Harris, J.E. and Wilkins,A.J. (1982) Remembering to do things: A theoretical framework and an illustrative experiment. *Human Learning* **1**, 123–136.

Koriat, A., Ben-Zur, H. and Druch, A. (1990) The contextualisation of input and output events in memory. *Psychological Research* **53**, 260–270.

Kruse, W., Eggert-Kruse, W., Rampmaier, J., Runnebaum, B. and Weber, E. (1991) Dosage frequency and drug-compliance behavior-a comparative study on compliance with a medication to be taken twice or four times daily. *European Journal of Clinical Pharmacology* **41**, 589–592.

Kuhl, J. (1983) *Motivation, conflict and action control.* Heidelberg: Springer.

Kuhl, J. (1986) Motivation and information processing: A new look at decision-making, dynamic change and action control. In R.M. Sorrentino and E.T. Higgins (eds) *Handbook of motivation and cognition: foundations of social behavior.* Chichester: Wiley.

Kvavilashvili, L. (1987) Remembering intention as a distinct form of memory. *British Journal of Psychology* **78**, 507–518.

Kvavilashvili, L. and Ellis, J.A. (1996) Varieties of intention: some classifications and distinctions. In M. Brandimonte, G.O. Einstein and M.A. McDaniel (eds) *Prospective memory: theory and applications.* Mahwah, NJ: Lawrence Erlbaum.

Leirer, V.O., Morrow, D.G., Pariante, G.M. and Doksum, T. (1989) Increasing influensa vacination adherence through voice mail. *Journal of the American Geriatric Society* **37**, 1147–1150.

Lewis, K.P., Ellis, J.A. and Milne, A. (1996) Prospective memory: self-initiated retrieval or 'cognitive' organisation. Presented at the 2nd International Conference on Memory, July, Terme, Padua, Italy.

McDaniel, M.A. and Einstein, G.O. (1993) The importance of cue familiarity and cue distinctiveness in prospective memory. *Memory* **1**, 22–42.

McKenney, J.M., Munroe, W.P. and Wright, J.T. (1992) Impact of an electronic medication compliance aid on long-term blood pressure control. *Journal of Clinical Pharmacology* **32**, 277–283.

Maylor, E.A. (1990) Age and prospective memory. *Quarterly Journal of Experimental Psychology* **42**, 471–493.

Maylor, E.A. (1993) Minimised prospective memory loss in old age. In J. Cerella, J. Rybash, W. Hoyer and M.L. Commons (eds) *Adult information processing: limits on loss.* San Diego: Academic Press.

Maylor, E.A. (1996) Does prospective memory decline with age ? In M. Brandimonte, G.O. Einstein and M.A. McDaniel (eds) *Prospective memory: theory and applications.* Mahwah, NJ: Lawrence Erlbaum.

Meacham, J.A. and Columbo, J.A. (1980) External retrieval cues facilitate prospective remembering in children. *Journal of Educational Research* **73**, 299–301.

Meacham, J.A. and Dumitru, J. (1976) Prospective remembering and external retrieval cues. *Abstracted in the JSAS Catelog of Selected Documents in Psychology* **6**, 65 *(Ms. No. 1284).*

Meacham, J.A. and Leiman, B. (1975) Remembering to perform future actions. Paper reprinted in U. Neisser (ed.) (1982) *Memory observed: remembering in natural contexts.* San Francisco: Freeman.

Morrell, R.W., Park, D.C. and Poon, L.W. (1989) Quality of instruction of prescription drug labels: Effects on memory and comprehension in young and old adults. *The Gerontologist* **29**, 345–353.

Morrell, R.W., Park, D.C. and Poon, L.W. (1990) Effects of labelling techniques on memory and comprehension of prescription information in young and old adults. *Journals of Gerontology: Psychological Sciences, Special Issues* **45**, 166–172.

Nides, M.A., Tashkin, D.P., Simmons, M.S., Wise, R.A., Li, V.C. and Rand, C.S. (1993) Improving inhaler adherence in a clinical trial through the use of the nebuliser chronolog. *Chest* **104**, 501–507.

Ortony, A., Clore,G.L. and Collins, A. (1988) *The cognitive structure of emotions*. Cambridge: Cambridge University Press.

Park, D.C. and Kidder, D.P. (1996) Prospective memory and medication adherence. In M.Brandimonte, G.O. Einstein and M.A. McDaniel (eds) *Prospective memory: theory and applications*. Mahwah, NJ: Lawrence Erlbaum.

Park, D.C., Morrell, R.W., Frieske, D. and Kincaid, D. (1992) Medication adherence behaviors in older adults: effects of external cognitive supports. *Psychology and Aging* **7**, 252–256.

Passolunghi, M.C., Brandimonte, M.A. and Cornoldi, C. (1995) Encoding modality and prospective memory in children. *International Journal of Behavioural Development* **18**, 631–648.

Patten, G.W.R. and Meit, M. (1993) Effect of aging on prospective and incidental memory. *Experimental Aging Research* **19**, 165–176.

Somerville, S.C., Welman, H.M. and Cultice, J.C. (1983) Young children's deliberate reminding. *Journal of Genetic Psychology* **143**, 87–96.

Tanke, E.D. and Leirer,V.O. (1993) Use of automated telephone reminders to increase elderly patients' adherence to tuberculosis medication appointments. *Proceedings of the Human Factors and Ergonomics Society 37th Annual Meeting* 193–196.

Vortac, O.U., Edwards, M.B. and Manning,C.A. (1995) Functions of external cues in prospective memory. *Memory 3,* 201–219.

West, R.L. (1988) Prospective memory and aging. In M.M. Gruneberg, P.E. Morris and R.N. Sykes (eds) *Practical aspects of memory: current research and issues*. Chichester: Wiley.

6

Health Promotion: Empowering Choice

Keith Tones

This chapter differs from others in this book. Other chapters involve a more formal review of the factors influencing adherence to a number of conditions and thus reflect a long established tradition of what used to be called compliance research. This chapter, by contrast, takes a critical look at the very notion of adherence to health promotion. Its central tenet is that health promotion and adherence are fundamentally incompatible. Although at first sight, this might appear to be a somewhat idiosyncratic perspective, it actually reflects the philosophy of World Health Organisation (WHO) and represents what is rapidly becoming the orthodox view. Readers might be excused for doubting this assertion since health promotion is still an essentially contested concept and, in practice, the term frequently describes activities which belong to a traditional model of health education with its relatively narrow goal of preventing disease by persuading individuals to adopt prescribed behaviours and lifestyles. Nonetheless, it is the broader WHO definition, with its emphasis on empowerment, which is adopted here. I will, therefore, comment briefly on the key principles of health promotion and its association with current challenges to the hegemony of medicine. This will be followed by a detailed examination of the psychosocial and environmental factors which influence and support people's decision making in relation to health and illness. Such an analysis forms the basis of an educational diagnosis which is an essential precursor to the development of effective health promotion programmes. The focus will not be on adherence to prescriptions for prevention and the adoption of prudent lifestyles but rather on the ways in which people may be helped to co-operate with both lay and professional health workers.

HEALTH PROMOTION AND THE CHALLENGE TO MEDICINE

The argument for a traditional model of health education has been well rehearsed. Since it had become increasingly apparent that many if not most of the diseases which were responsible for the major burden of morbidity and premature mortality in contemporary society were either proving unresponsive to curative medicine or incurring excessive and escalating costs, prevention seemed to offer the prospect of a cost effective solution. Moreover, since human behaviour is involved in the aetiology and management of the disease process, health education seemed to be the method of choice to persuade individuals to adopt prudent lifestyles and use the medical services appropriately in order to achieve these various preventive goals. Following Talcott Parson's (1951; 1979) formulation of the sick role, patients would be excused normal duties but would be expected to fulfil their part of the bargain by striving to get better and complying with the recommendations of the medical practitioner. Admittedly, the sick role concept has been challenged (Ssasz and Hollender, 1956; Freidson, 1961) but it serves to characterise (and perhaps caricature) the relationship between doctor and patient.

Nonetheless, it was clear that the imbalance of power between patients and medical/health practitioners was logically inappropriate for those preventive enterprises which required patients and the public at large to "look after themselves". Compliance and initiative do not readily go hand in hand – and people were increasingly being expected to take responsibility for their own health. However, this power imbalance was deemed to be not only logically inconsistent but also ideologically incongruent with the emerging philosophy of health promotion in the form espoused by WHO and enshrined in the Ottawa Charter (WHO, 1986). Indeed, those who were committed to what is fast becoming a new orthodoxy of empowerment tend to ally themselves with a number of other social scientists and "new public health" practitioners in mounting a challenge to the hegemony of medicine. It is illuminating to consider the extent and variety of such challenges – and some of these are described below.

For instance, Kelleher et al. (1994) described the way in which the process of medicalisation, "... led to doctors being cast more and more in the role of secular priests whose expertise encompassed not only the treatment of bodily ills but also advice on how to live the good life, and judgements on right and wrong behaviour" and then observed that "... the occupation of healing changed from being frequently seen as a rattlebag of quacks and rogues to a profession with considerable power, authority and status". They then proceeded to identify a number of diverse influences which threatened the supremacy of medicine. They cited Hunter's (1994) observations about the challenge from an increasingly powerful management culture in the UK health service. They also commented on the effect of the professionalisation of occupations allied to medicine – especially nursing (Witz, 1994) and the increasing threat of litigation (Dingwall, 1994). The important influence of the feminist movement was acknowledged (Doyal, 1994) and reference was also made to the anti-vivisectionist movement (Elston, 1994), the importance of *some* self help groups (Kelleher, 1994) and even the phenomenon of "trial by television" (Bury and Gabe, 1994). Williams and Popay (1994) describe the increasing recognition of the value of lay knowledge and Saks (1994) refers to the presence of alternatives to "scientific" medicine. Clearly the rise of consumerism might also contribute to the erosion of medical authority – perhaps rather cynically orchestrated by a new power elite of managers (Winkler, 1995).

It is, then, in the context of this scenario of debate and challenge, that Health Promotion has emerged to add its weight to the move towards demedicalisation and to assert the primacy of empowering individuals and creating "active empowered communities". At the same time, a quite fierce and radical attack has been launched on the *victim blaming* tendency which has become inextricably linked with the medical model and its associated emphasis on compliance. I will, therefore, give some brief consideration to the key features of health promotion and observe the ways in which health education might contribute to its ideological and practical goals.

PRINCIPLES AND PRACTICE OF HEALTH PROMOTION

Only a relatively cursory view of health promotion is possible here. For a more complete account of its ideological basis and its relationship to models of health education, see Tones and Tilford (1994); for a review of its principles and certain historical "landmarks", see also Baric (1994).

Health Promotion: a Challenge to Victim Blaming

Two of the important historical influences on the health promotion movement are the Canadian Government's report on the health of the nation (Lalonde, 1974) and the Alma Ata conference on Primary Health Care (WHO, 1978). Both, in their different ways, questioned the effectiveness of prevailing measures to handle national and international inequalities in health and the associated failure to prevent diseases which were eminently preventable. Both drew on a substantial literature which, inter alia, challenged what was considered to be both an inequitable and ineffective tendency to *blame the victim.*

According to the *Health Field Concept* incorporated in the Lalonde Report (Lalonde, 1974), health and illness are due to the interplay of four major influences: medical services, individual lifestyle, genetic predisposition and environmental circumstances. Perhaps arguably, the most important of these is the environment (physical, socio-economic and cultural) and, more certainly, the least important is the contribution of medical services. Logically, then, health promotion is any intervention which takes account of all four influences and develops programmes which orchestrates them so as to maximise the health of individuals. If, however, explanations of the causes of ill health – and subsequent interventions based on such causal analysis – focus primarily on individual lifestyle while ignoring the more important social and structural causes, then programme planners are guilty of blaming the individuals whose ill health results primarily from the environmental circumstances to which they have been exposed and which those planners have studiously ignored !

The term victim blaming, which has been espoused by health promotion, is not specific to health concerns but is considered by Ryan (1976) to be at the heart of general social problems. This is, perhaps, worth underlining since broader social measures may have a more substantial effect on health and illness than specific health programmes. A flavour of the thinking and the arresting polemical nature of the book is provided by the following quotation: " Being poor is stressful. Being poor is worrisome; one is anxious about the next meal, the next dollar, the next day. Being poor is nerve-wracking, upsetting. When you're poor, its easy to despair and it's easy to lose your temper. And all of this is because you're poor. Not because your mother let you go around with your diapers full of a bowel movement until you were four; or shackled you to the potty chair before you could walk. Not because she broke your bottle on your first birthday or breast-fed you until you could cut your own steak. But because you don't have any *money,"* Ryan (1976).

Putting this perspective in rather less florid terms, we should merely note how inequalities in health are considered to stem primarily from broader socio-economic factors and, therefore, health promotion places the pursuit of equity at the top of its agenda for change. A quotation from a recent study of health promotion in general practice in UK underlines the importance of taking account of the broader social determinants of health: " .... If there isn't enough money to pay for the rent or food or clothes, then you can't begin to think of other things. You have to have these things, like a roof over your head, a job for self-respect, a coat on your back and food in the stomach. I've got *good health*, I've not been in hospital, I don't take tablets, but that's not health to me. I'm sick because I have trouble paying my bills, I have trouble feeding the kids at times, so bodily I'm all right, but up here (in my head) I'm terrible, 'cos I worry and that's not health is it" ? (Durrant, 1993).

Health Promotion: Ideology and Anatomy

Five brief principles can be used to summarise the ideologically based principles of health promotion as encapsulated in two major publications by WHO – the discussion of the concept (WHO, 1984) and its promulgation in the Ottawa Charter (WHO, 1986).

- Health is a positive state; quality of life and not merely quantity is important. It is an essential commodity which people need in order to achieve a socially and economically productive life.

- Equity should be the most important concern of health promotion: progress towards the achievement of *Health for All* will depend on the extent to which inequalities in health within and between nations can be addressed.
- Health is not merely an individual responsibility. It is unethical to seek to cajole individuals into adopting healthy habits whilst at the same time failing to take account of the social and structural determinants of health. *Healthy Public Policy* is an essential precursor to creating an environment in which *the healthy choice is the easy choice.*
- Since substantial policy change typically involves a major challenge to existing power bases, health promotion is essentially a political activity. Health promotion must therefore generate political consciousness; it must mobilise communities if it is to take its place as a significant part of the *"New Public Health"* movement.
- Health is too important to be left to medical professionals and so, medical services must be redefined and reoriented. Moreover, since a wide range of public services also contribute to public health, an important task for health promotion is to raise awareness of the potential contribution which might be made by these various services – such as transport and housing. Medical services such as primary care and hospitals should be designed to be maximally accessible to and meet the real needs of the populace. In all this, *the focus of the relationship between health service and client should be on empowerment, on co-operation rather than compliance.*

The Contribution of Health Education

Health Promotion has, with some justification, been labelled an essentially contested concept – although the WHO version described above is acquiring some of the cachet of orthodoxy. However, it is quite usual – certainly in practice – for the term health promotion to be used interchangeably with health education. Indeed, the so-called health promotion "clinic", which at one time formed part of the UK primary care imperative had more in common with the victim blaming preventive health education model described at the beginning of this chapter than with the WHO approved model. Health education is viewed here as a quite distinct process and although its ideology is entirely consistent with the five principles listed above, it makes a particular and partial contribution to achieving health promotion aims. More technically, it may be defined thus: "health education is any intentional activity which is designed to achieve health or illness related learning, i.e. some relatively permanent change in an individual's capability or disposition. Effective health education may, thus, produce changes in knowledge and understanding or ways of thinking; it may influence or clarify values; it may bring about some shift in belief or attitude; it may facilitate the acquisition of skills; it may even effect changes in behaviour or lifestyle" (Tones and Tilford, 1994).

Central to the definition of health promotion which is used here – and which will be used in relation to the discussion of the Health Action Model below (Tones, 1987; Tones and Tilford, 1994) – is the symbiotic and synergistic relationship between education and policy development and implementation. Indeed, a short hand way of describing health promotion is incorporated in the following simple "formula":

Health Promotion = Health Education X Healthy Public Policy

In short, education alone is unlikely to have a substantial impact on health related behaviour and on the psychosocial factors underlying it unless it operates within a generally supportive environment. "Healthy public policy" – to use the nomenclature popularised by the Ottawa Charter – is often necessary to facilitate individual decision making and complement educational activities. Conversely, an oppressive or negative environment at macro or micro level will inhibit health and illness related learning and action. On the other hand, although various forms of lobbying and advocacy might contribute to the creation of health and social policy that is conducive to healthy choices, our contention here is that the consciousness raising function of education (following the Freirean model of critical consciousness raising and praxis) is a prerequisite for the implementation of policy – particularly policy which challenges dominant ideology and the self interest of powerful political lobbies and pressure groups (Freire, 1972). For a further discussion of this and related issues, see Tones and Tilford (1994).

I have, thus far, commented on the problematical relationship between adherence and the more voluntaristic ideals of health promotion; I have listed key features of health promotion and re-iterated the assertion that its goal – and, importantly, the criterion for judging its success – is to empower and gain the co-operation of clients rather than their compliance. It is, therefore, worth noting at this juncture that, perhaps paradoxically, the preventive goals of traditional approaches to health education are more likely to be achieved by adopting the empowerment model with its emphasis on co-operation rather than compliance. I will now consider how certain specific empowering techniques might relate to a number of psychosocial and environmental factors governing health and illness related choices. In this discussion, the focus will be on health behaviour and primary prevention – although the model and its underpinning health promotion philosophy is equally applicable to the analysis of the factors determining illness behaviour and secondary and tertiary prevention – and, of course, to more holistic and positive outcomes such as the enhancement of self-esteem or the attainment of mental health.

THE HEALTH ACTION MODEL: A DESIGN FOR HEALTH PROMOTION

Although there is a plethora of models which are widely used to provide a framework for research and, more rarely, for the development of educational programmes, the model selected here was devised as an attempt to provide a comprehensive framework for explicating the key psychological, social and environmental factors determining and sustaining health or illness related actions. The original focus was on health education (Tones, 1979) but subsequently greater emphasis was placed on those factors which might support the translation of behavioural intention into the routine adoption of behaviours in accordance with the emerging philosophy and practice of health promotion (Tones, 1987; Tones and Tilford, 1994). Figure 1 provides an overview of the model.

Behavioural intention – or intention to undertake a particular health or illness related action – operates as a kind of interface between a number of psychological factors which influence the nature and strength of that intention and a number of factors which make it more or less likely that the intention will be translated into

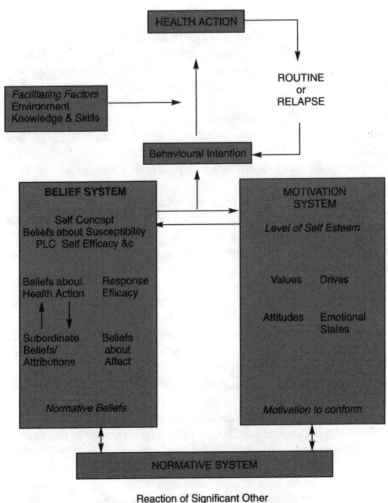

FIGURE 1 The Health Action Model

practice. The definition of belief follows Fishbein's formulation, i.e. it is "... a probability judgement that links some object or concept to some attribute. (The term "object" and "attribute" are used in a generic sense and both terms may refer to any discriminable aspect of an individual's world. For example, I may believe that PILL (an object) is a DEPRESSANT (an attribute). The content of the belief is defined by the person's subjective probability that the object-attribute relationship exists (or is true)" (Fishbein, 1976).

Perhaps the most common function of health education is to influence beliefs in an attempt to ensure that the subjective probability matches the objective probability (or in the case of some scare tactics to ensure that the subjective probability is an exaggerated version of objective reality – in which case, it would certainly not be consistent with the empowering goal of health promotion!)

The Motivational System within the Health Action Model (HAM, Tones, 1987; Tones and Tilford, 1994) seeks to identify the most important affective elements which influence health actions and includes values and attitudes, drives and emotional states. Again, following Fishbein, attitudes are defined in relation to: "... a person's location on a bipolar evaluative or affective dimension with respect to some object, action, or event. An attitude represents a person's general feeling of favourableness or unfavourableness toward some stimulus object...". Again, the relationship between belief and attitude envisaged by the HAM is similar to Ajsen's and Fishbein's (1980) conceptualisation: "Each belief links the object to some attribute; the person's attitude toward the object is a function of his evaluations of these attributes". The Normative System, on the other hand, enables an analysis to be made of important social influences – ranging from the effect of interpersonal pressure to the more general contribution of social norms.

One of the truisms of social and health psychology is the existence of a gap between attitude or intention and practice. HAM seeks to bridge the gap by paying particular attention to the factors which facilitate the translation of "good intentions" into practice – or which, conversely, erect barriers which prevent the achievement of these good intentions. Two broad categories of facilitating or inhibiting factor are identified. The first – and often most substantial of these factors – is the environment in which the health action is to be practised. It might, merely comprise the immediate social or physical environment in which, say, graduates from smoking cessation groups have to maintain their new non smoking status; alternatively it might comprise the cluster of negative circumstances associated with areas of multiple deprivation and which characterise the "underclass" whose poor health and excess mortality create such concern for public health medicine.

Even when the environment is generally favourable, a number of personal competencies and skills may be necessary to ensure the successful transition from behavioural intention to practice. Individuals may merely need knowledge – e.g. of how to access contraceptive services. Alternatively, they may require psychomotor or social interaction skills – for instance the skills to use and dispose of a condom appropriately and, more importantly, the assertiveness and communication skills needed to negotiate condom use with a partner.

In most circumstances, of course, the client and health professional alike will hope that the new "healthy" behaviour will become routinised – and form an integral part of the client's lifestyle. However, the experience of a healthy lifestyle may well prove disappointing, inconvenient or downright unpleasant – and result in relapse and a return to the former, unhealthy way of living. Prochaska and DiClemente's Transtheoretical Model (1986) provides a specialist perspective on relapse and usefully demonstrates how progress from behavioural intention ("contemplation") to final adoption will often involve a cyclical process of *Behavioural Intention – Action – Relapse – Behavioural Intention* before the new behaviour becomes routinised or finally rejected. The HAM accepts the importance of diagnosing a client's readiness to change and the subsequent use of appropriate counselling or *"motivational interviewing"* (Rollnick *et al.*, 1992). However, it also specifies the provision of supportive "self regulatory" skills (e.g. Kanfer and Karoly, 1972) and anticipatory guidance prior to the adoption of the potentially problematic behaviour. The "precontemplation stage" of Prochaska and DiClemente's "revolving door" of course forms a major part of HAM and comprises those beliefs, motives and social pressures which lead to "contemplation" or indeed maintain the attitudinal status quo. I will now consider one of the most important determinants of contemplation – client beliefs.

The Belief System

The importance of identifying and influencing beliefs has already been mentioned. I have also noted how professional and lay beliefs can conflict; indeed Tuckett *et al.* (1985) argued that failure to take account of patients' "theories of illness" was a major source of both patient dissatisfaction and lack of commitment to the doctor's recommendation. We should also note people's capacity to hold contradictory beliefs and Blaxter (1993), for instance, has convincingly demonstrated how individuals are often capable of, "... *holding in equilibrium ideas which might seem opposed*". She describes, for example, apparently contradictory beliefs held by her study sample about the environmental origins of their illness experience together with a simultaneous acceptance of their personal culpability – or as Blaxter put it, they acknowledged that their social circumstances were "... the ultimate cause, in the story of the deprived past, of their current ill health, but at the same time (they accepted) their own responsibility for *who they were;* the inevitability of ill health, given their biographies, but at the same time guilt if they were forced to *give in* to illness".

Standard survey instruments, of course, are extremely limited in teasing out such complex and, sometimes, latent beliefs; it is, however, essential to construct a sophisticated picture and use this as a basis for developing an equally sophisticated health promotion programme.

As may be seen from Figure 1, the Belief System incorporates a set of beliefs about the specific health action in question together with related subordinate beliefs. These subordinate beliefs typically comprise attributions of cause (causal attributions) – such as those described by Blaxter. They also include broader "theories of illness" and various "myths" about the nature of a disease such as cancer. For example, cancer is often associated with a variety of negative images: it may be viewed metaphorically as sinister, invasive, uncontrollable. The commonly held *"seed and trigger"* theory reflects a causal explanation in which everyone is considered to have the seeds of cancer distributed throughout their bodies merely waiting for some trigger – a knock or blow, emotional upset – almost any event – to trigger the disease. Such explanations and images, not surprisingly, create a level of pessimism which may result in delay in seeking medical advice, denial of symptom significance or lead to a general scepticism about the value of any preventive measure. Pessimism is thus a kind of superordinate belief in a hierarchy of which causal attributions form a kind of foundation. The implication of a hierarchical order of beliefs for practice is, quite clear: a truly radical strategy must address underlying influences rather than merely focus on their manifestations. This axiom applies whether we are considering the socio-environmental determinants of action or, as in this case, psychological variables. This latter point may be illustrated by considering a limitation of the Health Belief Model (HBM, e.g. Becker, 1984).

The HBM does not figure as a separate entity within the Belief System primarily because of the confusion of belief proper with affect. For instance, beliefs about the seriousness of a condition and beliefs about the likely costs and benefits of a given health action are more usefully considered as proxy measures for attitudes, values or even drives or emotional states. They simply refer to an individual's assessment that a particular action is likely to lead to a positively or negatively evaluated outcome. It is this positive or negative *motivation* that actually energises the Behavioural Intention. On the other hand, the notion of *response efficacy*, primarily derived from Social Learning Theory (Rotter, 1966), is more conceptually sound. The calculation that a given health action will result in outcomes which are likely to lead to some positively (or negatively) valued state, is likely to generate motivation and *contribute* to intention to act.

The notion of *existential belief* merits some further comment in view of its relevance for the empowerment of health decision making. The term is used in accordance with Lewis' (1986) conceptualisation of *existential control*. It refers to a kind of creed – a philosophy of life – which is paralleled in the Motivation System by a related set of moral and religious values. There are, in short, individuals and even cultural groups who accept with apparent equanimity that they are not in control of their lives; nonetheless, provided that they can attribute meaning to this arrangement – and follow the Panglossian view that "all is for the best in the best of possible worlds", they might experience a kind of existential satisfaction which, in Western society, is normally associated with feelings of control. The associated fatalism is potentially significant for health promotion in that individuals or whole populations will be rather reluctant to adopt an empowered approach to health related decision making – or, at any rate, use it as an excuse for not changing unhealthy lifestyles.

The Belief System also acknowledges the importance of *beliefs about affect*. At first glance these beliefs are similar to the notion of response efficacy. However, whereas response efficacy is concerned with "calculations" about the likelihood of given actions resulting in positive or negative outcomes, the concept outlined here is concerned with beliefs about the affective state itself and is thus a kind of meta cognition. For instance, a belief that sexual intercourse will result in both feelings of pleasure and guilt might create a given level of intention to act – depending on which of the two motives were stronger. At the same time, though, the individual will conceptualise and develop subjective probabilities about *what the pleasure and guilt will be like*. These latter beliefs may generate their own motivational force or add to the already existing inclination to act. Marsh and Matheson (1983) illustrate this point empirically in their study of UK adult smokers' intentions to stop or maintain their habit. They showed how one of the key factors determining the likelihood of their giving up smoking was their belief about whether or not they would be able to cope with the loss of positive affect and/or the "withdrawal symptoms" they anticipated experiencing. More extensively and perhaps radically, Davies (1992) has emphasised the importance of beliefs about the drive-like state of addiction, suggesting that attributions of addiction exaggerate the pharmacological power of drugs and militate against "will power" – or, in the parlance of this chapter, empowered decision making.

The Motivation System

The Motivation System is viewed as an affective complex comprising basic drive-like forces, such as hunger or thirst, together with various emotional states. It also comprises values and values systems together with the attitudes they generate. A full discussion of these constructs is beyond the scope of this chapter and should need little further elaboration. I will, however, comment briefly on the relevance of drives and emotional states to health promotion programmes and explore the inter-relationship of Belief System and Motivation System in the context of some unpublished research undertaken by the author on the subject of choice of infant feeding.

It is not profitable to enter into a discussion about the "instinctive" features of breast feeding. However, to the extent that breast feeding can result in "prolactin induced nurturance" or give rise to quasi orgasmic experiences (Newton and Newton, 1967), then it would be reasonable to describe the affective force as "drive-like". Clearly, *intention* to breast feed would, in such a case, be influenced only by anticipation (i.e. a belief about affect) although *maintenance of* the practice might be affected. On the other hand, there is clear evidence for an opposite effect since "embarrassment" is frequently considered to be the most significant reason for women not electing to breast feed (Martin, 1978). The term is, of course, rather vague and will range from a relatively mild concern for modesty to rather more deep-seated anxieties. Some indications of this latter state is provided by quotes from the Salber, Stitt and Babbott (1958) study and observations from the sample of 305 women in the unpublished study by the author. Comments included such observations as: *"... It's an animal thing to do." "... The idea makes me feel quite sick." "... You feel like a cow being milked." "...I find it rather disgusting."* Sixty seven per cent of the sample of 305 mothers, to which reference was made above, believed that women would be embarrassed about breast feeding and 60% believed this would be an important deterrent.

Before considering the interaction of beliefs and motives, it is worth noting in passing that the state of *dissonance*, which was a major focus of Festinger's (1957) work, features as an emotional state, albeit not necessarily very prominently, in the Motivation System. For some women, the dissonance which might be created in a woman who has decided not to breast feed her baby despite believing that it is better than bottle feeding for the health of her baby would be akin to feelings of guilt and might even cause her to reverse her intention – particularly if she has high self-esteem. An alternative way of reducing dissonance, of course, is to convince oneself that bottle is just as good as breast ! This is a not uncommon result of the interaction of belief and affect which we will now consider.

Interactions between Belief and Affect

I observed earlier one example of the interdependence of belief and affect when reference was made to beliefs *about* affect. More commonly – and consistent with the Theory of Reasoned Action (Ajsen and Fishbein, 1980) – one would expect beliefs to generate action through the mediation of attitudes. The view here is that beliefs about response efficacy will indeed contribute to intention to act provided that the responses are judged to be efficacious in achieving desired goals. The hypothesised mechanism is shown in Figure 2

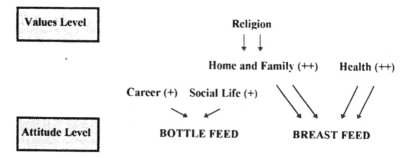

FIGURE 2   Relationship between Values and Attitudes

below in respect of decision to breast or bottle feed. Certain values are assumed to generate one or more attitudes which, other things being equal, will contribute to the selection of one or other type of feeding for the baby.

This contention is further illustrated by the study of 305 expectant mothers who were interviewed before and after they gave birth to their children. Table 1A below summarises their *salient* beliefs (i.e. those beliefs which were spontaneously produced as opposed to the *latent* beliefs which resulted from probing and closed questions).

Table 1A   Beliefs of 305 women about Breast Feeding

Positive Beliefs	Percent of Sample
Better for baby's health	64%
More convenient	44%
More 'natural'	31%
Improves bonding with baby	25%
Specific disease prevention/health benefit for baby	18%
Cheaper	17%
More hygienic/less risk of infection	12.5%
Better for health of mother	8%
Baby more contented	7%
Better for maternal figure/breasts	6%
More enjoyable for mother/Relaxing	6%

The beliefs shown in Table 1A all refer to the beliefs about the positive features of breast feeding and represent the responses of the sample as a whole – *whether they intended to breast feed or not.* The sample also had a number of salient beliefs about the anticipated costs of breast feeding and these are at Table 1B.

Respondents also provided their beliefs about *bottle* feeding but these observations are not included here due to limited space.

Table IB   Beliefs about Anticipated Costs

Negative Beliefs	Per cent of sample
Embarrassing	29%
Inconvenient – social life	13%
General inconvenience	11.5%
Uncomfortable	11.5%
Tiring	9%
"Messy"	7%
Cannot judge quantity of milk available	7%
Inconvenient – return to work	less than 1%

Table II   Evaluations of Key Attributes of Breast or Bottle Feeding

Anticipated Outcome	Mean Scale Score (Importance attached to Outcome) **	% Associating Outcome with Type of Feeding		Assumed Contribution to Likelihood of Breast Feeding $$
		Bottle	Breast	
Baby's Health	5.0	1%	56%	+++
Enhanced Bonding	4.5	1.5%	65.5%	+++
More Likelihood of Obese Baby	3.95	62%	7.5%	+++
Benefits for Maternal Figure	3.52	8%	46.5%	++
Cheaper	2.45	1%	95%	?
General convenience	3.04	37%	54%	?
Benefits/Costs Breasts	2.83	1%/0.5%	9%/9%	?
Effect on Conjugal Role Sharing	3.96	0%	31%	—
Embarrassment	3.43	0%	67%	—
Discomfort	3.01	3%	68%	—
Social Inconvenience	2.73	5%	53.5%	−
Work Inconvenience	1.76	1%	39%	?

** High score is 5 and indicates high level of importance. Women were not asked to rate importance of baby's health as it was not conceivable that anyone would admit to not rating this less than '5' – and so a notional score of '5' was given.
$$ Plus sign indicates notional positive contribution to intention to breast feed and negative sign indicates converse. Three pluses given where evaluation is greater than '3' and proportion of sample is over 50%.

As we have noted, the extent to which any beliefs influence behavioural intention will depend on the positive or negative evaluation of the belief attributes. In addition to exploring salient beliefs, the study cited above asked the sample of expectant mothers to rate the importance of what, according to current research, were supposedly the key determinants of feeding intention. These referred to not only the salient beliefs described earlier but also latent beliefs which were not spontaneously mentioned by the sample.

Table II provides a nice example of the value-expectancy dimension of HAM showing how both belief strength and strength of attitude derived from underlying values may contribute, inter alia, to intention to breast or bottle feed. The finding that both breast and bottle feeding was considered to be "convenient" by a quite high proportion of the sample also illustrates the need to deal with potential difficulties of ascertaining the direction of causality. It is normally assumed that beliefs contribute to attitude. However, it is important to reiterate that attitudes and motivation generally can contribute to belief: indeed the phenomenon of *"autistic thinking"* – believing what it is comfortable to belief (typically to reduce dissonance) is well known in both the literature and in everyday life. There is evidence from the research discussed here that the general label of "convenience" has little explanatory value but might reflect the tendency to rate *whatever* method of feeding is preferred as more convenient than the other.

A simple value expectancy calculation, in which the number of women holding a particular belief about the costs or benefits of either breast or bottle feeding is multiplied by a mean score on a five point scale of importance attached to each belief attribute, was used to assess the relative overall benefits of the two approaches to infant feeding. Breast feeding received more plaudits but unfortunately for breast feeding advocates, it was also perceived as having considerably more disadvantages. In fact breast feeding was considered to have 7.25 times the benefits of bottle feeding but incur approximately two and one half times the costs !

The Normative System

The Normative System describes the direct and indirect effects of different degrees of social pressure on individuals' intention to act. Again, following Fishbein's (1976) model, it operates by means of an interacting belief and motivation system. Individuals have a given level of certainty about the attitude of people in their social world and also a given level of motivation to conform to what they perceive to be the wishes of other people and social norms more generally. In HAM, social pressure is considered to be exerted with decreasing force from the relatively powerful influence of *"significant others"* – i.e. key referents interacting on a face to face basis with the individual – to the more attenuated impact of general social norms which are conveyed indirectly through mass media. In relation to choice of infant feeding then, the likelihood of influence will depend on (i) the nature and strength of women's beliefs about the prevalence and therefore the "normality" of breast feeding and the likely reaction of other people such as friends, family and health professionals and (ii) on the extent to which they are motivated to conform and comply with the perceived preferences of the significant others.

Harfouche (1970) describes rather dramatically the potential effect of socialisation and general normative pressure on women's feeding intentions in a particular Islamic culture. "Lactation management and breast-feeding as an act and way of life are acquired in the home. The pattern has a familial transmission; girls usually identify with their mothers, and after marriage they try to comply with the wishes of their in-laws and husbands".

The importance of normative pressure and associated sanctions is well illustrated by the same author describing the mother's role. Breast milk is, *"... God's special gift to the infant ... It is the best food and there is nothing like it.."* For the mother, *"... Nursing is a duty; a mother who does not nurse denies her baby's right.."* In fact, she is, *".... stingy, lazy, negligent, lacks affection like a step mother ... No lactation, no affection."*

In Western culture, health promoters have to consider a different and more indirect kind of *"norm sending".* This too is concerned with the social construction of women and their role. More particularly though, it has to do with the ways in which mass media, for example, portray gender – and especially the ambiguous and often conflicting messages about the breast as both a signal of sexual gratification and at the same time a mammary gland. This latter function, ironically, may create the embarrassment which I have shown to be a deterrent to the adoption of breast feeding.

In relation to the current study of choice of infant feeding methods, suffice it to say that professional norms were overwhelmingly perceived as favouring breast feeding. Both mothers and husbands/partners were the most important significant others – particularly the partner. It is interesting to note, however, that although there was a tendency for referents to be perceived as supporting the woman's choice of feeding and 21% of the sample claimed that the husband had influenced her decision (13% in the case of mothers), only a minority denied that the influence had been very great. Moreover, nearly 50% claimed that they would be either "not at all concerned" or "not very concerned" if their partner were to disapprove of the way she intended to feed her baby (the equivalent figure for "mother" was 82.5%).

Self Efficacy and Anticipated Costs

Reference was made above to beliefs about discomfort in relation to choice of feeding method. I also noted earlier how the actual experience of negative consequences of a health action can result in relapse. It is also clear that *anticipated* negative consequences can weaken the very intention to act. A substantial proportion of the sample of women identified a number of sources of anticipated discomfort associated with breast feeding (in rank order: soreness; engorgement; general discomfort; problems with nipples; biting) – together with a general concern about problems with milk supply. Such anticipated difficulties militate against a particularly important belief which is shown in Figure 2 as one of a number of *beliefs about self*. This is the concept of self efficacy which has been identified by Bandura (1982; 1986) as one of the more powerful indicators of the likelihood of individuals adopting behaviours of any kind. See Horne and Weinman, Chapter 2, for a discussion of self-efficacy. Self efficacy is also of central importance to the definition of empowerment – which I will now consider.

HEALTH PROMOTION: EMPOWERING HEALTH ACTIONS

A central tenet of this chapter is that health promotion is not so much concerned with adherence but rather with facilitating choice and gaining client co-operation. It is important, therefore, that we give some consideration to the translation of rather vague and ideological aims into more specific operations. However, only a limited discussion of empowerment is possible here. For more detailed analyses, see Tones (1992), Tones and Tilford (1994) and Tones (1995).

Empowerment, Values and Voluntarism

There are many who would consider the adoption of breast feeding as primarily an example of health behaviour designed to prevent a number of diseases and disorders in baby and, perhaps, mother. It is, however, equally or more legitimate to argue that this smacks of medicalisation and mothers should be free to choose whatever mode of feeding appeals most to them. However, if the promotion of safer sexual behaviours to prevent HIV and AIDS is considered, the situation is much more clear cut. It would certainly be nonsensical to argue that health promotion is concerned merely to help people decide whether or not they wished to infect themselves and other people. Health promoters are, of course, concerned with the public health and the well-being of individuals; they would also wish to maintain as far as possible the principles of voluntarism – the right to choose. On the other hand, they would clearly advocate certain choices and disapprove of others. Empowerment, therefore, is not value free and is not about merely inviting people to choose their own path to health or illness – quite the reverse. In fact, a major principle embodied in the approach described here is that empowerment will increase the likelihood of individuals making healthy choices and thus achieving the goals of preventive medicine. Indeed, I have already noted the high rate of non compliance using traditional educational approaches; an empowerment approach can hardly achieve worse results! In part, any success resulting from an empowerment approach must be ascribed to the enhancement of individuals' confidence in achieving desired outcomes; more importantly perhaps, an active empowered community might attain preventive outcomes by addressing the underlying causes of ill health – such as the inequalities whose association with health problems have already been mentioned. We must, however, have a detailed understanding of the empowerment process if we are to influence health choices and so I will now give some thought to operationalising empowerment within the framework of the HAM.

Operationalising Empowerment

A preliminary requirement for making empowered choices is, of course, possession of appropriate knowledge. Knowledge, it is said, is power: but power is much more than knowledge. Knowledge needs to be supplemented by the acquisition of decision making skills which are envisaged here as comprising the capacity to clarify values and utilise problem solving tactics such as those identified as "problem solving" by Gagne (1985) and "vigilant decision making" by Janis and Mann (1977).

A second and more important feature of empowerment relates to the two elements of the Belief and Motivational Systems described in terms of beliefs about self and self-esteem. In short, the self concept (the complete set of knowledge and beliefs about self) incorporates certain critical empowering beliefs about control. The relevance of beliefs about perceived locus of control (PLC) for "healthy decision-making" is well known (e.g. Wallston and Wallston, 1978): a perceived *internal* locus of control, i.e. the belief that one's actions *in general* – and the gains and losses ensuing from those actions – result from one's own efforts rather than the intervention of fate, chance, powerful others or the intrinsically chaotic nature of life. See Horne and Weinman, Chapter 2 for a description of the model. Self efficacy beliefs have already been mentioned. These are *specific* beliefs and refer to the extent to which individuals are capable of achieving some particular objectives – such as coping with the demands of breast feeding, or buying and negotiating use of a condom with a partner.

A number of other more specific beliefs which are conducive to the empowerment goal have also been identified. These include *cognitive control* (the provision of information which enables the intellectual management of, typically, aversive events); *decisional control* (the provision of an opportunity to make actual choices based on real rather than tokenistic consultation); *behavioural control* (the possession of a variety of skills needed for the actual exercise of control).

Self-esteem is a complementary feature of the self concept and it refers to the extent to which the individual values the attributes which make up the self concept. Just as we form attitudes to any aspect of our world in accordance with our value system, we develop attitudes to ourselves. The sum of these attitudes defines our self-esteem. The central relevance of self-esteem for empowered decision making is based on the following rationale: presumably if people possess a good measure of self worth, they are more likely to respond to the exhortation *"look after yourself"*; individuals having high self-esteem are more likely to have the courage of their convictions and an associated capacity to resist normative and interpersonal pressures; they are more likely to handle threat in a realistic and productive manner rather than resorting to defensive avoidance; those having high self-esteem will experience more dissonance if they fail to adopt those healthy but problematic behaviours which they believe they ought to adopt !

Reciprocal Determinism: Support and the Environmental Dimension

I have already argued that environmental factors play a major (if not *the* major) part in determining whether or not people are in a position to "choose health". Bandura (1982;1986) has described this interactive process of individual with environment as *reciprocal determinism.* Following this formulation, empowerment involves two complementary actions: the empowerment of individuals to help them negotiate the environment in an effective way and engineering changes in the environment in order to reduce barriers to the negotiation process. As I have noted, the implementation of "healthy public policy" is necessary to achieve the latter goal; the former goal is primarily the concern of education. Health education would be concerned to influence the beliefs about control mentioned above and one of the most powerful ways to doing this is to provide individuals with the skills they need to achieve success. These skills or "action competences" (Tones, 1994) would be many in number and range from the provision of psychomotor skills – such as training in breast feeding or teaching how to use and dispose of a condom. They might also include general social interaction skills such as assertiveness or the capacity to communicate with a partner about emotional issues. Possession of such competences would influence efficacy beliefs and thus influence intention to act (or, using Prochaska and DiClemente's term, move the individual from "precontemplation" to "contemplation"). The skills also form part of the facilitating factors identified in HAM: i.e. those conditions necessary to increase the likelihood of individual intention being translated into successful outcome.

Figure 1 categorised these supportive factors in terms of knowledge, skills and environment. As noted earlier in the chapter, they include the self regulatory skills needed to anticipate and forestall relapse as well as the action competences to which reference was made above. All we need to add here is the observation that while health education might supply the knowledge and skills, policy decisions would often be necessary to ensure that the environment is one in which the healthy choice is the easy choice. For instance, knowledge and skills in relation to condom use are irrelevant if condoms are not accessible. More importantly, if at risk, sexually active individuals are locked into a multiply deprived setting which generates alienation and learned helplessness, knowledge and skills would be irrelevant : the group in question would never leave the precontemplation phase!

Health Promotion: Strategies and Methods

Finally, we can comment on the implications of the analysis that this chapter has provided for the delivery of interventions. Only the sketchiest observations can be made about these implications which derive directly from the psychosocial and environmental factors which, I have argued, govern people's co-operation with recommended health actions. For a more complete review, see Tones and Tilford (1994). I should, though, reiterate the importance of the *health education x healthy public policy* "formula" and make the following assertions:

- Because specific health and illness outcomes – such as adoption of safer sex practices or breast feeding – ultimately depend on general policy (e.g. to manage poverty) and general psychological characteristics (such as the possession self-esteem and general lifeskills), then *"horizontal"* programmes, which address fundamental causes , rather than *"vertical"* programmes, which target specific diseases, offer the best hope for success (Tones, 1993)
- A "healthy alliance" between a variety of different "settings" will maximise chances of success. A "settings *approach"* – e.g. a "health promoting hospital" – routinely incorporates policies which seek to empower individuals and ensure that the whole ethos of the setting is congruent with its health education and health care goals.

- The settings approach should be supported by appropriate use of mass media – whose major function is potentially one of critical consciousness raising and advocacy rather than behaviour and attitude change (Tones, 1996).
- At the micro level, educational methods and the minutiae of the face-to-face consultation should be sufficiently sophisticated to take account of the complex psychosocial and environmental determinants of health actions. Personnel should have the necessary educational skills – and have empowerment in mind (Tones, 1997).

REFERENCES

Ajsen, I and Fishbein, M. (1980) *Understanding attitudes and predicting social behavior*. New Jersey: Prentice-Hall.

Bandura, A. (1986) *Social foundations of thought and action: a social cognitive theory*. New Jersey: Prentice-Hall.

Bandura, A. (1982) Self-efficacy mechanism in human agency. *American Psychologist* **2**, 122–147.

Baric, L. (1994) *Health promotion and health education in practice: module 2, the organisational model*. Cheshire: Barns Publications.

Becker, M.H. (1984) (ed.) *The health belief model and personal health behavior*. New Jersey: Charles B Slack: Thorofare.

Blaxter, M. (1993) What is health ? In B. Davey, A. Gray, and C. Seale (eds) *Health and disease: a reader*. Buckingham: Open University Press.

Bury, M. and Gabe, J. (1994) Television and medicine: medical dominance or trial by media? In J. Gabe, D. Kelleher, and G. Williams (eds.) *Challenging medicine*. London: Routledge.

Davies, J.B. (1992) *The myth of addiction: an application of the psychological theory of attribution to illicit drug use*. Switserland: Harwood.

Dingwall, R. (1994) Litigation and the threat to medicine. In J. Gabe, D. Kelleher, and G. Williams (eds.) *Challenging medicine*. London: Routledge.

Doyal, L. (1994) Changing medicine? Gender and the politics of health care. In J. Gabe, D. Kelleher and G. Williams (eds.) *Challenging medicine*. London: Routledge.

Durrant, K. (1993) *The creative arts and the promotion of health in community settings*. Unpublished MSc dissertation, Leeds Metropolitan University.

Elston, M.A. (1994) The anti-vivisectionist movement and the science of medicine. In J. Gabe, D. Kelleher, and G. Williams (eds.) *Challenging medicine*. London: Routledge.

Festinger, L. (1957) *A theory of cognitive dissonance*. New York: Harper and Row.

Fishbein, M. (1976) Persuasive communication. In A.E. Bennett (ed.) *Communication between doctors and patients*. Oxford University Press/Nuffield Provincial Hospitals Trust.

Freidson, E. (1961) *Patients' views of medical practice*. New York: Russell Sage.

Freidson, E. (1970) *Profession of medicine*. New York: Dodd, Mead.

Freire, P. (1972) *Pedagogy of the oppressed*. Harmondsworth: Penguin.

Gagne, R.M. (1985) *The conditions of learning and theory of instruction*. New York: Holt-Saunders.

Harfouche, J.K. (1970) The importance of breast feeding. *Journal of Tropical Paediatrics Monograph* **10**, 133–175.

Hunter, D. (1994) From tribalism to corporatism: the managerial challenge to medical dominance. In J. Gabe, D. Kelleher, and G. Williams (eds) *Challenging medicine*. London: Routledge.

Jaco, E.G. (1979) *Patients, physicians and illness: a source book in behavioral science and health (3rd ed)*. New York: Free Press.

Janis, I.L. and Mann, L (1965) *Decision making*. New York: Free Press.

Janis, I.L. and Mann, L (1977) *Decision making*. New York: Free Press.

Kanfer, F.H. and Karoly, P (1972) Self-control: a behavioristic excursion into the lion's den. *Behavior Therapy*, **3**, 398–416.

Kelleher, D. (1994) Self-help groups and their relationship to medicine. In J. Gabe, D. Kelleher, and G. Williams (eds) *Challenging medicine*. London: Routledge.

Kelleher, D., Gabe, J. and Williams, G. (1994) Understanding medical dominance in the modern world. In J. Gabe, D. Kelleher, and G. Williams (eds) *Challenging medicine*. London: Routledge.

Lalonde, M. (1974) *A new perspective on the health of Canadians*. Ottawa: Goverment of Canada.

Lewis, F.M. (1997) The concept of control: a typology and health related variables. *Advances in Health Education and Promotion* **2**, 277–309.

Marsh, A. and Matheson, J. (1983) *Smoking attitudes and behaviour.* London: HMSO.

Martin, J. (1978) *Infant feeding 1975: attitudes and practices in England and Wales.* London: HMSO.

Newton, N.R. and Newton, M. (1967) Psychological aspects of lactation. *New England Journal of Medicine* **277**, 1179–1188.

Parsons, T. (1951) *The social system.* New York: Free Press.

Parsons, T. (1979) Definitions of health and illness in the light of American values and social structure. In E.G. Jaco (ed.) *Patients, physicians and illness. Third edition.* New York: Free Press.

Prochaska, J., and DiClemente, C. (1986) Toward a comprehensive model of change. W.R. Miller and N. Heather (eds.) *Treating addictive behaviors: processes of change.* New York: Plenum.

Rollnick, S., Heather, N. and Bell, A. (1992) Negotiating behaviour change in medical settings: the development of brief motivational interviewing. *Journal of Mental Health* **1**, 25–37.

Rotter, J.B. (1966). Generalised expectancies for internal versus external control of reinforcement. *Psychological Monographs* **80**, 1–28.

Ryan, W. (1976) *Blaming the victim.* New York: Vintage Books.

Saks, M. (1994) The Alternatives to medicine. In J. Gabe, D. Kelleher, and G. Williams (eds.) *Challenging medicine.* London: Routledge.

Salber, E.J., Stitt, P.G. and Babbott, J.G. (1958) Patterns of breast feeding (I): factors affecting the frequency of breast feeding in the newborn period. *New England Journal of Medicine*, **259**, 707–713.

Ssasz, T.S. and Hollender, M.H. (1956) A contribution to the philosophy of medicine. The basic models of the doctor patient relationship. *Archives of Internal Medicine* **97**, 585–592.

Tones, B.K. (1979) Past achievement and future success. In I. Sutherland (ed) *Health Education: perspectives and choices.* London: Allen and Unwin.

Tones, B.K. (1987) Devising strategies for preventing drug misuse: the role of the health action model. *Health Education Research* **4**, 305–318.

Tones, B.K. (1992) Health promotion, empowerment and the concept of control. In D. Colquhoun (ed.) *Health education: politics and practice.* Geelong, Victoria: Deakin University Press.

Tones, B.K. (1993) The importance of horizontal programmes in health education (editorial), *Health Education Research* **4,** 455–459.

Tones, B.K. (1994) Health promotion, empowerment and action competence. In B.B. Jensen and K. Schnack (eds.) *Action and action competence as key concepts in critical pedagogy.* Copenhagen: Royal Danish School of Educational Studies.

Tones, B.K. (1995) Health education as empowerment. In *Health promotion today.* London: Health Education Authority.

Tones, B.K. (1996) Models of mass media: hypodermic, aerosol or agent provocateur ? *Drugs: Education, Prevention and Policy* **1,** 37.

Tones, B.K. (1997) Health education, behaviour change, and the public health. In R. Dettels and J. McEwen (eds.) *Oxford textbook of public health. Volume 2. The methods of public health. Third Edition..*

Tones, B.K. and Tilford, S. (1994) *Health education: effectiveness, efficiency and equity.* London: Chapman and Hall.

Tuckett, D., Boulton, M., Olson, C. and Williams, A. (1985) *Meetings between experts.* London: Tavistock.

Wallston, B.S. and Wallston, K.A. (1978) Locus of control and health: a review of the literature. *Health Education Monographs* **2,** 107–117.

World Health Organisation (1978) Report on the international conference on primary health care, *Alma Ata,* 6–12 September. Geneva: WHO.

World Health Organisation (1984) *Health promotion: a discussion document on the concepts and principles.* Copenhagen: WHO.

World Health Organisation (1986) *Ottawa Charter for health promotion: an international conference on health promotion.* Copenhagen: WHO.

Williams, G. and Popay, J. (1994) Lay knowledge and the privilege of experience. In J. Gabe, D. Kelleher, and G. Williams (eds.) *Challenging medicine.* London: Routledge.

Winkler, F .(1995) Transferring power in health care. In B. Davey, A. Gray, and C. Seale (eds.) *Health and disease: a reader.* Buckingham: Open University Press.

Witz, A. (1994) The challenge of nursing. In J. Gabe, D. Kelleher, and G. Williams (eds.) *Challenging medicine.* London: Routledge.

Zola, I.K. (1972) Studying the decision to see a doctor: review, critique, corrective. *Advances in Psychosomatic Medicine* **8**, 216–236.

Adherence in particular groups

7
Adherence to Treatment in Children

Mandy Bryon

Poor adherence to prescribed medical treatment regimens is extremely common in both child and adult populations (La Greca, 1990; Epstein and Cluss, 1982). Rates of non-adherence are clinically significant, reported at around 50% for most chronic conditions (Rapoff and Christopherson, 1982), although rates vary as a function of a range of variables such as method of measurement and complexity of treatment. Yet, it is a consistent finding that poor adherence is a major cause of concern for health professionals (HPs).

The consequences of inadequate treatment practice on health can be serious in both the immediate and long-term. Yet, many children will not readily adhere to treatment even in the face of life-threatening conditions. Numerous studies have found that the severity of a disease does not play a part in determining adherence, these include a range of chronic illnesses such as cystic fibrosis (Gudas, Koocher and Wypij, 1991; Passero, Remor and Salomon, 1981; Abbott *et al.*, 1994), asthma (Lemanek, 1990), seizures (Hazsard, Hutchinson and Krawiecki, 1990) and cancer (Phipps and DeCuir-Whalley, 1990).

Advances in medical technology are likely to increase the problem of poor adherence as treatment regimens become more complex and new treatments become available for previously incurable diseases. Geiss *et al.* (1992) document the extensive daily routine necessary for the management of cystic fibrosis. The regimen is time-consuming and lifelong, but has resulted in life expectancy increasing substantially over the past ten years. A similar situation has occurred in diabetes management (Reid and Appleton, 1991). Bone marrow transplantation has now become a routine and increasingly successful treatment for a range of childhood malignancies, but the necessary regimen is intensive and painful (Phipps and DeCuir-Whalley, 1990).

To understand why poor adherence is so prevalent it may be useful to outline some of the daily regimens expected of certain diseases. Children with cancer may have experienced surgery, chemotherapy and radiation therapy, often in combination. They may have been subjected to regular painful treatments at clinic visits such as injections, wound cleaning or even bone marrow aspirations. Home treatment includes oral medications, daily mouth care to prevent oral sores and hygienic care of the central catheter line (Manne *et al.*, 1993).

The daily management of insulin-dependent diabetes mellitus involves daily insulin injections, often several times per day. These injections may comprise more than one type of insulin and, therefore, require skilled preparation. Blood glucose monitoring by finger prick between two and four times per day is necessary as insulin requirements vary throughout the day. A minimum of daily exercise is necessary to reduce insulin requirements, and dietary restrictions are also imposed (Johnson *et al.*, 1992; Reid and Appleton, 1991). For a review of diabetes in adults, see Warren and Hixenbaugh, Chapter 16.

The treatment of cystic fibrosis likewise involves several components. Medication includes pancreatic enzyme replacements taken with all food and drink plus vitamins and antibiotics. Chest physiotherapy must be administered several times per day to clear secretions and thus avoid infection. Exercise is necessary. Dietary recommendations require a high calorie intake irrespective of appetite, which often is poor due to digestive difficulties. Some children will also need nebulised antibiotics or drugs to thin accretions of mucus in the airways (Geiss *et al.*, 1992).

This chapter reviews research in an attempt to discover why some children demonstrate poor adherence even in the face of life-threatening disease. Inconsistent measurement and methodology across studies have made it difficult to demonstrate causal links between hypothesised stressors and adherence behaviour. The findings have been categorised into five potential influences on adherence, demographic, disease, child, knowledge, and family. These influences are examined in order that any predictors of poor adherence to treatment can be identified.

CONCEPTUALISING ADHERENCE

In recent years the term adherence with treatment has been preferred to compliance with treatment. The reason for this is that "adherence" implies some element of wilful intention, whereas "compliance" implies submission to the direction of others (Koocher, McGrath and Gudas, 1990). Studies of apparently non-adherent behaviour have discovered the problem comprises more than a failure to "do as one is told". Poor adherence can result from a multitude of causes.

This finding can lead to confusions in the conceptualisation of adherence when attempting to study the behaviour. Few studies (except perhaps those presenting case reports) compare the behaviours of individual patients with the explicit instructions given by their physician. Most assume a typical treatment regimen has been prescribed for the particular disease. However, regimens differ from physician to physician and from time to time. Therefore, finding a simple outcome behaviour which would apply over a range of patients and diseases would be difficult if not impossible.

An additional confound is that discrepancies have been found between the patient and physician in their understanding or memory of prescribed treatment instructions. Page *et al.* (1981) found that only 18% of recommendations reported by physicians were accurately recalled by patients. Reid and Appleton (1991) document an interesting finding which suggests that parents and physicians may have different goals for the daily regimen. Marteau *et al.* (1987) suggested that for children with diabetes the parents' aim was to avoid a hypoglycaemic attack whilst the physician's aim was to limit the potential long term negative consequences of the illness. These different aims would involve different priorities and emphasis of the daily treatment.

Typically, treatment protocols for chronic illness are complex. They comprise several different daily components and some of these vary according to situation-specific problem-solving requirements. For example, it may be necessary to alter the amount of insulin according to blood sugar level as evidenced by prior finger pricks in a diabetic regimen. The management of many chronic diseases relies on parents to judge their child's symptoms in order to administer a prescribed drug or to seek medical attention. Obviously, certain regimens involve technical skills such as injection. Johnson *et al.* (1982) found considerable error in the skills of patients with diabetes and their carers in an observational study. The participants were not aware of their skill deficits.

Often patients are judged to be non-adherent if their health status is poor. Johnson (1994) warns that this assumes a direct link between adherence behaviour and health status. Sanders *et al.* (1991) found that physicians were more likely to rate a child with cystic fibrosis as having poor adherence if the child had poor lung capacity and growth. There must be cautious conclusions drawn from studies of adherence to treatment since, as yet, no causal links can be made between health behaviours and health status.

MEASURING ADHERENCE IN CHRONIC ILLNESS

Direct Methods

Obviously, the methods used for measurement of adherence need to be taken into account when making cross-study comparisons. Methods have varied from the direct to the indirect. Direct methods involve assessment of the amount of prescribed medication found in body fluids. For example, assessment of the level of medication ingested from blood samples to determine the presence and level of theophylline-based compounds for children with asthma (Rylance and Moreland, 1980) and glycosylated haemoglobin to estimate blood glucose control over the previous 6–8 week period for children with diabetes (Anderson *et al.*, 1990).

Direct observation of administration of a procedure has been extensively used in measures of adherence for children with diabetes. Delameter *et al.* (1989) used direct observation to assess self-monitoring of blood glucose, Johnson *et al.* (1982) used the method for assessment of injecting insulin.

Whilst these methods appear objective, they are not without limitation. Laboratory drug essays are expensive, invasive and often the results show a summary of pharmaceutical residue in the body which may not accurately reflect the drug taking behaviour. Different children may have different rates of metabolism and these may also vary in the same child over time especially during a growth spurt, e.g. puberty. Even direct observation has potential observer bias. Johnson (1994) warns of the difficulty of reliably measuring complex health behaviours occurring daily in the patients' natural environment.

Indirect Methods

Indirect methods refer to reported rates of adherence. Studies have obtained measures from child, parent or HP. There are conflicting reports as to whether or not there is any agreement from the three different sources. Gudas *et al.* (1991) report high correlations between parent, child and HP for each part of the treatment regimen in children with cystic fibrosis. La Greca (1990), however, claims that parents are found to over-report adherence. Unfortunately, the method of data collection as well as the targeted person reporting has also varied. Gudas *et al.* (1991) had parent, child and physician rate the same aspects of adherence on a five-point Likert scale. Johnson *et al.* (1992) used their 24 hour recall method whereby parents and children were interviewed separately about the treatment regimen completed during the previous day. Geiss *et al.* (1992) had physicians complete a rating scale of adherence behaviours immediately following an outpatient visit, whilst Csajkowski and Koocher (1987) rated adherence according to the ease of which each aspect of the child's regimen was completed during an inpatient admission. Of course ratings by HPs are also subject to bias as they know the child's history both in terms of their physical status and previous complaints of poor adherence.

Other indirect measures used are questionnaires which may also assess knowledge of the disease. Koocher and Csajkowski (1984) have developed a measure to assess adherence, the Medical Compliance Incomplete Stories Test (MCIST) which they hope will allow some standardisation across studies. The instrument consists of separate scenarios in which the character is faced with a dilemma as to whether or not to follow medical advice. The participant must predict the outcome for the character in each of the stories.

Clearly, it is necessary to measure adherence by means of a variety of sources in order to reduce bias. What will produce informative data will be studies which correlate estimates of adherence with measures of health status.

MALADJUSTMENT OF CHILDREN WITH CHRONIC ILLNESS

In the face of the repeatedly traumatic experiences of children with chronic illness, is it only to be expected that they will be maladjusted? Nolan and Pless (1986) in their review of research which examined the impact of chronic illness on psychological well-being, concluded that many chronically ill children were at significant risk for emotional disturbances of many kinds. Their review criticised the definitions and methodology in most studies. As a result, they concluded that it was impossible to know clearly the types of risk, the types of children or the aspects of the disease which give rise to maladjustment.

Eiser (1994) suggests a significant shift in the assumptions underlying contemporary psychological theories in this field: "The most fundamental shift has been from a perspective which emphasises *dying from* to one which acknowledges the difficulties in *living with*... a related shift is from a perspective which is deficit-centred, and concerned with maladjustment, to one which is more optimistic, and focused on coping, adjustment and adaptation".

Thus, it would be inaccurate to consider the child with a chronic illness to be maladjusted simply because we perceive their lifestyle to be emotionally and behaviourally disturbed. Instead, we must construe the chronically ill child's daily treatment regimen as a series of stressors with which the child and family must cope. In order to understand why a child may fail to adhere to treatment, it is necessary to identify aspects of the regimen, the child, and the family which may predict risk for poor adherence.

POTENTIAL INFLUENCES ON ADHERENCE

Given the differences in measurement techniques and prescribed medical regimens, it is possible to identify groups of factors which are believed to influence adherence behaviours across disease types. Researchers have attempted to account for the effects of similar psychosocial factors. In order to make sense of the findings, it may be fruitful to categorise potential influences. These can be grouped into five global headings; demographic, disease/regimen issues, child psychological factors, knowledge and family factors.

Demographic

There are conflicting results regarding the extent to which certain demographic characteristics account for the variance in adherence. In virtually all studies, gender has not been found to influence adherence in bone-marrow transplants (Phipps and DeCuir-Whalley, 1990); diabetes (Jacobson *et al.*, 1990); seizures (Hazsard *et al.*, 1990); cystic fibrosis (Abbott *et al.*, 1994); and asthma (Lemanek, 1990).

The only study to document a gender difference is that of Csajkowski and Koocher (1987) who found more girls than boys with cystic fibrosis show poor adherence. This finding may not be spurious, however, as a difference between the sexes was found in the emotional adjustment of adolescents with cystic fibrosis (Simmons *et al.*, 1985). Boys were found to exhibit more behaviour problems than girls who were found to deny illness-related stress.

Race also has not been found to account for any differences in rates of adherence. Similarly, socio-economic status has not been identified generally except, to the author's knowledge, in two studies. Gudas *et al.* (1991) investigating levels of perceived adherence in cystic fibrosis found children in lower socio-economic groups to be at greater risk for poor adherence. Manne *et al.* (1993) found lower socio-economic status to be associated with more frequent appointment cancellations, late arrival times and more delays in reporting negative symptoms.

Age is the variable which accounts for the largest proportion of variance in almost all studies. Generally, adolescent children are more likely than younger children to be reported as poor adherers themselves, by their parents and by HPs. This finding is consistent irrespective of disease type, in studies of diabetes (Jacobson *et al.*, 1990; Hauser *et al.*, 1990; Johnson *et al.*, 1992; Johnson *et al.*, 1990; Anderson *et al.*, 1990; Kovacs *et al.*, 1992; and Bond, Aiken and

Somerville, 1992) or studies of cystic fibrosis (Gudas *et al.*, 1991; Geiss *et al.*, 1992; Csajkowski and Koocher, 1987). Most studies suggest this finding to be a result of the rebellion against authority which marks this stage of development. Interestingly, younger children had the most reported problems with adherence to treatments for cancer regimens (Manne *et al.*, 1993; Phipps and DeCuir-Whalley, 1990). Both studies link this finding with parenting style and the type of treatment which has immediate aversive effects such as pain and vomiting.

Although age is an important consideration, it must not be assumed that all adolescents deliberately reduce their levels of adherence. Many diseases become increasingly difficult to manage at this time of rapid growth and hormonal change. Shifts in responsibility for aspects of regimen may be subject to miscommunication (Anderson *et al.*, 1990). It is also important that chronological age is not equated with developmental and intellectual capacity (La Greca, 1990).

Disease/Regimen Issues

Differential Rates of Adherence

Passero *et al.* (1981) examined the rates of adherence reported by patients for different aspects of their cystic fibrosis daily regimen. The results indicated a differential adherence rate ranging from 90% full adherence with prescribed medication to 70% partial or non-adherence to dietary recommendations. This variance in adherence according to different aspects of the treatment protocol has been documented for other chronic diseases such as seizures (Hazsard *et al.*, 1990), and diabetes (Reid and Appleton, 1991). Perhaps patients are more likely to adhere to the recommendations made by physician than those made by an allied profession such as dietician or physiotherapist. It is worth examining in more detail the reasons for these differential rates in adherence behaviour.

Noxious Treatments

Phipps and DeCuir-Whalley (1990) and Manne *et al.* (1993), in their studies of children with cancer, found less adherence with aspects of treatment that had aversive side-effects such as vomiting. Children with diabetes are reported to have more difficulties with finger prick blood glucose measures which are initially perceived as painful. The implication here is that poor adherence results from learned or anticipated aversive associations with aspects of the treatment protocol.

Interference with Daily Lifestyle

Gudas *et al.* (1991) in their study of adherence behaviour in children with cystic fibrosis, found that aspects of the regimen for which there were higher reported rates of poor adherence involved family disagreements, required advance planning or interfered with activities of daily living. This finding is supported by Csajkowski and Koocher (1987) who found adherence rates were higher for children whose daily lifestyle was not disrupted by the daily regimen of cystic fibrosis. Perhaps excessive and time-consuming treatments or those which illustrate the difference between the sick and healthy child are the ones for which some chronically ill children have the least commitment.

Complexity

Complex daily regimens which involve frequently altered dosages of medication, require considered judgements or involve complicated drug delivery systems such as nebulisers, have been associated with lower rates of adherence (Johnson *et al.*, 1982; Voyles and Menendez, 1983). It has been suggested that the combination of chronicity and a complex regimen would predict poor adherence (Varni and Wallander, 1984). Similarly, reduced rates of adherence have been found when the number of drugs or dosages increases beyond four per day (Blackwell, 1979).

Symptom Relief Versus Prophylaxis

The treatment of many chronic illnesses incorporates aspects which have prophylactic effects, that is, their action is to prevent or reduce likelihood of future exacerbations of the illness. By definition, these treatments do not have immediate or noticeable benefit. Phipps and DeCuir-Whalley (1990) found that aspects of the treatment regimen which had immediate symptom relief resulted in higher rates of adherence. Abbott *et al.* (1994) studied adherence in adults with cystic fibrosis. Patients who reported immediate benefits following implementation of a treatment were more likely to show good adherence as rated by self and HP. Lemanek (1990) reports findings from studies by Becker *et al.* (1978) and Smith *et al.* (1986) which found inconsistent effects on symptom relief of the same drug in treatment of asthma. This had consequences for rates of adherence. Those participants who experienced the differential effects of the drug were the least adherent as they had doubts about the necessity of this daily medication.

Patient-Professional Relationship

The quality of the relationship between patient and HP has been found to account for variance in adherence with treatment. Adolescents were found to be more likely to adhere with recommendations if they found the physician to be caring (Hanson *et al.*, 1988). Parent satisfaction with the child's medical care for treatment of seizures was positively correlated with adherence (Hazsard *et al.*, 1990).

Child Psychological Factors

Psychological Adjustment

Research into the psychological effects of chronic illness on children continues to discover a vulnerability for emotional, educational and behavioural difficulties. The trend nowadays, however, is to document how children adjust to and cope with the stresses that a chronic illness brings rather than assess rates of psychopathology. In an overview of the effects of chronic illness on children and their families, Midence (1994) concludes: "As a group, most of these children do not demonstrate elevated levels of psychological maladjustment and seem to cope well with their illness. Similarly, their families generally are functioning well and demonstrate remarkable resiliency. A simple or direct relationship between chronic illness and poor psychological functioning does not seen to exist".

Investigators of adherence behaviour have examined the child's adjustment as an influence on varying rates and, likewise, have generally found no effects. Geiss *et al.* (1992) were concerned to measure adjustment patterns of patients attending a centre for treatment of cystic fibrosis. Mothers rated their children on the Personality Inventory for Children (Wirt *et al.*, 1980). Results indicated that all scores fell within the normal range, thus indicating no psychopathology. Similarly, as part of an investigation of the correlates of medical adherence for boys with haemophilia (D'Angelo *et al.*, 1992) parents completed the Child Behaviour Checklist (CBCL; Achenbach and Edelbrock, 1983). Results indicated that all participants had ratings within the normal range.

Self-Esteem and Optimism

Self-esteem was not found to be a predictor of adherence to treatment by West, DuRant and Pendergrast (1993) nor for Kovacs *et al.* (1992) in their longitudinal assessment of risk for psychiatric disorder in children with diabetes. The measures used in these studies were investigator devised questionnaire or interview thus difficulties with clear definitions and methodology must be considered.

Although these studies did not find an effect of self-esteem, level of optimism reported by children with a chronic illness appears to correlate positively with rates of adherence. Gudas *et al.* (1991) found optimism to be a predictor of good adherence when examining perceptions of adherence in children with cystic fibrosis. They found an interaction between age and optimism; older children who were highly optimistic were more adherent than children who were less optimistic. Interestingly, level of optimism did not correlate with perceived disease severity. That is, children who had severe and deteriorating health status were just as likely to have high levels of optimism as children with better health status.

Health Locus Of Control

It has been reported that children with a chronic illness and their parents are more likely to attribute control of the illness to chance and powerful others (Perrin and Shapiro, 1985). Several researchers have hypothesised that health locus of control (e.g. Wallston and Wallston, 1978) would explain variance in adherence behaviour. Children who believe they have some control over their health would be more likely to adhere to treatment than those who feel dependent on luck or events beyond their control. However, no correlation was found between health locus of control and adherence levels in seizure patients (Hazsard *et al.*, 1990) or for adherence to dental appointments (West *et al.*, 1993). It is noteworthy that Hazsard and colleagues admit to flaws in their measurement as they had constant ceiling effects and were unable to discriminate any differences children may have perceived for amount of self- versus physician control over their illness.

Jacobson *et al.* (1990) in contrast used the Nowicki and Stickland (1973) measure of health locus of control as part of a battery to assess the effects of coping on adherence to a diabetic regimen. They found scores to be predictive of adherence, that is, patients who experienced themselves as more in control of situations exhib- ited greater adherence to their treatments. It is interesting that those researchers who adapted the locus of control measure to health attitudes produced negative results whilst using the measure in its original form to rate perceptions of self-control per se, produced positive correlations. Many children with chronic illness do not perceive themselves as sick or ailing and so it would be more mean- ingful for them to complete normalised attitude questionnaires. Eiser (1990) advocates a move towards researchers construing children with a chronic illness as ordinary people in exceptional circum- stances rather than as being deviant.

Coping Strategies

Another frequently raised hypothesis is that children who cope better with their illness will show better adherence to treatment. "Coping" is defined as " . . . the responses emitted when an individual is confronted with problematic situations" (Varni and Wallander, 1988). The difficulty here, however, is the possibility that "coping" and "adherence" are confounded, do we perceive a child who adheres to all aspects of regimen as a child who demonstrates good coping strategies? The results of these studies depend heavily on how coping has been operationalised in their measures.

Again, there seems to be no consistent method of measuring coping in the literature on adherence. All researchers incorporate their own constructs into questionnaires or interview. Csajkowski and Koocher (1987) identified several coping behaviours which were assumed to assist adolescents to adapt to their life situation. These included active participation in school, openness with peers about their illness, active responsible attitude towards medical self-care and recognising the severity of the illness. Here it can be clearly seen that coping and adherence measures will be confounded. Not surprisingly, children who were rated as good at coping were also rated as adherent to regimen during inpatient admission.

An alternative definition of coping was employed by Jacobson *et al.* (1990) in their investigation of the influence of coping on adherence among children with diabetes. Here coping referred to the relevance of problem-solving strategies generated by children to given demands. The measure looked at the specific action and the regulation of the effects of that action. Action was assessed by locus of control and adaptive strengths (e.g. stress tolerance, persistence and commitment) regulation was assessed by ego defence mechanisms obtained from systematic analyses of responses to interview (e.g. acting out, turning against self). All aspects of coping were significantly associated with adherence behaviour, but when each aspect was analysed separately using a stepwise regression, only level of ego defence was significant. Thus, those children who were better at self-monitoring and regulation generally, not just for their illness, were more adherent with treatment. Obviously, cognitive capacity would be a confounding variable in this analysis but the effects were found when controlling for age. The researchers conclude that coping strategies predict level of adherence and these patterns were maintained at a four year follow-up. The longitudinal design of this study allowed traits to be assessed over time. Good and bad coping styles were found to persist which suggests that it may be possible to predict from "personality style" children at risk of poor adherence.

Attempts to test the utility of an objective measure of competency/ coping in predicting medical regimen adherence has been found to be reliable across chronic diseases. The MCIST was completed by adolescents with cystic fibrosis (Csajkowski and Koocher, 1987) and boys with haemophilia (D'Angelo *et al.*, 1992). Both studies found good correlations with the subscales of the MCIST and adherence rated by medical professionals. Two subscales in particular had high predictive value, these were the compliance/coping subscale and the health optimism subscale. Whilst the MCIST offers hope as a standardised assessment tool for adherence both these studies had a flaw in their method of professional rating of adherence. These ratings were completed during an inpatient admission. It has been documented above that adherence rates vary according to the extent to which the treatments interfere with daily lifestyle. The hospital setting would therefore have greatly reduced the stressors in the natural environment.

The identification of child personality features which may predict adherence behaviours has been fraught with difficulty. Definitions and measurements have been mostly subjective. Obviously, more consistent measurement across and within disease type will help with clarity.

Knowledge

It would be expected that knowledge about illness would lead to greater adherence. However, a recognition of the severity of a disease or the consequences of poor adherence does not necessarily improve adherence behaviour. Beliefs about positive health care can be held without the participant engaging in those behaviours (Counte and Christman, 1981).

Knowledge of illness and reasons for treatment have been found to correlate positively with adherence to daily physiotherapy in children with cystic fibrosis (Gudas *et al.*, 1991) and asthma management (Rubin, Bauman and Lauby, 1989). It has been suggested that level of cognitive maturity is the important factor and this should not be equated with age. Gudas *et al.* (1991) report that formal operational thinkers are more likely to adhere with treatment than pre-operational or concrete operational thinkers. A teaching programme aimed at helping children with diabetes conceptualise their illness in a more formal operational manner was reported to improve adherence (Ingersoll, Orr and Herrold, 1986). There is not a simple relationship between knowledge of disease and adherence. Adherence certainly does not improve with ever increasing understanding of the illness. Instead, it appears that there is an optimum level of knowledge which helps adherence but beyond this further information does not have any effect (Rubin *et al.*, 1989).

There is an assumption amongst HPs that age equates with knowledge and this in turn equates with responsibility and skill. The competence of skilled disease management in older children has been questioned, however, (Mazse *et al.*, 1984; Clarke and Warren, 1989). In fact, more and more research indicates that adolescents given total self-responsibility for disease management make more errors and are less adherent than those who continue to have parental involvement (Anderson, 1995).

Cognitive maturity of the individual child rather than amount of knowledge of the disease appears to be a key predictor of adherence with treatment (Wallander, 1993). Lemanek (1990) suggests that although adolescents are more knowledgeable than younger children, mothers are the most knowledgeable group (Johnson *et al.*, 1992). Thus, mother and child, irrespective of age, working together may have a better prospect of good adherence.

Family Factors

It makes sense that a family will be greatly affected by the diagnosis of a chronic and/or life-threatening illness in a child. Indeed, there exists a wealth of research documenting the impact (Kronenberger and Thompson, 1990; Patterson, 1988; Hauser *et al.*, 1885; Wertlieb, Hauser and Jacobson, 1988). Revaluation of the plans and expectations parents held for the sick child must occur as well as practical management of treatment and appointments. However, the emotional stress which diagnosis brings does not necessarily lead to family dysfunction or psychopathology amongst family members (Eiser, 1990; Midence, 1994). Of interest here is whether there are any aspects of family functioning which facilitate or impede adherence with treatment. There are, as yet, fewer papers addressing these issues.

Geiss *et al.* (1992) examined the impact of psychosocial variables on rates of adherence with treatment for children with cystic fibrosis. Standardised measures were used: The Personality Inventory for Children (Wirt *et al.*, 1980); the Beck Depression Inventory (Beck *et al.*, 1979); the Social Isolation Scale (Beach, Arias and O'Leary, 1986) and the Marital Adjustment Test (Locke and Wallace, 1959). All scores were in the normal range supporting the contention that studies should research the particular resources families utilise for coping with intermittent stress (Drotar, 1981).

Geiss *et al.* (1992) did find some significant correlations of psychosocial variables and adherence with treatment. When mothers reported low marital satisfaction and less adult contact, their children were found to have higher rates of adherence with treatment. The implications of these findings may be that a mother in such a situation becomes more involved with her child's care. Conversely, the stress of achieving the demands of the daily regimen may have resulted in the breakdown of adult relationships for the mother. This latter hypothesis has implications for HPs in considering the demands and expectations placed on families by the daily treatment regimens. It may be that prescribed treatments must be acceptable for the whole family well-being and not just the sick child.

Several studies reviewed by Hauser *et al.* (1990) find certain aspects of family functioning to be associated with rates of adherence behaviour among children with diabetes. These include: family support, cohesion, expressiveness, conflict and organisation. In particular, higher family cohesion, greater expressiveness and better organisation have been found to correlate with good initial adjustment following diagnosis (Galatser *et al.*, 1982; Hanson, Henggler and Burghen, 1987; Schafer, McCaul and Glasgow, 1986; Shouval, Ber and Galatser, 1982). Miller-Johnson *et al.* (1994) found that parent-child conflict was associated with poor adherence and inadequate metabolic control in children with diabetes.

Hauser *et al.* (1990) administered the Family Environment Scale (Moos and Moos, 1981) to children with diabetes and their parents annually, for four years. Adherence with diabetic regimen was rated by health providers. Initial good adherence was predicted by parents' perception of family cohesiveness. Family conflict adversely affected adherence in the long and short term. Good family organisation resulted in better adherence initially, but was not significant in the long term. Whilst these results are intuitively appealing it must be remembered that these findings are correlational not causal. As such, the direction of influence is not clear. It may be that the child's good adherence behaviour makes the family feel cohesive, whereas poor adherence causes conflict. Thus, the child's health behaviour may affect the responses made to the questionnaire.

Parent-Child Relationship

Mothers of sick children have often been accused of being overprotective or enmeshed with their child (Kucia *et al.*, 1979; Gustaffson *et al.*, 1987). Dadds *et al.* (1987) have suggested that parenting skills within and between all families vary according to many variables such as the particular setting, mood of parent, observers present etc. Manne *et al.* (1993) examined the role of parenting style on adherence behaviours for children with cancer. They report that parents who were observed to let more undesirable behaviours (as defined by the researchers) go by without consequence were more likely to have children with poor adherence. In this study, most adherence problems were noted in children who were visibly most healthy. Parents of such functionally active children were less likely to keep appointments or report negative symptoms. Other research has suggested that adherence is poorer when parents underestimate the severity of their child's illness (Gordis, Markowitz and Lilienfeld, 1969).

Schobinger *et al.* (1993) analysed mother-child speech samples for critical remarks. They found more critical remarks made by mothers of children with asthma than controls. The most critical mothers had children with greater problems of adherence. Thus, a child having a chronic illness does not necessarily interfere with the parent-child relationship. However, when problems are observed that child is more likely to display poor adherence.

Sharing Of Responsibility

Another aspect of family functioning which has been found to influence adherence is the sharing of responsibility for treatment amongst family members. Transfer of responsibility for treatment from parent to child as the child approaches adolescence is common practice. Children of that stage of development have been assumed to be keen to gain independence and control over their affairs. Recently, developmental theorists have argued that it is a mistaken belief that the stage of adolescence is marked by a strive for independence and distance from parents. Instead there is a move towards interdependence with parents. This stage in a young person's development, therefore, requires some renegotiation of responsibilities for the child and parents, not just increased responsibility for the child alone (Baumrind, 1987).

The fact that a youngster has the cognitive capacity to master a skilled treatment technique does not mean they will willingly carry out that task competently (Ingersoll *et al.*, 1986). Responsibility for treatment was not found to affect adherence in adolescents with cystic fibrosis (Gudas *et al.*, 1991) or those with diabetes (Anderson *et al.*, 1990). In both cases, children showed poor adherence irrespective of level of responsibility ascribed. Gudas *et al.* (1991) further postulate that the process of redefining roles and responsibilities during adolescence may involve some need for the youngster to assert their individual style. For the child with a chronic illness, this may be achieved by readjusting their medical routine. This may not necessarily mean the youngster is compromising their health. The child may not be complying with parental authority, but they are adhering to treatment.

DISCUSSION OF RESEARCH FINDINGS

Despite the difficulties with measurement of medical adhérence and the variations in treatment regimens across disease type, there has been some agreement in the research findings. Although no causal links have been defined and thus it is not possible to answer definitively the question of why children do not adhere to treatment, it is possible to examine the factors found to correlate with poor adherence and identify some areas of risk.

A common finding is that rates of adherence deteriorate as children get older. Adolescence has the peak rates for poor adherence irrespective of diagnosis: for diabetes (Jacobson *et al.*, 1990); for cystic fibrosis (Gudas *et al.*, 1991); for asthma (Voyles and Menendez, 1983); for seizures (Hazsard *et al.*, 1990). It has also been documented that age per se is not the important factor but the nature of the developmental stage of adolescence which may be the issue.

Two particular features of this stage may play a part in the poor adherence seen in some children with a chronic illness. Firstly, it is expected by parents and health providers that children of this age should assume more self-responsibility for their treatment and health. In some cases the child does not want this independence but would rather maintain some interdependence with parents (Baumrind, 1987). In addition, many adolescents do not share the long term view of health care held by parents and professionals and are reluctant to engage in time consuming daily procedures for which they gain no immediate effects (Phipps and DeCuir-Whalley, 1990; Gudas *et al.*, 1991).

Secondly, a function of this developmental stage is to achieve successful separation from parents in order to become a self-sufficient adult. The stage is marked by the testing of opinion and rebellion against authority (Baumrind, 1987). It can be hypothesised that the disease may be a convenient emotional battleground. Some adolescents may refuse to administer a procedure simply because a parent has reminded them of the required task. The parent can be perceived as interfering and mistrustful of the youngster.

As has been suggested by Gudas *et al.* (1991), the adaptation of a prescribed medical regimen may not necessarily constitute poor adherence. Some youngsters may believe that their daily regimen could be altered to better fit their lifestyle. There have been consistent reports from all studies indicating differential adherence rates with different aspects of treatment regimens. Those aspects which cause most disruption to family life or require most planning are least adhered with, sometimes with parental approval (Gudas *et al.*, 1991; Csajkowski and Koocher, 1987).

Peers have a major influence on the social and emotional functioning of children. There is no evidence that having a chronic illness necessarily adversely affects peer relationships, but some children with a chronic illness will have poor friendships. Those with friendship problems generally suffer from an illness which affects physical appearance, or one that has the greatest impact on lifestyle (Spirito, DeLawyer and Spark, 1991).

During adolescence those feelings of being "different" may reduce a youngster's willingness to become involved with their peer group. Elkind (1967) described adolescence as the period of the "imaginary audience" whereby the youngsters consider themselves to be constantly under public scrutiny. Thus, the child with a chronic illness may become acutely aware of the abnormality their disease may bring. Some children may respond by a withdrawal from peer group contact, for which they blame their illness and consequently fail to adhere with treatment as an attack on the diagnosis. Some adolescents minimise the differences from their peers which they perceive their illness to cause. Accordingly, they may control the administration of treatment in public or may even deny their diagnosis.

In general, researchers who have looked for evidence of psychopathology in the child with a chronic illness to explain poor adherence have found none. Scores on standardised measurement tools tend to be within the normal range (Geiss *et al.*, 1992; D'Angelo *et al.*, 1992). There is evidence that certain psychological characteristics of children put them at risk of poor adherence.

It must be stressed, however, that the measures which have shown significant correlations with adherence have not been adapted for children with a chronic disease. Children who are generally pessimistic in their outlook, who express feelings of impotence regarding their illness, who tend to use defensive styles such as "acting out", "turning against self" and " ascetism", who show uncreative problem-solving skills are more likely to demonstrate problems with adherence than children with converse personality traits (Jacobson *et al.*, 1990; Csajkowski and Koocher, 1987).

The role of the family in influencing adherence rates is not conclusive. Not surprisingly, families which are cohesive and have low conflict, as perceived by both parent and child, correlated with good treatment adherence (Hauser *et al.*, 1990). Parents who show some difficulties with behaviour management generally have children who show poor adherence (Manne *et al.*, 1993).

Thus, a checklist of stressors which may help the clinician in remedial or preventative input can be tentatively assembled. Koocher *et al.* (1990) described three typologies of non-adherence in cystic fibrosis. They used Flanagan's "critical incident technique" (Flanagan, 1954) to identify key elements which foster adherence. Patients were asked to describe specific incidents which had produced favourable or non-favourable outcomes for their medical status. The first typology is "inadequate knowledge" where non-adherence ensues as a result of lack of information or inadequate understanding. This may be the fault of the patient or the health providers. The second typology is "psychosocial resistance" where such factors cause active non-adherence, e.g. struggles with authority figures, cultural pressures, striving for normality or a chaotic home environment. The third typology is "educated non-adherence" where the child makes a choice to give up or change aspects of their regimen with full understanding of the consequences of their decision. This behaviour has been termed elsewhere as "adaptive non-adherence" (Deaton, 1985). Although the typologies described by Koocher and colleagues have not been subject to empirical validation, they do cover many of the aspects found to account for poor adherence in the experimental studies reported above.

CONCLUSION

It has been suggested that some children may have a personality type which, in the face of chronic disease, makes them less likely to cope with daily treatment management. These traits may be particularly evident during the adolescent stage of development since this is the period when most poor adherence is noted. Aspects of independence, responsibility and peer relationships may affect adherence with treatment. Treatment regimens that are complex and time-consuming emphasise the difference between a chronically ill child and their healthy peers. It would not be surprising to find that all children with a chronic illness fail to adhere with treatment on occasions.

In the face of little evidence to link health behaviours with health outcome (Johnson, 1994) it is important to consider the expectations of health providers in their prescriptions of medical regimens. Children are torn between striving to live a normal life, often at the insistence of medical teams, whist being constantly reminded of their abnormality by their daily treatment regimen (Pless and Nolan, 1991). The findings of Geiss *et al.* (1992) which correlate low marital satisfaction and maternal isolation with the highest adherence rates may be a warning of the stress regimens place on families.

Reid and Appleton (1991) refer to the potential use of a model of risk and resistance (Wallander *et al.*, 1989) in understanding the various dilemmas and choices facing a child with a chronic illness. The model accounts for the range of factors (person, disease, environment) which interact in varying degrees of adaptation or maladjustment. The research findings from studies of poor adherence would suggest that a chronically ill child with tendencies to "act out" their emotional turmoil, who has poor problem-solving resources, who has a noticeable and time-consuming treatment regimen, who is struggling through adolescence with difficult parental relationships, who is influenced by peers and comes from a family where conflict is high is at risk for poor adherence with treatment. The risk resistance model would allow assessment of the degrees to which any of these factors were present for any given child. The model also avoids the temptation to look only at the child for the cause of poor adherence.

Suggestions for Further Research

To understand why children might fail to adhere to their treatment regimen even in the face of life-threatening disease, further research needs to examine the ways in which psychosocial adjustment both influences and is influenced by disease management.

It would be particularly useful to understand why adherence rates begin to deteriorate during adolescence. Do previously adherent children give up this behaviour following experience of reduced return for their efforts as their physical condition worsens? Can potential poor adherers be identified by personality assessment long before the behaviour is exhibited? A more systematic examination of the hypothesised typical features of adolescence and correlations with adherence behaviour would be useful. This would require that traits such as "rebelliousness", "seeking of autonomy", "stroppiness" etc. be operationalised to allow measurement. More efforts at delineation of typologies of non-adherence along the lines of Koocher *et al.* (1990) would be fruitful in the development of clinical assessment tools perhaps using single case methodology. The use of longitudinal designs will be invaluable for identification of predictors of poor adherence.

The development of validated psychometric techniques such as the Medical Compliance Incomplete Stories Test (Koocher and Csajkowski, 1984) would greatly reduce the problem of inconsistent measurement when trying to make cross-study comparisons. Finally, more systematic research of the causal links between health behaviour and health outcome would clarify the requirements of treatment regimes and, therefore, the expectations HPs have of children and families for adherence with treatment.

REFERENCES

Abbott, J., Dodd, M., Bilton, D. and Webb, A.K. (1994) Treatment compliance in adults with cystic fibrosis. *Thorax* **49,** 115–120.

Achenbach, T.M. and Edelbrock, D.S. (1983) *Manual for the Child Behaviour Checklist and Revised Behavior Profile.* Burlington, VT: University of Vermont Press.

Anderson, B.J. (1995) Childhood and adolescent psychological development in relation to diabetes. In C.J.H. Kelnar (ed) *Childhood and Adolescent Diabetes..* London: Chapman & Hall.

Anderson, B.J., Auslander, W.F., Jung, K.C., Miller, J.P. and Santiago, J.V. (1990) Assessing family sharing of diabetes responsibilities. *Journal of Pediatric Psychology* **15,** 477–492.

Baumrind, D. (1987) A developmental perspective on adolescent risk taking in contemporary America. In C.E. Irwin (ed) *Adolescent social behavior and health*. San Francisco: Jossey-Bass.

Beach, S.R.H., Arias, I. and O'Leary, K.D. (1986) The relationship of marital satisfaction and social support to depressive symptomatology. *Journal of Psychopathology and Behavioral Assessment* **8**, 305–316.

Beck, A.T., Rush, A.J., Shaw, B.F. and Emery, G. (1979) *Cognitive therapy of depression*. New York: Guilford Press.

Becker, M.H., Radius, S.M., Rosenstock, I.M., Drachman, R.H., Schuberth, K.C. and Teets, K. (1978) Compliance with a medical regimen for asthma: a test of the health belief model. *Public Health Reports* **93**, 268–277.

Blackwell, B. (1979) The drug regimen and treatment compliance. In R.B. Haynes, D.W. Taylor, and D.L. Sackett (eds) *Compliance in health care*. Baltimore: Johns Hopkins University Press.

Bond. G.G., Aiken, L.S. and Somerville, S.C. (1992) The health belief model and adolescents with insulin-dependent diabetes mellitus. *Health Psychology* **11**, 190–198.

Clarke, C.F. and Warren, S. (1989) Accuracy of home blood glucose monitoring in children with insulin-dependent diabetes mellitus. *Practical Diabetes* **6**, 156–157.

Counte, M.A. and Christman, P.L. (1981) *Interpersonal behaviour and health care*. Boulder CO: Westview.

Csajkowski, D.R. and Koocher, G.P. (1987) Medical compliance and coping with cystic fibrosis. *Journal of Child Psychology and Psychiatry* **28**, 311–319.

D'Angelo, E., Woolf, A., Bessette, J., Rappaport, L. and Ciborowski, J. (1992) Correlates of medical compliance among hemophilic boys. *Journal of Clinical Psychology* **48**, 672–680.

Dadds, M.R., Sanders, M.R., Behrens, B.C. and James, J.E. (1987) Marital discord and child behavior problems: a description of family interactions during treatment. *Journal of Consulting and Clinical Psychology* **16**, 192–203.

Deaton, A.V. (1985) Adaptive non-compliance in pediatric asthma: the parent as expert. *Journal of Pediatric Psychology* **10**, 1–14.

Delameter, A.M., Davies, S.G., Bubb, I.J., Santiago, J.V. and White, N.H. (1989) Self monitoring of blood glucose by adolescents with diabetes: technical skills and utilisation of data. *The Diabetic Educator* **15**, 56–61.

Drotar, D. (1981) Psychological perspectives in chronic childhood illness. *Journal of Pediatric Psychology* **6**, 211–218.

Eiser, C. (1990) Psychological effects of chronic disease. *Journal of Child Psychology and Psychiatry* **31** , 85–98.

Eiser, C. (1994) Making sense of chronic disease: the eleventh Jack Tisard memorial lecture. *Journal of Child Psychology and Psychiatry* **33**, 1373–1389.

Elkind, D. (1967) Egocentrism in adolescence. *Child Development* **38**, 1025–1034.

Epstein, L.H. and Cluss, P.A. (1982) A behavioural medicine perspective on adherence to long-term medical regimens. *Journal of Consulting and Clinical Psychology* **50**, 960–971.

Flanagan, J.C. (1954) The critical incident technique. *Psychological Bulletin* **51**, 327–358.

Galatser, A., Amir, S., Karp, M. and Laron, Z. (1982) Crisis intervention program in newly diagnosed diabetic children. *Diabetes Care* **5**, 414–419.

Geiss, S.K., Hobbs, S.A., Hammersley-Maercklein, G., Kramer, J.C. and Henley, M. (1992) Psychosocial factors related to perceived compliance with cystic fibrosis treatment. *Journal of Clinical Psychology* **48** , 99–103.

Gordis, L., Markowitz, M. and Lilienfeld, A. (1969) Why parents don't follow medical advice: a study of children on long-term anti-streptococcal prophylaxis. *Journal of Pediatrics* **75**, 957–968.

Gudas, L.J, Koocher, G.P. and Wypij, D. (1991) Perceptions of medical compliance in children and adolescents with cystic fibrosis. *Developmental and Behavioral Pediatrics* **12**, 236–242.

Gustaffson, P.A., Kjellman, N.-I.M., Ludvigsson, J. and Cederblad, M. (1987) Asthma and family interaction. *Archives of Disease in Childhood* **62**, 258–263.

Hanson, C.L., Henggler, S.W. and Burghen, G.A. (1987) Social competence and parental support as mediators of the link between stress and metabolic control in adolescents with insulin-dependent diabetes mellitus. *Journal of Consulting and Clinical Psychology* **55**, 529–533.

Hanson, C.L., Henggler, S.W., Harris, M.A., Mitchell, K.A., Carle, D.L. and Burghen, G.A. (1988) Associations between family members' perceptions of the health care system and the health of youths with insulin-dependent diabetes mellitus. *Journal of Pediatric Psychology* **13**, 543–554.

Hauser, S.T., Jacobson, A.M., Lavori, P., Wolfsdorf, J.I., Herskowitz, R.D., Milley, J.E., Bliss, R., Wertlieb, D and Stein, J. (1990) Adherence among children and adolescents with insulin-dependent diabetes mellitus over a four-year longitudinal follow-up: II. Immediate and long-term linkages with the family milieu. *Journal of Pediatric Psychology* **15**, 527–542.

Hauser, S.T., Jacobson, A., Wertlieb, D., Brink, S. and Wentworth, S. (1985) The contribution of family environment to perceived competence and illness adjustment in diabetic and acutely ill adolescents. *Family Relations* **34**, 99–108.

Hazsard, A., Hutchinson, S.J. and Krawiecki, N. (1990) Factors related to adherence to medication regimens in pediatric seizure patients. *Journal of Pediatric Psychology* **15**, 543–555.

Ingersoll, G.M., Orr, D.P. and Herrold, A.J. (1986) Cognitive maturity and self-management among adolescents with insulin-dependent diabetes mellitus. *Journal of Pediatrics* **108**, 620–623.

Jacobson, A.M., Hauser, S.T., Lavori, P., Wolfsdorf, J.I., Herskowitz, R.D., Milley, J.E., Bliss, R., Gelfand, E, Wertlieb, D. and Stein, J. (1990) Adherence among children and adolescents with insulin-dependent diabetes mellitus over a four-year longitudinal follow-up: I. The influence of patient coping and adjustment. *Journal of Pediatric Psychology* **15**, 511–526.

Johnson, S.B. (1994) Health behaviour and health status; concepts, methods and applications. *Journal of Pediatric Psychology* **19**, 129–141.

Johnson, S.B., Freund, A., Hansen, C.A. and Malone, J. (1990) Adherence health-status relationships in childhood diabetes. *Health Psychology* **6**, 606–631.

Johnson, S.B., Kelly, M., Henretta, J.C., Cunningham, W.R., Tomer, A. and Silverstein, J.H. (1992) A longitudinal analysis of adherence and health status in childhood diabetes. *Journal of Pediatric Psychology* **17**, 537–553.

Johnson, S.B., Pollak, R.T., Silverstein, J.H., Rosenbloom, A.L., Spillar, R., McCallum, M. and Harkavy, J. (1982) Cognitive and behavioural knowledge about insulin dependent diabetes among children and their parents. *Pediatrics* **69**, 708–713.

Koocher, G.P. and Czajkowski, D.R. (1984*) The Medical Compliance Incomplete Stories Test (MCIST).* Unpublished manuscript. The Children's Hospital, Boston, MA.

Koocher, G.P., McGrath, M.L. and Gudas, L.J. (1990) Typologies of non-adherence in cystic fibrosis. *Developmental and Behavioural Pediatrics* **11**, 353–358.

Kovacs, M., Goldston, D., Obrosky, S.D. and Iyengar, S. (1992) Prevalence and predictors of pervasive noncompliance with medical treatment among youths with insulin-dependent diabetes mellitus. *Journal of the American Academy of Child and Adolescent Psychiatry* **31**, 1112–1119.

Kronenberger, W.G. and Thompson, R.J. (1990) Dimensions of family functioning in families with chronically ill children: a higher order factor analysis of the Family Environment Scale. *Journal of Clinical Child Psychology* **19**, 380—388.

Kucia, C., Drotar, D., Doershuk, C., Stern, R., Boat, T. and Matthews, L. (1979) Home observation of family interaction and childhood adjustment to cystic fibrosis. *Journal of Pediatric Psychology* **4**, 189–195.

La Greca, A.M. (1990) Issues in adherence with paediatric regimens. *Journal of Pediatric Psychology* **15**, 423–436.

Lemanek, K. (1990) Adherence issues in the medical management of asthma. *Journal of Pediatric Psychology* **15**, 437–458.

Locke, H.J. and Wallace, K.M. (1959) Short marital adjustment and prediction tests: their ability and validity. *Marriage and Family Living* **21**, 251–255.

Manne, S.L., Jacobsen, P.B., Gorfinkle, K., Gerstein, F. and Redd, W.H. (1993) Treatment adherence difficulties among children with cancer: the role of parenting style. *Journal of Pediatric Psychology* **18**, 47–62.

Marteau, T.M., Johnson, M., Baum, J.D. and Bloch, S. (1987) Goals of treatment in diabetes: a comparison of doctors and parents of children with diabetes. *Journal of Behavioral Medicine* **10**, 33–48.

Mazze, R.S., Shamoon, H., Pasmantier, R., Lucido, D., Murphy, J., Hartmann, K., Kuykendall, V. and Lopatin, W. (1984) Reliability of blood glucose monitoring by patients with diabetes mellitus. *American Journal of Medicine* **77**, 211–217.

Midence, K. (1994) The effects of chronic illness on children and their families: an overview. *Genetic, Social and General Psychology Monographs* **120**, 309–326.

Miller-Johnson, S., Emery, R.E., Marvin, R.S. and Clarke, W. (1994) Parent-child relationships and the management of insulin-dependent diabetes mellitus. *Journal of Consulting and Clinical Psychology* **62**, 603–610.

Moos, R.H. and Moos, B.S. (1981) *Family Environment Scale Manual*. Palo Alto: Consulting Psychologists Press.

Nolan, T. and Pless, I.B. (1986) Emotional consequences and correlates of birth defects. *Journal of Pediatrics* **109**, 210—216.

Nowicki, S. and Stickland, B. (1973) A locus of control scale for children. *Journal of Consulting and Clinical Psychology* **40**, 148–154.

Page, P., Verstraete, D.G., Robb, J.R. and Etzwiler, D.D. (1981) Patient recall of self-care recommendations in diabetes. *Diabetes Care* **4**, 96–98.

Passero, M.A., Remor, B. and Salomon, J. (1981) Patient-reported compliance with cystic fibrosis therapy. *Clinical Pediatrics* **20**, 264–268.

Patterson, J. (1988) Chronic illness in children and the impact on families. In C. Chilmas, E. Nunnaly, and F. Cox (eds) *Chronic illness and disability*. Beverley Hills: Sage.

Perrin, E. and Shapiro, E. (1985) Health locus of control beliefs of healthy children, children with a chronic physical illness and their mothers. *Journal of Pediatrics* **107**, 627–633.

Phipps, S. and DeCuir-Whalley, S. (1990) Adherence issues in pediatric bone marrow transplantation. *Journal of Pediatric Psychology* **15**, 459–475.

Pless, I.B. and Nolan, T. (1991) Revision, replication and neglect – research on maladjustment in chronic illness. *Journal of Child Psychology and Psychiatry* **32**, 347–365.

Rapoff, M.A. and Christopherson, E.R. (1982) Compliance of pediatric patients with medical regimens: A review and evaluation, in R.B. Stuart (ed) *Adherence, compliance and generalisation in behavioural medicine*. New York: Bruner/Masel.

Reid, P. and Appleton, P. (1991) Insulin dependent diabetes mellitus: regimen adherence in children and young people. *The Irish Journal of Psychology* **12**, 17–32.

Rubin, D.H., Bauman, L.J. and Lauby, J.L. (1989) The relationship between knowledge and reported behaviour in childhood asthma. *Journal of Developmental and Behavioural Pediatrics* **10**, 307–312.

Rylance, G.W. and Moreland, T.A. (1980) Drug level monitoring in pediatric practice. *Archives of Disease in Childhood* **55**, 89–98.

Sanders, M.R., Gravestock, F.M., Wanstall, K. and Dunne, M. (1991) The relationship between children's treatment-related behaviour problems, age and clinical status in cystic fibrosis. *Journal of Paediatric Child Health* **27**, 290–294.

Schafer, L.C., McCaul, K. and Glasgow. (1986) Supportive and non-supportive family behaviors. *Diabetes Care* **9**, 179–185.

Schobinger, R., Florin, I., Reichbauer, M. and Lindemann, H. (1993) Childhood asthma: Mothers' affective attitude, mother-child interaction and children's compliance with medical requirements. *Journal of Psychosomatic Research* **37**, 697–707.

Shouval, R., Ber, R. and Galatser, Z. (1982) Family social climate and the health status and adaptation of diabetic youth. In Z. Laron (ed) *Psychological aspects of diabetes in children and adolescents.* Basel, Switzerland: Karger.

Simmons, R.J., Corey, M., Cowen, L., Keenan, N., Robertson, J. and Levison, H. (1985) Emotional adjustment of early adolescents with cystic fibrosis. *Psychosomatic Medicine* **47**, 111–121.

Smith, N.A., Seale, J.P., Ley, P., Shaw, J. and Bracs, P.U. (1986) Effects of intervention on medication compliance in children with asthma. *Medical Journal of Australia,* **144**, 119–122.

Spirito, A., DeLawyer, D.D. and Stark, L. (1991) Peer relations and social adjustment of chronically ill children and adolescents. *Clinical Psychology Review,* **11**, 539–564.

Varni, J.W. and Wallander, J.L. (1984) Adherence to health-related regimens in pediatric chronic disorders. *Clinical Psychology Review* **4**, 585–596.

Varni, J.W. and Wallander, J.L. (1988). Pediatric chronic disabilities: hemophilia and spina bifida as examples. In D. Routh (ed) *Handbook of Pediatric Psychology.* New York: Guilford Press.

Voyles, J.B. and Menendez, R. (1983) Role of patient compliance in the management of asthma. *Journal of Asthma* **20**, 411–418.

Wallander, J.L. (1993) Special section editorial: Current research on pediatric chronic illness. *Journal of Pediatric Psychology* **18**, 7–10.

Wallander, J.L., Varni, J.W., Babani, L., Banis, H.T. and Wilcox, K.T. (1989) Family resources as resistance factors for psychological maladjustment in chronically ill and handicapped children. *Journal of Pediatric Psychology* **14**, 157–174..

Wallston, B.S. and Wallston, K.A. (1978) Locus of control and health: a review of the literature. *Health Education Monographs* **2**, 107–117.

Wertlieb, D., Hauser, S.T. and Jacobson, A. (1988) Adaptation to diabetes: behaviour symptoms and family context. *Journal of Pediatric Psychology* **11**, 463–479.

West, K.P., DuRant, R.H. and Pendergrast, R. (1993) An experimental test of adolescents' compliance with dental appointments. *Journal of Adolescent Health* **14**, 384–389.

Wirt, R., Lachar, D., Klinedinst, J. and Seat, P. (1980) *Multi-dimensional description of child personality: A manual for the Personality Inventory for Children.* Los Angeles: Western Psychological Services.

8

Adherence in Pregnancy

Deborah Rosenblatt

"Women when pregnant should lead a regular and temperate life carefully avoiding whatever is to disagree with the stomach; they should breathe a free open air; their company should be agreeable and cheerful; their exercise should be moderate, and adapted to their particular situation; they should, especially in the early months when the connection between ovum and womb is feeble, avoid crowds, confinement, every situation which renders them under any disagreeable restriction; agitation of body from violent or improper exercise....and whatever disturbs either the body or mind" (Hamilton, 1781).

WHAT IS ADHERENCE IN PREGNANCY AND WHY IS IT AN ISSUE?

Pregnancy has always been a special time in a woman's life, with prescriptions and expectations regarding her behaviour. For those women who are fit and well it may also herald a unique period in which regular consultations with health professionals (HPs) are scheduled. The roles, beliefs and behaviours of mothers-to-be in relation to the expectations and instructions of obstetric and midwifery staff will form the basis of this chapter on adherence. Unlike the relatively simple situation of taking a drug for a particular medical problem, pregnancy encompasses changes in lifestyle and often "advice" from many, occasionally contradictory, sources. Unless there is a documented medical problem women these days see themselves as going through a normal process supported by knowledgeable HPs. In early pregnancy a woman's source of information may include a pamphlet about health and lifestyle ("eat a healthy diet"), detailed instructions from her General Practitioner (GP) regarding her own health ("avoid gaining much more weight"), advice from a friend with three children ("you don't look too fat to me"), or a specific medical instruction at the antenatal clinic ("you have gestational diabetes and will require a special diet"). Although maternity pamphlets assume that all pregnant women will act on the advice, it may be either too general or inappropriate, or a mother may conclude that if it did not make a difference last time, it can be ignored this time (Jewell, 1990).

PREGNANT WOMEN AND HEALTH PROFESSIONALS

There are enormous system differences in the delivery of maternity care even within the Western world. In the UK until recently, women were referred by their GP to the local maternity hospital where they were "booked" under the care of a Consultant Obstetrician. Those women with particular risk factors would be seen regularly by an obstetrician, whose seniority was usually dictated by the degree of risk, including parity, past or current medical problems and sometimes social factors. Midwives, though highly trained and often more experienced than junior obstetric staff, were not perceived as the primary carers. Now, however, women are just as likely to be examined, informed, supported and nurtured by one of a team of midwives working autonomously (Department of Health, 1993). Care may be provided mainly in the GPs' surgery, or in an outpatient hospital clinic, or, occasionally, at home.

PROMOTING LIFESTYLE CHANGES IN PREGNANCY

Fitness, Nutrition, Alcohol and Smoking

HPs and written material usually advise moderate exercise in pregnancy but little data are available about women's behaviour in relation to general or specific instructions. An exception is a questionnaire study of delegates at a physical fitness conference who were asked about their knowledge of the American College of Obstetricians and Gynaecologists (ACOG) guidelines (Zeenah and Schlosser, 1993). Although 83% knew the recommendations, only 53% said that they had followed them during pregnancy. Those who had exceeded the guidelines, however, did not appear to have compromised their own infant's health. Thus, women may ignore official advice, particularly, perhaps, if they feel that they are fitter and more healthy than other women.

Perhaps because maternity staff are less didactic about diet in pregnancy, there are no recent reports on women's adherence. Orr and Simmons (1979) found that although almost all of the women felt that diet was important, and made the recommended changes, only one-third reported that adherence was a serious concern. Higgins, Frank and Brown (1994) asked 115 women to list the changes they had made in health behaviour during pregnancy. Eighteen different behaviours were identified, with 49% mentioning diet, exercise pattern, smoking, alcohol and vitamin intake. More information is needed, however, about what motivates individuals to do so and why.

Religion can be a factor too. A large Australian Study (6566 women) (Najman *et al.*, 1988) compared the pregnancy outcomes of three groups: members of religious sects (Christian sects), Christians who go to church regularly (Christian attenders) and infrequent attenders (lukewarm Christians). The most favourable group for mother's health and lifestyles, and baby's health at birth, were the sect members with the children of "lukewarm" Christians doing worst. This could be due to specific characteristics of the mother who goes to church or direct or indirect ("buffering") aspects of her beliefs, or the social support of others with shared values. However, religious "conviction" can have tragic consequences too. Failure of women of the Faith Assembly in midwest America to utilise antenatal care led to higher rates of perinatal mortality (Kaunitz *et al.*, 1984).

Depression also has a negative effect on health behaviours (Zuckerman *et al.*, 1989). In their sample of 1014 women, primarily poor and from minority groups, depression was associated with greater use of cigarettes, alcohol and cocaine. Many pregnant women are unaware of the teratogenic effects of alcohol during pregnancy and continue to drink. Waterson and Murray-Lyon (1990) compared the efficacy of different mediums for "delivering the message" to stop drinking, including a standard Health Education Association leaflet, the leaflet plus personal advice and reinforcement, and, in a second trial, the use of a short video. There was a 60–70% adherence rate to the advice in each condition, with a slight advantage for the doctor and the video over the leaflet only.

Smoking in pregnancy is associated with significant effects on the foetus, including intrauterine growth retardation and infant morbidity and mortality (Cnattingius, Haglund and Meirik, 1988). A number of studies have examined the reasons why women continue to smoke and evaluated the impact of intervention programmes. It is often assumed that educated, middle class clients are more likely to utilise advice to minimise harm. However, in their sample from four private obstetric practices, Albrecht and Rankin (1989) found that the women who continued to smoked during pregnancy were highly educated (at least two years at college, 45% with a post-graduate qualification) and working in managerial or professional jobs. Differences in smoking rates were not explained by state or trait anxiety scores but those who smoked were also more likely to drink. Increased state anxiety was associated with low social support and higher trait anxiety with low scores on a personal resources measure. The authors suggest that this population may need different approaches to health promotion, including measures to reduce work-related stress and nursing interventions designed to enhance coping strategies.

It is not clear which methods are most effective in motivating pregnant women to make positive changes in their health behaviour, and whether the cost/benefit ratio is satisfactory. Windsor, Warner and Cutter (1988) found that a self-help correspondence course to reduce smoking in pregnancy was cheap (equivalent to $11.75 per mother), and saved $3 for every $1 spent. A subsequent study (Windsor et al., 1993) extended the protocol to evaluate the impact of a health education guide to reduce smoking in 814 pregnant women. The design also included self-report measures and tests for cotinine levels in saliva at three points in the pregnancy. Two-thirds reported use of the guide, which was rated highly. However, adherence with the programme (defined as quitting for 4 plus days using 5 or more of the cessation measures) was not as successful. Black mothers were twice as likely to quit (13.2%) as Caucasian mothers (6.6%). By delivery, however, 84% of smokers and 35.2% of the "quitters" had relapsed. Valbø, Thelle, and Kolås (1996) also documented high relapse rates, 100% in the intervention group and 66% in the standard, while those who did quit were mainly light smokers (<10 p/day). Ershoff *et al.* (1990) were more successful with their self-help programme; 22.2% in the intervention group compared to 8.6% of controls stopped smoking and they were 45% less likely to deliver a low-birthweight infant, thus yielding a benefit/cost ratio for the Health Maintenance Organisation (HMO) of 2.8:1.

The problem, however, is that women who are motivated enough to participate in a self-help programme may be different from those who do not. Other options are classes, or individual consultation with HPs. Ershoff *et al.* (1990) believe that the most influential provider is the physician, but that five minutes of physician time would be as costly as their entire self-help programme. It may be that the interpersonal, rather than the programme elements are the important factor. Aaronson (1989) measured the effect of social support on abstinence from alcohol, cigarettes and caffeine during pregnancy in a sample of 529 women. Specific perceived and received support independently predicted all three behaviours, but general social support did not.

"Just Keep Taking Your Tablets." Adherence to Medication in Pregnancy

Surprisingly, little research has focused on this issue. One study attempted to ascertain the validity of reported adherence to medication during high risk pregnancy (Du Bard *et al.*, 1993). They studied 604 women participating in a double blind trial of low dose aspirin to prevent pre-eclampsia. Of the 303 women assigned to receive aspirin, 283 had a blood sample measure which was compared to the percentage of pills taken from bottles with variable numbers of tablets. Pill counts in the medium range were related to better biochemical effects than lower or higher counts, suggesting that when women reported a higher figure they were being deceptive, indicating poor adherence, while low counts reflected low biochemical effect.

In a population at high risk for foetal growth retardation (FGR), it is important to know whether maternal behaviours make any contribution to outcome. Goldenberg *et al.* (1992) studied 289 women of whom 29% had previously delivered a growth retarded infant. From the first antenatal visit they were provided with iron and folic acid tablets. A psychosocial score (including self-esteem, locus of control, anxiety, social support and stress) was determined, of whom 29% scored poorly. Women with higher psychosocial scores always demonstrated higher maternal serum folate levels, indicating that these maternal characteristics were related to adherence in taking the folate. However, in both groups (good vs bad psychological scores) folate itself was related to lower risk of FGR and increased birth weight.

In developing countries, where perinatal mortality and morbidity is high, a great deal of research has focused on women's apparently poor adherence to medication and nutritional supplementation. Galloway and McGuire (1994), however, demonstrated that patient factors were less significant than program problems. For instance, inadequate political and financial support often leads to insufficient service delivery, including poor provider-user dynamics, lack of supplies, and training and motivation of the health workers. These then interact with patient factors, such as a belief that supplements will lead to big babies and make delivery more difficult and dangerous. Choosing an appropriate "medium" is also important, particularly for women with low literacy skills. A Mexican health team (Alcalay, Ghee and Scrimshaw, 1993) significantly improved adherence by using a variety of approaches (posters, leaflets, calendars, radio songs) to change both attitudes and behaviour.

ISSUES AT DIFFERENT STAGES OF PREGNANCY

Screening

Lumley and Astbury (1989) suggest that women are not only bombarded with advice during pregnancy, but come under extensive pressure before they have even conceived. This may particularly affect those who see adherence to professionals as important or the: "worried well, those with strong beliefs about nutrition, exercise or wellness, and increasingly those who see pre-conceptional care as the right and proper way to go about becoming a parent".

Ultrasound is now a routine procedure in early pregnancy in order to date the foetus, to identify multiple pregnancies and malformations and to locate the placenta. Most women are very keen to have this "window into the womb" but there is at least one organisation (AIMS) which campaigns against its use. However, no studies were identified by the author regarding attendance for ultrasound appointments, or whether adherence with health advice based on ultrasound findings (e.g. identification of small baby or malposition) differs from that based on other investigations. However, in a randomised trial of the advantage of early ultrasound on mother-infant bonding, Lumley (1990) detected a short-term effect on health behaviours, including decreased smoking, alcohol consumption and more visits to the dentist.

Toxoplasmosis (an infection carried by cats) is not part of the screening programme in the UK, but experience in France suggests that the take-up rate for screening is affected by knowledge (Wallon *et al.*, 1994). In fact, of their sample of 806 women, most of those at risk were ill-informed: only 3% knew the main routes of contamination, 63% believed that vaccination was possible, and 11% believed that they had already been vaccinated. Thus, screening programmes must ensure that women have accurate information in order to modify their own behaviour and to opt into appropriate services.

Blumfield (1996) argues that "denial in the form of neglect of routine tests should alert family doctors that this expectant mother needs extra support and counselling". However, for non-routine testing, attendance may be low because of the fear of discovering a problem (Reid and Garcia, 1989). A multi-disciplinary study in Leeds assessed the effect of specific forms of non-directive information on the take-up of prenatal testing in the UK (Thornton *et al.*, 1995). Their randomised controlled trial allocated 1,691 women to either an individual session with a research midwife, class participation or the standard discussion with an obstetrician. Women were less likely to attend the classes than an individual appointment. Even though women who received the extra information demonstrated greater understanding and satisfaction it did not affect their decisions about testing. Group assignment did not, for instance, determine the uptake of ultrasound (99%) but cystic fibrosis testing was higher in "controls" (79%) than for the individual sessions or classes. The expectation that group discussion could facilitate understanding, knowledge and hence take-up suggests that the issue of who chooses prenatal diagnosis is not simply about the way in which the information or options are presented or discussed.

Use of Antenatal Care: Models of Behaviour

A great deal of literature is available on antenatal care but information on adherence is not always presented. Special problems are likely to be associated with low uptake of antenatal care by women who are poor and from minority groups. St. Clair and Anderson (1989) interviewed a large sample of low-income, inner-city women in the postnatal period about their recent pregnancy to assess the relationship between social networks, advice and behaviour. Women had received up to 211 (median of 20) pieces of advice from as many as 19 (median of 5) household members, relatives and friends. Although most of the advice was appropriate, the rationale was not always understood and some was potentially dangerous. If women are more likely to trust relatives then they may ignore, or only partially follow, advice from maternity staff, especially if it is conflicting. In an American study (Melson, 1989) of 80 black and 82 white women the best predictors of positive health behaviours were socio-economic status of the father, social support, general well-being and intrinsic motivation. Acceptance of the pregnancy and feelings of general well-being were related to earlier uptake of antenatal care.

A number of studies have used psychological models, especially the Health Belief Model (HBM, e.g. Becker and Rosenstock, 1984) to investigate the reasons why women do not attend antenatal care. See Horne and Weinman, Chapter 2 for a description of the HBM. Some of the "barriers" identified are financial (including the cost of appointments, treatments, medications, hospitalisation, loss of earnings), transport difficulties, compromise to job status by taking time off, and childcare issues (Toomey, 1985). However, Leatherman, Blackburn and Davidhizar (1990) found that although insufficient money was named most frequently (81%), motivational issues accounted for nearly half of the variance, including women's beliefs that appointments were not really necessary, that there had been no previous problems, and that they felt so good that early attendance was unnecessary. The authors suggest that emphasis should be on educating women to realise that antenatal care is necessary. It could be argued, however, that without a financial support system, motivation will not be enough to ensure either access or a better outcome. It is likely that such determinants are partly defined by the health care system (e.g. whether care is free or subsidised) and, unfortunately, comparative studies of adherence across different health systems are not available.

In some cases, such barriers may prevent the take-up of service, in other cases they act as a delay factor, which may equally, or to a lesser extent, impair outcome. Bueche (1993) applied the model to beliefs about prenatal care, nutrition, smoking and alcohol use. However, their 106 item questionnaire identified only 3 constructs and could not distinguish susceptibility and seriousness.

Tinsley *et al.* (1993) reviewed work on the contribution of locus of control (Rotter, 1966) and specific pregnancy beliefs to predict adherence in 62 women during the 3rd trimester. See Horne and Weinman, Chapter 2 for a description of the model. However, it is still not clear how these beliefs are translated into positive health behaviours. They suggest that tailoring advice to the woman's orientation may be more effective, such that those with an "internal" locus of control would do better with a participative style and those with a "powerful others" orientation would respond to the more traditional didactic approach. Earlier work by Faragalla (1983) indicated that health locus of control and perceived benefits did not predict better prenatal care, and Desmond, Price and Losh (1987) failed to demonstrate differences in the health locus of control in smokers vs. non-smokers. However, the more specific Fetal Health Locus of Control Scale (Labs and Wurtele, 1986) demonstrated that non-smokers had high "internality" scores as did women who reported less caffeine consumption. They concluded that women's beliefs about their own influence on pregnancy outcomes do lead to better self-care, and that prevention tailored to an individual woman's locus of control could be more effective than general advice. Women who felt in control of their pregnancy and the perinatal period were less likely to use drugs and to smoke, but the "chance" and "powerful others" factors did not predict adherence.

Further work (Reisch and Tinsley, 1994) demonstrated opposite predictions for utilisation of antenatal care by impoverished women. Their samples were mainly Latino (57.7%), Euro-American (30.6%) and Afro-American (10%) women, of whom half had not completed secondary school. Those women with an external locus of control were 3 times more likely to receive adequate care than those with an internal locus of control, and 7½ times more likely if antenatal care was perceived as important. The authors suggest that trusting "powerful others" is more effective because only the professionals can really access the necessary services for them. However, Porter and Macintyre (1989) argue that the majority of women attend antenatal clinics because of a possible non-specific benefit and also because they would feel guilty if they did not. The emphasis should be on ensuring that care is both clinically and psychosocially beneficial.

Changing Styles of Antenatal Care

Over the last decade there has been a chorus of dissatisfaction with antenatal care from pregnant women, their midwifery attendants and community support groups. These complaints include impersonal care, long waiting times, and unnecessary investigations. Although the intent of recent initiatives has been to make women feel more autonomous and involved, the expected consequences should also be greater knowledge and understanding of pregnancy and motivation to follow any advice given – " to do what the doctors and midwives say". Two recent multicentre studies in the UK addressed some of these issues. Tucker, Hall and Howie (1996) randomised 1765 low-risk women from 51 general practices to either routine "obstetrician-led" care or clinics run by GPs or midwives. There were positive benefits for those in the GP and midwifery-led groups, including greater continuity of care, fewer routine visits, and fewer antenatal admissions.

Sikorski *et al.* (1996) also used a randomised controlled trial (RCT) design with 2974 women to investigate the impact of reducing the traditional schedule of 13 antenatal visits to a new style of care involving only 6–7 visits. Women in the new system reported greater continuity of care, less conflicting advice, fewer scans and fewer day admissions. Unfortunately, however, they also felt that the opportunities to talk to staff were fewer and they reported more worries about the baby during pregnancy and concerns about how they would cope after delivery. However, it is notable that at least 26.3% of eligible women chose not to enter the trial, primarily because they felt that fewer visits would deprive them of extra reassurance and the opportunity to talk. Thus, ironically, patient non-adherence to "group" assignment may also potentially bias pregnancy research using psychosocial adjustment as a dependent variable.

The need to improve outcome in socially deprived women has also led to home visiting programmes by nurses (USA) or midwives (UK). These are expensive services, and few studies have included sufficient women or a randomised design to evaluate their effectiveness.

One multi-disciplinary project in a semi-rural area in New York (Olds *et al.,* 1986) included parent education, enhancement of the women's existing support system, and accessibility to a range of community services. The women were either teenagers (47%), unmarried (62%) and/or in social classes IV or V; only 15% had no risk factors while 23% had all three. Participation rates were high and the only women who dropped out of the program had either moved or miscarried. By the end of the pregnancy those in the visited group were significantly more knowledgeable about community services, attended childbirth classes more often, improved the quality of their diets, and smoked fewer cigarettes. A contemporary study (Elster *et al.,* 1987) demonstrated that parent education also increased new mothers' attention to parenting and their knowledge of the care of newborns. Home visiting has also been shown to enhance communication with family and friends (Dineen *et al.,* 1992), perhaps because the natural setting empowers women to share their feelings and concerns.

Antenatal Classes And Instruction

Most North American and Western European healthcare systems offer some form of pregnancy and parenting instruction, although these are sometimes limited to primiparae, and not all include the father. Attendance at such classes may enhance adherence because of the opportunity to hear answers to questions posed by other couples, skilled facilitation of discussion, the social interaction, and – if they meet throughout the pregnancy – the opportunity to develop friendships and supportive networks. For instance, the majority of mothers who participate in the antenatal classes run by the National Childbirth Trust, an educational charity, maintain their friendships through the postnatal period and often longer. Data are available from a number of countries about the perceived value of antenatal classes. In a Finnish study, 75% of mothers felt that courses improved their knowledge but those who were already well-informed rated them as inadequate, out of date and poorly presented. Few of the women, however, believed that classes reduced anxiety (Rautava, Erkkola and Sillanpaa, 1990). Printed materials seem to be more effective in women of higher socio-economic status (SES) while television and video programs were preferred by those with a poorer educational background (Aaronson, 1989).

Birth and the Postpartum Period

Even if women do attend antenatal classes they do not always adhere to instructions during labour and delivery. Lindell and Rossi (1986) noted that women could recount the instructions about breathing, but did not necessarily use the techniques when they were instructed to "do what was most comfortable". "Birth plans" are a powerful tool for enhancing labour and delivery by giving the mother information to make choices and reflect with her midwife. An Australian study (Moore and Hopper, 1995) found that 95% of those who had used a birth plan would encourage others to do so. The plan enabled them to ask for what they wanted (89%), and also improved their understanding (93%) and communication with staff. The take-up rate for the postnatal check is almost universal in the UK; 91% of a sample of 1278 women attended (Bick and MacArthur, 1995). Those who did not attend cited "busyness", "forgetfulness", "embarrassment", and "not perceiving the need".

Increasingly, HPs believe that it is beneficial to breastfeed babies. This can only be achieved by better staff adherence to international guidelines, especially those of the joint initiative of WHO and UNICEF which was launched as the Baby Friendly Hospital Initiative (BFHI) in 1989 (World Health Organisation, 1989). This "Ten Steps to Successful Breastfeeding" programme was designed to reward maternity facilities which support breastfeeding. It could be argued, however, that adherence may be easier to some aspects (e.g. providing information) than in changing attitudes (of both mothers and staff) and actually achieving good breastfeeding. For instance, having a written policy, training staff and informing women about the benefits is probably easier to implement than helping them breastfeed within a half-hour of birth and withholding food, drink and pacifiers (dummies) unless medically indicated. The last of these "Ten Steps" – fostering the establishment of breast feeding support groups and referring mothers – will depend as much on staff and mothers' attitudes toward peer support, and availability of help out of hours.

Wright, Rice and Wells (1996) put the "Ten Steps" program into practice by reviewing and improving existing policies, including education for doctors, nursing staff and students. Staff significantly increased the number of infants put to the breast in the first hour (1990 = 24.8%; 1993 = 63.2%) thus bringing the mean time to first feed down from 3.3 hours to only 0.7 hours. However, staff remained constrained by: a) policies of a 4-hour separation after delivery; b) putting infants in the nursery at night and c) the difficulty of removing formula samples from the free gift packs distributed within the hospital. Generally the increase in breastfeeding has been more marked in Caucasian, better educated mothers. However, a large state funded programme in the USA (Grossman *et al.,* 1989) attempted to increase breast-feeding among single, poor women with little education. Sixty nine percent of those who planned to breastfeed did so, but they were still more likely to be older, better educated, have good health habits and take advantage of antenatal care. The fact that those who chose breastfeeding also made a significantly greater number of antenatal visits suggests they were committed to enhancing their infants' welfare in general, rather than just feeding.

An innovative project in a deprived inner city area in Scotland has begun to address the low breastfeeding rate of 12–16% compared to the affluent areas where it is 60 - 70% at seven days (Gribble, 1996). Instead of traditional HPs, the project uses local mothers who have breastfed successfully. Other countries have made efforts to enable all women to breastfeed. In an Italian study (Romito and Saurel-Cubrizolles, 1996) of primiparous working mothers, 87% had put the baby to the breast in hospital, and 38% breastfed for at least 24 weeks. Even once they resumed work, 31% still continued. The positive correlation between employment and continued breastfeeding remained after controlling for socio-demographic variables.

Cultural beliefs can also enhance the reasons for breastfeeding. For instance, the Navajo say that "a bottle-fed infant becomes too detached from the mother and cow's milk infuses the child with the faculties of animals – undesirable ones presumably!" (Phillips and Lobar, 1990).

HIGH-RISK PREGNANCY

Adolescents

In 1992, in the UK, 7% of all births were to teenagers, about 48,000 (Ineichen and Hudson, 1994). In the USA 18% of all firstborns infants were to teenagers, equalling 0.5 million new teenage mothers (Flanagan *et al.*, 1995). Adolescents often fail to initiate health care and by the time they are assessed they may have missed the opportunity to initiate measures associated with good outcome (e.g. diet, smoking and drinking). Smoking rates in one sample were high (28.5% in those aged 12–15, and 41.4% in those 16–19) (Amini *et al.*, 1996). Pregnant adolescents are likely to have particular factors that compromise their ability and motivation to adhere to the recommendations or requests of HPs. These include knowledge level, family support, approachability of HPs, suspicion of outsiders and fear of ridicule. A study in Virginia (Julnes *et al.*, 1994) compared two types of perinatal care for disadvantaged pregnant adolescents – a traditional multidisciplinary program with HPs and a community-based program using lay visitors (the Resource Mothers Program). The new initiative was more effective in involving the most high-risk teens (under 17 years: 75.5% vs. 45.6%), and promoting earlier care (53.1% vs. 32.6%, before 4 months).

However, although such programs are effective for both mother and child, the take-up rate generally is very low. Lee and Grubs (1993) compared teens who booked antenatal care in the first trimester compared to those who delayed until the third trimester. Analysis of interviews, however, did not identify differences in knowledge about diet, exercise and self-care that would explain the delay. Health behaviours included 62 nutrition and self-care activities by the "early care" girls, and 14 by the 12 "late care" girls, particularly for healthy foods. Increased sleep and rest time was also reported. Family members contributed to the development of self-care practices in both the early care (94%) and late care groups (83.3%). The authors suggest that the "late bookers" felt more "in tune" with their bodies so did not feel the need for physician care, and that the desire for self-care indicated a greater internal locus of control. Stevens-Simon, O'Connor and Basford (1994) showed that incentives for adolescents to follow health recommendations can be successful. Simply by the promise of a baby carrier, they increased postnatal attendance, especially in multiparous teenagers, school non-attendees and those who had not used antenatal services.

Substance Use

Illicit use of drugs is an increasing problem and one which has significant implications for pregnancy and parenthood. The first step in offering appropriate counselling and intervention is accurate and non-judgmental history taking. Klein, Friedman-Campbell and Tocco (1993) emphasise the process of interviewing, especially using questions which acknowledge that many people use "mood altering" substances. They even suggest that the practitioner's own experience of substance use (e.g. family) can increase empathy. A study of 30 drug-using women in the north of England (Lewis, Klee and Jackson, 1995) highlighted a number of difficulties that such women face in being a "good mother". They had many incorrect beliefs about conception, pregnancy and childbirth, for instance failing to use contraception because of the belief that methadone and street drugs prevent pregnancy. Female addicts may come from dysfunctional families, resulting in a learned sense of failure that presents as low self-esteem, feelings of inadequacy and powerlessness (Daghestani, 1988).

De Petrillo and Rice (1995) examined the relationship between patient characteristics and adherence with urine toxicology requests. Not surprisingly, those who entered the programme earlier were more likely to decrease their opiate and cocaine use and to provide urine specimens for analysis. Elk *et al.* (1994) studied cocaine users receiving intensive counselling, contingency management or baseline visiting who did not succeed in reducing their drug use in the first four weeks. They found that those who were adherent at entry to the treatment programme were more likely to attend appointments and remain drug-free. Killeen, Brady and Thevos (1995) looked more closely at the possible reasons for non-adherence in cocaine users during pregnancy and the postpartum period. The women had high rates of psychiatric problems, with many also presenting with personality disorder. Those women defined as "treatment compliant" (attendance at 50% or more aftercare appointments) had lower psychiatric scores and better employment records. In addition, 73% of the sample reported a history of victimisation, with the "non-compliant" women more likely to have been abused in childhood. Thus, adherence can probably only be improved in this population by providing community support and treatment for the mental health problem.

Substance use is not confined to the West. Mikhail *et al.* (1995) documented poorer maternal-foetal attachment scores during pregnancy in methadone users in the Soviet Union. He suggests that the mother's lesser affiliation with her infant could lead to poor adherence to pregnancy advice. Physical abuse, alcohol and drug use also clearly compromise positive health behaviours. They often co-exist, either because the woman turns to drugs and alcohol to help her cope, or because her partner has a drug problem himself. McFarlane, Parker and Soekeen (1996) examined the convergence of these problems in a sample of African (414), Hispanic (412) and Caucasian (377) Americans, yielding an physical abuse rate during pregnancy of 16%. A significant association between smoking and physical abuse was evident in both African-American (33.7% vs. 49.5%) and Caucasian women (46.6% vs. 59.6%). Alcohol and/or illicit drug use was higher in all 3 groups but significant only in the African-American women (20.8% vs. 42.1%). The nurse practitioner authors suggest that by helping a woman to focus on strategies for safety and abuse prevention, she may be able to reduce her substance use.

HIV and AIDS

A recent review of the International AIDS Conference in Vancouver (Sherr, in press) highlights some themes relevant to adherence and includes data from the USA, Europe and developing countries. The first area is the relative lack of data about the woman's perspective on interventions. This would include the complex mechanisms underlying the decision to be tested, to return for the results, to be part of an intervention, and to follow a given regimen. We know more about how many women adhere than why women do not come or refuse to come when they are asked. Rates for testing were very high – between 80 - 90% from Thailand to Africa, in sample sizes up to 15,000. Abreu (in press) in Puerto Rico demonstrated an increase from 40% in 1992–3 to 60% in 1994–6. In an African sample (Cartoux, in press) the reasons for refusal included "husband's advice" (43%), fear of AIDS (37%) and a further 20% which included lack of interest, or other/no reason. Being married accounted for a three-fold refusal rate in one centre, as did not wanting the pregnancy.

However, not everybody returns for their results. Of those in Cartoux's African sample 61% returned spontaneously and 21% after an HIV nurse visited; 18% failed to return, of whom the youngest were least adherent. In Dabi's (in press) West African sample 45–80% returned. Adherence rates to treatment with AZT (an anti-retroviral agent) are also very high: 100% in Argentina and 85% in

Puerto Rico, 91.5% in Spain (Martinez-Tejada, in press) and 94% in New York (Landsberger, in press). Seventy percent of Seal's (in press) sample said that they would follow the drug protocol unless they detected any doubt from the doctor. The best predictor of adherence was previous use of AZT without side-effects. However, there are also numerous other factors that make care unavailable or unlikely to be taken up, including drug use, low education, and being single (Shakarishvili, in press). Additionally, services and personal factors sometimes interact to compromise treatment. Of the 125 infected women in Bryson's (in press) New York study only 49 were detected during pregnancy, only 37% chose AZT and even fewer received the medication. In a small sample of mostly black adolescents, Lawrance, Levy and Rubinson (1990) found a significant relationship between perceived vulnerability, self- efficacy and preventative behaviours to avoid high risk.

Diabetes

Diabetes mellitus is a complex condition, with particular implications during pregnancy. Some of the potential problems are initial acceptance of the condition, knowledge about practical aspects, management of dietary restrictions and fears about self -injection. See Warren and Hixenaugh, Chapter 16 for a review of diabetes in adults. Zarzycki *et al.* (1994) found that pregnant women with diabetes had high levels of knowledge about the condition – more so than women who were not pregnant – and 82% did accept the whole management programme. One concern during pregnancy is whether post-prandial or pre-prandial monitoring is more reliable, and if so, whether the timing makes a difference to adherence. Data indicated that testing after meals improved both glycaemic control and subsequent risks and that women were equally adherent with the two protocols. Langer *et al.* (1995) explored determinants of adherence in a multicultural sample of women with diabetes and ways to improve adherence. Women completed 60–70% of necessary tests, with no differences between the Caucasian, Mexican-American and Afro-American samples. Regardless of socio-economic status or ethnic origin, adherence was improved by interacting positively with the women, and providing them with memory reflectance meters and education about diabetes.

Books for the expectant mother often present adherence as a certain pathway to an optimal outcome, in this case to the controlling of diabetes: "I can't stress it enough: strict adherence to the diet, insulin requirements, self-testing procedures and doctors' orders. If you have gestational diabetes, you can return your chances of having a good outcome to your pregnancy almost to normal by doing everything that's required of you to keep your condition in check" (Rich, 1991). Such books can be very helpful in informing women about problems and solutions and empowering them to ask questions that, in turn, may motivate them to manage their condition more effectively. However, they may also set up unrealistic expectations and hence frustration if a medical condition does not improve or the infant is affected.

Preterm Labour, Hospital Admission and Bed Rest

It has also been suggested that particular "lifestyle" factors might be associated with preterm labour such that preventative programmes could be implemented to reduce the risk (Freda *et al.*, 1990). After screening for 12 adverse lifestyle factors, women received counselling and were taught to recognise symptoms and modify their behaviour. Women who were able to decrease the activity or stress had a lower rate of preterm birth. Blankson, Goldenberg and Keith (1994) investigated the reasons for missed appointments in high-risk antenatal patients after an initial evaluation indicated a rate of 30–40%. Of 118 women available for telephone interview, the most common reasons given were access to a telephone, high mobility, poor knowledge of their condition and limited understanding about the reason for referral or the potential benefits of clinic attendance. Nearly three quarters were aware of their diagnosis, but only 30% perceived it as a threat. Those who could identify their diagnosis gave a positive assessment of their antenatal care, and were less likely to blame lack of transport for missed appointments. This suggests that greater attention needs to be paid to better service delivery strategies, but also to improving women's perception of the severity of the problem and when, and how, to seek urgent treatment. Nonetheless, 18.2% of women who delivered at <32 weeks gestation were advised to rest for at least a week; the reasons included first trimester bleeding (3.9%), hypertension (4.8%), early/

false labour (4.8%), and oedema (5.2%). Eleven percent of all patients spent at least one week in hospital.

Bedrest is the cornerstone of high-risk pregnancy management in the USA, and is used in nearly 20% of all pregnancies for conditions as diverse as threatened abortion, preterm labour, oedema and chronic hypertension. Women who are hospitalised during pregnancy may also feel powerless and unable to participate in their own care. For instance, 68% of the women in Kirk's (1994) Manchester sample reported that they always had to ask for information, they were not involved in decision-making (54%), received conflicting information and had not received as much as they would have liked (34%).

A comprehensive review of adherence with bedrest for "high risk" pregnancy (Josten *et al.*, 1995) included data on 326 women with various conditions – primarily preterm labour, bleeding or high blood pressure. About two-thirds reported following the advice and one third did not. Adherence was worse in those prescribed total bed rest. Primary reasons given for non-adherence were childcare (62%), "not feeling sick" (40%), household demands (35%) and lack of partner/family support (17%). These rates are higher than in the few randomised control trials but less than the 50% of Monahan and DeJoseph (1991). Those least likely to follow the protocol were also more likely to continue to drink alcohol. However, the authors also acknowledge that since behaviour was self-reported, their adherence may be an overestimate. Crowther (1995) concludes from a number of studies that since there is no well-controlled evidence for bedrest, the views of women who experience such complications should be taken into consideration.

Being admitted to hospital for a high-risk pregnancy can have undesirable effects on health behaviour, quite apart from the reason for admission. Kirk (1994) reported that 81% of the mothers increased their smoking, 50% of those doubled it, and 75% were already smoking before 9.00 am! In Thompson's (1993) study women also reported more smoking, and for longer periods, often attributing it to boredom.

In the USA, "prevention of prematurity" programs have focused on teaching women to identify preterm labour so that interventions could be used to prevent delivery. Brustman *et al.* (1990) investigated whether women were accurate and assiduous in doing so. Thirty eight women carried out the protocol for two 60 minute sessions daily over 21 days, but only identified 10% of contractions, with 35% under-reporting, only 5% over-reporting and no change over time. Neither motivation, adherence, or level of education correlated with their perceptions of uterine activity, suggesting that patient factors are not responsible for the poor outcome.

A high risk pregnancy may result in an infant with medical problems, usually due to prematurity. It is routine in America for preterm infants to be discharged home on cardio-respiratory monitors to "prevent" sudden infant death syndrome. Silvestri *et al.* (1995) used an automatic recording system to document the level of parental adherence and factors that might affect such adherence. Of the 67 study infants, parents used the monitors for an average of 15.5 hours with 75% monitored for more than 10.5 hours and 25% for more than 21 hours. However, since previous studies indicate that 57–80% of infant deaths are associated with non-adherence to proper technique (Meny, 1988; Kelly, 1988), instruction and discussion of potential problems as well as continued support for families may boost effective surveillance even higher.

ADHERENCE IN OBSTETRIC, NURSING AND MIDWIFERY STAFF

Although pregnant women are expected to follow the doctor or midwife's orders health care staff do not always do so. Yoong *et al.* (1992) examined obstetricians' adherence to departmental protocols for maternity care. In their care of 2000 pregnant women only 23.5% (3673 of an expected 15,658) of the prescribed actions were performed. Even for the 63 most clinically significant risk factors, only 28.3% of the doctors initiated appropriate action. Staff were most assiduous in counselling about alcohol (100%) and advising reduction in heavy (10+ cigarettes) smokers. The failure of medical staff to follow protocols for screening can also have significant consequences. For instance, although 1% of antenatal patients were positive for hepatitis B, 42% of these were missed, and two years later the rate was little different. Of equal concern, however, is the number of " unnecessary rituals" that obstetricians continue to perform, including x-ray pelvimetry after Caesarean section (Sharif and Hammadieh, 1993) and routine vaginal examination (Neelamkavil, 1993).

A Norwegian study examined GPs' adherence with their national guidelines for maternity care over a 12 month period (Backe and Jacobsen, 1994). Adherence was lower in male doctors, and those from a single-handed practice. However, as reflected in the detection of major disorders, there was no relationship between the complication score and outcome. In developing countries, clear guidelines for risk management and referral to specialist care can be thwarted by non-human factors, such as weather and problems with transport. However, in an examination of 5060 pregnancies in Zaire, Dujardin *et al.* (1995) found only a 33% referral rate in spite of favourable conditions. The two crucial factors were geographical accessibility of hospital care and the mother's perception of risk. Although patient education might improve earlier self-referral, this underscores the fact that optimal outcome cannot always be assured.

Few studies have examined patient adherence to requests for involvement in research or medical student teaching. Magrane, Gannon and Miller (1996) surveyed 222 American maternity patients and 67 medical students about the primary reasons for acceptance or refusal of student participation in interpartum care in hospital. Sixty-one percent of the mothers cited the importance of contributing to student education. Reasons for refusal included concern about potential errors by students. This was mentioned by 30% of patients and 22% of the students. Other reasons included a desire to limit numbers in the delivery room, imposition on the woman's time and the need for repetition of activities. Women felt that student participation should be requested rather than assigned, and more women (83%) than students (48%) felt that the issue should not be pursued after initial refusal. Most (87%) women did not want the student present at the time of request compared to 45% of the students, who did not seem to acknowledge that it may be inappropriate to be there.

CONCLUSION: IMPLICATIONS FOR ENHANCED PRACTICE

The literature on pregnancy demonstrates that women want to do the best for their baby and are able to make changes to their lifestyle and follow advice from HPs. However, the reasons why some do not are complex and probably determined by the interplay of health beliefs, personal values, socio-economic factors, and family and community support. It is also clear that some vulnerable groups do not, or perhaps cannot, adhere and that their lifestyle may alienate those professionals who are best placed to serve them. At worst, a prejudiced, unsympathetic consultant might make a drug addict feel that she is unworthy to have a baby and thus decrease her likelihood of utilising care that might prevent neonatal complications, and accessing support to improve her mothering skills. At best, a supportive midwife might help a pregnant teenager to "turn her life around" by liaising with her parents, the school, social services and adolescent peer support networks. Also important are the changes in the maternity services, not just in the organisation of hospital and community care, but ostensibly in the shift from an "expert-centred" system to a "woman centred" approach in which the "consumer" is offered real choices about where and how to have her baby.

Differences across cultural groups, health systems and styles of care require further study. For instance, there is clearly a polarisation of maternity services in the USA and Australia between those women who have a private obstetrician / gynaecologist and those in public care settings. The obstetrician-gynaecologist in America is likely to have been the primary physician for a woman, and may have known her since adolescence. Such familiarity and trust may enhance adherence. In the UK, women lack this continuity in their "reproductive career" unless their GP is on the "maternity list" and is willing and available to provide the kind of delivery she wishes. However, as midwives take more responsibility for maternity care in the community, families are likely to benefit from the integration of GPs, health visitors and hospital care. Bryce (1990) suggests that "women probably feel more at ease discussing emotional problems with their midwife than with their doctor because the midwife has a perceived lower authority status than the doctors, often appears less busy and is generally of the same sex". However, improving information is essential too. As Reid and Garcia (1989) note, research studies "point to a high degree of compliance among pregnant women, but also a considerable lack of comprehension about the reasons for what they were asked to do". If the clarion call for "evidence-based practice" in medicine results in fewer unnecessary procedures, then at least women will feel that the advice they are asked to follow has been properly evaluated, carefully chosen and likely to be effective.

There are still some areas that have received scant attention. For instance, we know more about the contribution of education and social class to adherence than about the influence of family support or maternal personality and outlook. It may also be that previous experience is crucial – both in terms of satisfaction with the pregnancy, delivery and postpartum outcome, and also the perception of having control over events and a sense of achievement – sometimes against the odds.

Perhaps the most important issue in adherence is whether it has future implications. As Reading (1983) reminds us, since women have extended contact with HPs during pregnancy, this "...may be a time of optimum receptivity for behavioural change and that attempts should be made to encourage mothers to maintain the gains made during pregnancy after the birth". If the new mother sees herself as an autonomous individual who has made use of new experiences, she may apply those to other health care problems later in her life.

REFERENCES

Aaronson, L.S. (1989) Perceived and received support: effects on health behavior during pregnancy. *Nursing Research* **38**, 4–9.

Albrecht, S.A. and Rankin, M. (1989) Anxiety levels, health behaviors, and support systems of pregnant women. *Maternal-Child Nursing Journal*, **18**, 49–60.

Abreu, E. *in press.* Presented at the 10th International Conference on AIDS (1996) cited in Sherr, L. Pregnancy and childbirth. *AIDS Care.*

Alcalay, R., Ghee, A. and Scrimshaw, S. (1993) Designing prenatal care messages for low-income Mexican women. *Public Health Reports* **108**, 354–362.

Amini, S.B., Catalano, P.M., Dierker, L.J. and Mann, L.I. (1996) Birth to teenagers: Trends and obstetric customs. *Obstetrics and Gynecology*, **87**, 668–674.

Backe, B. and Jacobsen, G. (1994) General practitioners' compliance with guidelines for antenatal care. *Scandinavian Journal of Primary Health Care* **12**, 100–105.

Becker, H.M. and Rosenstock, J.M. (1984) Compliance with medical advice. In A. Mathews and A. Steptoe (eds) *Health care and human behaviour.* London, Academic Press.

Bick, D.E. and MacArthur, C. (1995) Attendance, content and relevance of the six week postnatal examination. *Midwifery* **11**, 69–73.

Blankson, M.L., Goldenberg, R.L. and Keith, B. (1994) Noncompliance of high-risk pregnant women in keeping appointments at an obstetric complications clinic. *Southern Medical Journal* **87**, 634–638.

Blumfield, W. (1996) Life after birth. *Journal of the Royal Society of Health* **116**, 176–179.

Brustman, L.E., Langer, O., Anyaegbunam, A., Belle, C. and Merkatz, I.R. (1990) Education does not improve patient perception of preterm uterine contractability. *Obstetrics and Gynecology (suppl.)* **76**, 97S–101S.

Bryce, R. (1990) Social and midwifery support. In *Balliere's Clinical Obstetrics and Gynaecology* **4**, 77–88.

Bryson, Y. *in press* Presented at the 10th International Conference on AIDS (1996) cited in Sherr, L. Pregnancy and childbirth. *AIDS Care.*

Bueche, M.N. (1993) Commentary on patient attitudes concerning health behaviors during pregnancy: initial development of a questionnaire. *Nursing Scan in Research* **6**, 15–16.

Cartoux, M. *in press* Presented at the 10th International Conference on AIDS (1996), Cited in Sherr, L. Pregnancy and childbirth. *AIDS Care.*

Cnattingius, S., Haglund, B. and Meirik, O. (1988) Cigarette smoking as a risk factor for late fetal and early neonatal death. *British Medical Journal* **297**, 258–261.

Crowther, C.A. (1995) Commentary: bedrest for women with pregnancy problems: Evidence for efficacy is lacking. *Birth* **22**,13–14.

Dabi, F. *in press* Paper presented at the 10th International Conference on AIDS (1996), cited in Sherr, L. Pregnancy and childbirth. *AIDS Care.*

Daghestani, A. (1988) Psychological characteristics of pregnant women addicts in treatment. In I.J. Chasnoff (ed) *Drugs, alcohol, pregnancy and parenting.* UK: Kluwer Academic Publishers.

Department of Health. (1993) *Changing childbirth*, London: HMSO..

Desmond, S.M., Price, J.H. and Losh, D.P. (1987) Multidimensional health locus of control of pregnant women who smoke. *Psychological Reports* **60**, 191–194.

DePetrillo, P.B. and Rice, J.M. (1995) Methadone dosing and pregnancy: impact on program compliance. *International Journal of Addiction* **30**, 207–217.

De Vries, R. (1989) Caregivers in pregnancy and childbirth. In: I. Chalmers, M. Enkin and M.J.N.C. Keirse (eds) *Effective care in pregnancy and childbirth*. New York: OUP.

Dineen, K., Rossi, M., Lia-Hoagberg, B. and Keller, L.O. (1992) Antepartum home-care services for high-risk women. *Journal of Obstetric, Gynecological, and Neonatal Nursing* **21**, 121–125.

Du Bard, M.B., Goldenberg, R.L., Copper, R.L. and Haut, L. (1993) Are pill counts valid measures of compliance in clinical obstetric trials? *American Journal of Obstetrics and Gynecology* **165**, 1181–1182.

Dujardin, B., Clarysse, G., Criel, B., De Brouwere, V. and Wangata, N. (1995) The strategy of risk approach in antenatal care: evaluation of the referral compliance. *Social Science and Medicine* **40**, 529–535.

Elk, R., Schmitz, J., Manfredi, L., Rhoades, H., Andres, R. and Grabowski, J. (1994) Cessation of cocaine use. *Addictive Behaviour* **19**, 697–702.

Elster, A.B., Lamb, M.E., Tavare, J. and Ralston, C.W. (1987) The medical and psychosocial impact of comprehensive care on adolescent pregnancy and parenthood. *Journal of the American Medical Association* **258**, 1187–1192.

Ershoff, D.H., Quinn, V.P., Mullen, P.D. and Lairson, D.R. (1990) Pregnancy and medical cost outcomes of a self-help prenatal smoking cessation program in a HMO. *Public Health Reports* **105**, 340–347.

Faragalla, T.H. (1983) *The relationship between Health Locus of Control, perceived benefits, and adherence to a prescribed prenatal care regimen*. Unpublished dissertation: New York University..

Flanagan, P.J., McGrath, M.M., Meyer, E.C. and Garcia Coll, C.T. (1995) Adolescent development and transitions to motherhood. *Pediatrics,* **96**, 273–277.

Freda, M.C., Anderson, H.F., Damus, K., Poust, D., Brustman, L. and Merkatz, I.R. (1990) Lifestyle modification as an intervention for inner city women at risk for preterm birth. *Journal of Advanced Nursing* **15**, 364–372.

Galloway, R. and McGuire, J. (1994) Determinants of compliance with iron supplementation: supplies, side effects, or psychology. *Social Science and Medicine* **39**, 381–390.

Gerstein, H.C., Simpson, J.R., Atkinson, S., Taylor, D.W. and Vander-Meulen, J. (1995) Feasibility and acceptability of a proposed infant feeding intervention trial for the prevention of type I diabetes. *Diabetes-Care* **18**, 940–942.

Goldenberg, R.L., Tamura, T., Cliver, S.P., Cutter, G.R., Hoffman, H.J. and Copper, R.L. (1992) Serum folate and fetal growth retardation: A matter of compliance? *Obstetrics and Gynecology* **79**, 719–22.

Gribble, J. (1996) An alternative approach. *New Generation* **15**, 12–13.

Grossman, L.K., Larsen-Alexander, J.B., Fitzsimmons, S.M. and Corders, L. (1989) Breastfeeding among low-income, high-risk women. *Clinical Pediatrics* **28**, 38–42.

Hamilton, A. (1781) Treatise on midwifery. Cited in Carter, J. and Duriez, T. (1996) *With child: birth through the ages.* Edinburgh: Mainstream Publishing Company.

Higgins, P., Frank, B. and Brown, M. (1994) Changes in health behaviors made by pregnant women. *Health Care for Women International* **15**, 149–156.

Ineichen, B. and Hudson, F. (1994) *Teenage pregnancy.* London: National Children's Bureau..

Jewell, D. (1990) Pre-pregnancy and early pregnancy care. *Antenatal Care* **4**, 1–23.

Josten, L.E., Savik, K., Mullett, S.E., Campbell, R. and Vincent, P. (1995) Bedrest compliance for women with pregnancy problems. *Birth: Issues in Perinatal Care*, **22**, 1–12.

Julnes, G., Konefal, M., Pindur, W. and Kim, P. (1994) Community-based perinatal care for disadvantaged adolescents: evaluation of the Resource Mothers Program 1. *Journal of Community Health,* **9**, 41–53.

Kaunitz, A., Spence, C., Danielson, T., Rochat, R and Grunes, D. (1984) Perinatal and maternal mortality in a religious group avoiding obstetric care. *American Journal of Obstetrics and Gynecology* **150**, 826–831.

Kelly, D.H. (1988) Home monitoring for the sudden infant death syndrome: the case for. In P.J. Schwartz, D.P. Southall and M. Valdes-Dapena, M. (eds) *The suddent infant death syndrome: cardiac and respiratory mechanisms and interventions.* New York: New York Academy of Sciences.

Killeen, T.K., Brady, K.T. and Thevos, A. (1995) Addiction severity, psychopathology and treatment compliance in cocaine-dependent mothers. *Journal of Addiction Disorders* **14**, 75–84.

Kirk, S.A. (1994) The needs of women hospitalized in pregnancy. In S. Robinsoon and A.M. Thomson (eds) *Midwives, research and childbirth*. London: Chapman and Hall.

Klein, R.F., Friedman-Campbell, M. and Tocco, R.V. (1993) History taking and substance abuse counselling with the pregnant patient. *Clinical Obstetrics and Gynecology* **36**, 338–346.

Labs, S.M. and Wurtele, S.K. (1986) Fetal health locus of control scale: development and validation. *Journal of Consulting and Clinical Psychology* **54**, 814–819.

Landsberger, E. *in press* Presented at the 10th International Conference on AIDS (1996), cited in Sherr, L. Pregnancy and childbirth. *AIDS Care*.

Langer, O., Langer, N., Piper, J.M., Elliott, B. and Anyaegbunam, A. (1995) Cultural diversity as a factor in self-monitoring blood glucose in gestational diabetes. *Journal of Association for Academic Minority Physicians*, **6**, 73–77.

Lawrance, L., Levy, S.R. and Rubinson, L. (1990) Self-efficacy and AIDS prevention for pregnant teens. *Journal of School Health* **60**, 19–24.

Leatherman, Blackburn, D. and Davidhizar, R. (1990) How postpartum women explain their lack of obtaining adequate prenatal care. *Journal of Advanced Nursing* **15** , 256–267.

Lee, S.H. and Grubs, L.M. (1993) A comparison of self-reported self-care practices of pregnant adolescents. *American Journal of Primary Health Care* **18**, 25–29.

Lewis, S., Klee, H. and Jackson, M. (1995) Illicit drug users' experiences of pregnancy. An exploratory study. *Journal of Reproductive and Infant Psychology*, **13**, 219–227.

Lindell, S.G. and Rossi, M.A. (1986) Compliance with childbirth education classes in second stage labor. *Birth* **13**, 96–99.

Lumley, J. (1990) Through a glass darkly: ultra-sound and prenatal bonding. *Birth: Issues in Perinatal Care and Education* **17**, 214–217.

Lumley, J. and Astbury, J. (1989) Advice for pregnancy. In I. Chalmers, M. Enkin, and M. Kierse (eds) *Effective care in pregnancy and childbirth*. Oxford University Press.

Lumley, J. and Brown, S. (1993) Attenders and non-attenders at childbirth education classes in Australia: how do they and their births differ? *Birth: Issues In Perinatal Care and Education* **20**, 123–131.

Magrane, D. Gannon, D.N.M. and Miller, C.T. (1996) Student doctors and women in labor: attitudes and expectations. *Obstetrics and Gynecology* **88**, 198–302.

Martinez-Tejada, B. *in press* Presented at the 10th International Conference on AIDS (1996), cited in Sherr, L. Pregnancy and childbirth. *AIDS Care.*

McFarlane, J., Parker, B. and Soekeen, C. (1996) Physical abuse, smoking and substance use during pregnancy: prevalence, interrelationships, and effects on birth weight. *Journal of Obstetric and Gynecological Nursing* **25**, 313–320.

Melson, J.S. (1989) The relationship of client characteristics to health behaviors and weeks gestation at the first prenatal visit in Black and White women receiving prepaid, uniform health care. *Unpublished thesis.*

Meny, R.G., Blackmon, L., Fleischmann, D. Gutberlet, R. and Naumberg, E. (1988) Sudden infant death and home monitors. *American Journal of Disorders of Childhood* **142**, 1037–1040.

Mikhail, M.S., Youchah, J., DeVore, N., Ho, G.Y. and Anyaegbunam, A. (1995) Decreased maternal-fetal attachment in methadone-maintained pregnant women: a preliminary study. *Journal of Association for Academic Minority Physicians* **6**, 112–114.

Monahan, P.A. and DeJoseph, J.F. (1991) The woman with preterm labor at home: a descriptive analysis. *Journal of Perinatal and Neonatal Nursing*, **4**, 12–20.

Moore, M. and Hopper, U. (1995) Do birth plans empower women? Evaluation of a hospital birth plan. *Birth* **22** 29–36.

Neelamkavil, P. (1993) Letter. *British Medical Journal* **307**, 1065.

Najman, J.M., Williams, G.M., Keeping, J.D., Morrison, J. and Anderson, M.J. (1988) Religious values, practices and pregnancy outcomes: a comparison of the impact of sect and mainstream Christian affiliation. *Social Science and Medicine*, **26**, 401–407.

Olds, D.L., Henderson, C.R. Jnr, Tatelbaum, R. and Chamberlin, R. (1986) Improving the delivery of prenatal care and outcomes of pregnancy: a randomized trial of nurse home visitation. *Pediatrics* **77**, 16–28.

Orr, R.D. and Simmons, J.J. (1979) Nutritional care in pregnancy: the patients view. II. Perceptions, satisfaction and response to dietary advice and treatment. *Journal of the American Diatetic Association* **75**, 131–136.

Phillips, S. and Lobar, S. (1990) Literature summary of some Navajo child health beliefs and rearing practices within a transcultural nursing framework. *Journal of Transcultural Nursing* **1**, 13–20.

Porter, M. and Macintyre, S. (1989) Psychosocial effectiveness of antenatal and postnatal care. *Midwives, Research and Childbirth* **1**, 72–94.

Rautava, P., Erkkola, R. and Sillanpaa, M. (1990) The Finnish family competence study: new directions in antenatal education. *Health Education Research* **5**, 353–359.

Reading, A. (1983) *Psychological aspects of pregnancy.* Harlow: Longman Group Ltd.

Reid, M. and Garcia, J. (1989) Women's views of care during pregnancy and childbirth. In I. Chalmers, M. Enkin and M. Keirse (eds) *Effective care in pregnancy and childbirth,* New York: OUP.

Reisch, A. and Tinsley, N. (1994) Impoverished women's health locus of control and utilization of prenatal services. *Journal of Reproductive and Infant Psychology* **12**, 223–232.

Rich, L. (1991) *When pregnancy isn't perfect: A layperson's guide to complications in pregnancy.* New York: Dutton.

Romito, P. and Saurel Cubrizolles, M. (1996) Working women and breast feeding: the experience of first-time mothers in an Italian town. *Journal of Reproductive and Infant Psychology,* **14,** 145–156.

Rotter, J.B. (1966) Generalised expectancies for internal versus external control of re-enforcement. *Psychological Monographs* **90**, 1–28.

Seal, B. *in press* Presented at the 10th International Conference on AIDS (1996), cited in Sherr, L. Pregnancy and childbirth. *AIDS Care.*

Shakarishvili, A. *in press.* Presented at the 10th International Conference on AIDS (1996), cited in Sherr, L. Pregnancy and Childbirth *AIDS Care.*

Sharif, K.and Hammadieh, N. (1993) Letter. *British Medical Journal* **307**, 1065.

Sherr, L. *In press.* Pregnancy and childbirth. *AIDS Care.*

Sikorski, J., Wilson, J., Clement, S., Das, S. and Smeeton, N. (1996) A randomised controlled trial comparing two schedules of antenatal visits: the antenatal care project. *British Medical Journal* **312**, 546–553.

Silvestri, J.M., Hufford, D.R., Durham, J., Pearsall, S.M., Oess, M.A., Weese-Mayer, D.E., Hunt, C.E., Levenson, S.M., Corwin, M.J.

and Collaborative Home Infant Monitoring Evaluation. (1995) Assessment of compliance with home cardiorespiratory monitoring in infants at risk of sudden death syndrome. *Journal of Pediatrics* **127**, 384–388.

Stevens-Simon, C., O'Connor, P. and Basford, K. (1994) Incentives enhance postpartum compliance among adolescent prenatal patients. *Journal of Adolescent Health* **15**, 396–399.

St. Clair, P.A. and Anderson, N.A. (1989) Social network advice during pregnancy: Myths, misinformation, and sound counsel. *Birth: Issues in Perinatal Care and Education* **16**, 103–107.

St. Clair, P.A., Smeriglio, V.L., Alexander, C.A., Connell, F.A. and Niebyl, J.R. (1990) Situational and financial barriers to prenatal care in a sample of low-income, inner city women. *Public Health Reports* **105**, 264–267.

Thompson, A.M. (1993) If you are pregnant and smoke admission to hospital may damage your baby's health. *Journal of Clinical Nursing* **2**, 111–120.

Thornton, J.G., Hewison, J., Lilford, R.J. and Vail, A. (1995) A randomised trial of three methods of giving information aboutprenatal testing. *British Medical Journal* **311**, 1127–1130 .

Tinsley, B.J., Trupin, S.R., Owens, L. and Boyum, L.A. (1993) The significance of women's pregnancy related locus of control beliefs for adherence to recommended prenatal health regimens and pregnancy outcomes. *Journal of Reproductive and Infant Psychology* **11**, 97–102.

Toomey, B. (1985) *Factors related to early entry into prenatal care.* Ohio Department of Public Health. Columbus: Bureau of Maternal and Child Health.

Towler, J. and Fairbairn, G. (1988) Choice in childbirth. In G. Fairburn.and S. Fairburn.(eds) *Ethical issues in caring* Avebury.

Tucker, J.S., Hall, M.H., Howie, P.W., Reid, M.E., Barbour, R.S., du Florey, C. and McIlwaine, G.M. (1996) Should obstetricians see women with normal pregnancies: a multi-centre randomised controlled trial of routine antenatal care by general practitioners and midwives compared with shared care led by obstetricians. *British Medical Journal* **312**, 554–559.

Valbø, A., Thelle, D.S. and Kolås, T. (1996) Smoking cessation in pregnancy: a multicomponent intervention study. *Journal of Maternal-Fetal Investigation,* **6**, 3–8.

Wallon, M., Grandilhon, F. Payron, F. and Mojon, M. (1994) Toxoplasmosis in pregnancy. *Lancet* **344,** 541.

Waterson, E.J. and Murray-Lyon, I.M. (1990) Preventing fetal alcohol effects: a trial of three methods of giving information in the natenatal clinic. *Health Education Research* **5,** 53–62.

Wilde, J. (1989) Caesarean section: whose choice and for whom? In G.R. Dunstan and E.A. Shinebourne (eds) *Doctors' decisions: ethical conflicts in medical practice.* Oxford, Oxford University Press.

Windsor, R. Warner, K. and Cutter, G. (1988) A cost-effectiveness analysis of self-help smoking cessation methods for pregnant women. *Public Health Reports,* **103,** 83–89.

Windsor, R.A., Lowe, J.B., Perkins, L.L., Smith-Yoder, D., Artz, L., Crawford, M., Amburgy, K. and Boyd, N.R. (1993) Health education for pregnant smokers: its behavioral impact and cost benefit. *American Journal of Public Health,* **83,** 201–206.

World Health Organisation. (1989) *Protecting, promoting and supporting breastfeeding: The special role of maternity services.* Geneva:WHO/UNICEF.

Wright, A., Rice, S. and Wells, S. (1996) Changing hospital practices to increase the duration of breast feeding. *Pediatrics,* **97 (5),** 669–675.

Yoong, A.F.E., Lim, J., Hudson, C.N. and Chard, T. (1992) Audit of compliance with antenatal protocols. *British Medical Journal,* **305,** 1184–1186.

Zarzycki, W., Chalupczak, R., Zarzycka, B., Jakubczyk, D. and Kinalska, I. (1994) Acceptance and subjective evaluation of intensive insulin therapy and an educational program by pregnant women with insulin dependent diabetes. *Przegl-Lek* **51,** 339–342.

Zeanah, M. and Schlosser, S.P. (1993) Adherence to ACOG guidelines on exercise during pregnancy: effect on pregnancy outcome. *Journal of Obstetric, Gynecological and Neonatal Nursing* **22,** 329–335.

Zuckerman, B., Amaro, H., Bauchner, H. and Cabral, H. (1989) Depressive symptoms during pregnancy: Relationship to poor health behaviors. *American Journal of Obstetrics and Gynecology* **160,** 1107–1111.

9

Adherence and the Elderly

James C. McElnay and C. Rosaleen McCallion

THE AGEING PROCESS

There are currently over 57 million people resident in the UK. The relative proportion of elderly people (aged 65 years or over) in this population has increased considerably and the proportion aged over 80 years shows an even more dramatic rise. In the UK in 1971, 10.9% of the population were aged between 65 and 79 with 2.3% over 80. The projected percentages for 2001 are 11.4% and 4.3% respectively (Key data, 1995). These trends are also reflected in other European countries. In the USA, 12.6% of the population were aged 65 or over in 1990. This proportion is expected to rise to 22.9% by the year 2050 with the over 85 year old group increasing by a factor of 3.9 in this time scale (Kane, Ouslander and Abrass, 1994). It has been estimated that 85% of people over the age of 65 years suffer from one or more chronic illnesses and up to 87% of this latter group are prescribed at least one medication for their condition. In fact, 30–40% of all National Health Service prescriptions written in Britain are for elderly patients (who make up around 15% of the total population).

Ageing has been defined " ... as a process that converts healthy adults into frail ones, with diminished reserves in most physiological systems and an exponentially increasing vulnerability to most diseases and death" (Miller, 1994). It is difficult to distinguish between what constitutes natural ageing and what constitutes accelerated ageing due to disease processes among elderly patients.

Cross-sectional studies, comparing findings in elderly people with those in younger people, have helped to highlight changes associated with the ageing process. In certain organs, such as the kidneys, a subgroup of people appear to experience a gradual decline in function over time, roughly a 1% loss in function per year starting around the age of 30, while in others function remains constant well into old age (Kane *et al.*, 1994). Such changes will obviously have a profound effect on drugs which are dependent on the kidney for elimination. Age-related changes in the eye including decreased pupil size and growth of the lens leads to decreased accommodation, acuity, colour sensitivity and depth of perception (Kane *et al.*, 1994) which can lead to difficulties for elderly people in distinguishing between tablets which look similar.

It is important to note that ageing is a gradual process, with many changes commencing in early adulthood, although most do not manifest themselves until later life. In addition, everyone does not age at the same rate or in the same way. Frequently the process of ageing only becomes apparent when a particular organ is subjected to external stress, for example, elderly people may often have a normal resting pulse but cannot sufficiently increase cardiac output to cope with exercise. In this chapter, factors known to influence adherence of elderly people to prescribed medications are considered.

THE AGEING PROCESS AND DRUG ACTION (PHARMACODYNAMICS)

It is necessary to understand how the effect of ageing alters drug handling and drug action in elderly people in order to appreciate how these changes may influence adherence in this subgroup of the population. The pharmacodynamics of a drug relates to the type, intensity, and duration of effect of a given concentration of a drug at the site of action. There is good evidence that age-related changes occur with this parameter. Such effects relate either to changes in homeostatic reserve or to changes in specific receptors or target sites. Tessier (1993) has summarised the main clinically significant age-related changes in drug pharmacodynamics (Table 1).

Table 1 Some, clinically significant, age-related changes in pharmacodynamic responses in elderly patients (after Tessier, 1993)

Adverse clinical event	Drug	Age-related mechanism of change
Falls	Sedation-hypnotics Antihypertensives, Tricylic antidepressants, Neuroleptics, Diuretics	Impaired mechanism of maintaining postural control, Vasodilation Alpha-adrenergic blockade, Reduced baroreceptor activity, Volume depletion
Reduced intestinal motility, constipation, impaction, intestinal obstruction	Anticholinergics, Tricyclic antidepressants, Antihistamines	Anticholinergic effects enhanced
Disorientation, Delirium, Psychosis	Anticholinergics, Tricyclic antidepressants, Antihistamines, Benzodiazepines Amphetamines, Theophylline Beta-Agonists, levodopa	Anticholinergic effects enhanced Increased benzodiazepine receptor sensitivity, CNS stimulation
Urinary incontinence	Diuretics Anticholinergics, Tricyclic antidepressants, Antihistamines	Bladder filling exceeds capacity, Urinary outflow obstruction (especially males with BPH)
Oedema, worsening CSF	Corticosteroids, Saline laxatives/enemas	Sodium retention
Tardive dyskinesia Exptrapyramidal symptoms Symptoms	Neuroleptics, Metoclopramide	Depletion of CNS dopamine

BPH = benign prostatic hypertrophy CNS = central nervous system

THE AGEING PROCESS AND DRUG HANDLING (PHARMACOKINETICS)

Age-related changes in pharmacokinetics can lead to different drug responses in the elderly compared with younger adults. Table 2 summarises the main clinically significant age-related changes in drug handling. These changes can result in increased toxicity of drugs in elderly patients compared to younger patients unless appropriate dosage adjustments are performed. For example, due to decreased renal function (Table 2), clearance of many drugs including atenolol (cardio-selective ß-blocker) (Barber *et al.*, 1980) and digoxin (cardiac glycoside) (Cusack *et al.*, 1979) markedly declines. Thus age-related decreases in the terminal elimination (the final step involved in the removal of drugs from the body) of these drugs occurs. To avoid drug accumulation and resultant toxic effects, dosage adjustments need to be carried out (either decreased unit dose or increased dosage interval).

Table 2 Summary of age-related changes in pharmacokinetics

Factor	Physiological change in elderly patients	References
Absorption	decreased gastric acid secretion leading to decreased gastric acidity decreased pancreatic lipase activity decreased gastric emptying and gastrointestinal motility decreased gastric blood flow less effective active drug transport mechanisms atrophy of gastrointestinal mucosa decreased activity of intestinal and hepatic enzymes	Iber *et al.*, 1994; Bender, 1965; Warren, 1978; Farinati *et al.*, 1993
Distribution	Plasma albumin decreases plasma globulin increases plasma albumin concentrations lower in "sick" elderly	Greenblatt, 1979; Wallace *et al.*, 1976, Gunashera *et al.*, 1996
Elimination **-liver**	decreased liver size decreased liver blood flow decreased activity of microsomal P450	Woodhouse and James, 1990; Parker *et al.*, 1995; O'Malley *et al.*, 1971; Vestal *et al.*, 1975
-kidneys	decreased kidney sise decreased renal blood flow decreased glomerular filtration rate decreased number of nephrons decreased ability to conserve absorbed phosphate and acidify the urine	Davies and Shock, 1950; Miller *et al.*, 1952; Belmin *et al.*, 1994

THE INFLUENCE OF AGE-RELATED CHANGES IN PHARMACODYNAMICS AND PHARMACOKINETICS ON ADHERENCE

Many of the adverse clinical events highlighted in Table 1 may well contribute to adherence problems in elderly patients. For example, the enhancement of anticholinergic effects of many drugs such as the tricyclic antidepressants, may result in disorientation, delirium and psychosis in an elderly person (Table 1). Impaired cognitive function is known to be a significant factor in non-adherence in elderly patients (Norell, 1985; Conn *et al.*, 1994). In a survey of 315 elderly patients admitted to hospital, in those whose admission was judged to be due to non-adherence as either a definite/probable or contributing factor (n=21), forgetfulness was cited by 25% and confusion by 10% as the main cause of non-adherence (Col *et al.*, 1990). In this latter study the main cause of non-adherence was due to unpleasant side-effects (35%). Such effects are largely due to the alterations in pharmacokinetics and pharmacodynamics (Tables 1 and 2). For example, drugs with a narrow therapeutic index (narrow range between minimum therapeutic and minimum toxic serum concentrations), that are cleared via the kidneys, are more likely to cause adverse drug reactions (ADRs) in elderly patients, due to the age-related changes in the kidneys highlighted in Table 2. Digoxin has been identified as one of the most likely to cause ADRs resulting in hospitalisation (Miller, 1974; Caranasos *et al.*, 1974; McKenny and Harrison, 1976; Levy *et al.*, 1980; McElnay *et al.*, 1997). ADRs are known to account for up to 31% of hospital admissions of elderly people world-wide (Williamson and Chopin, 1980; Popplewell and Henschke, 1982; Grymonpre *et al.*, 1988; Col *et al.*, 1990; Smuker and Kontak, 1990; Jackson *et al.*, 1992; Lindley *et al.*, 1992; Nicolson *et al.*, 1994; Cunningham *et al.*, 1994; McElnay *et al.*, 1997).

INTENTIONAL NON-ADHERENCE

In a study conducted by Col *et al.* (1990), discussed earlier, it was also noted that, from a total of 103 patients who reported a history of non-adherence within the previous year, in 54% of the cases non-adherence was intentional. Of these patients 12.5% did not think that the drug was necessary and 9.4% stated that they disliked taking medicine. The fact that non-adherence to medical treatment in the elderly may well be intentional, has also been highlighted in other studies. Cooper *et al.* (1982) in a survey of 111 non-institutionalised elderly patients (aged 60 or over) found that 43% were non-adherent to the instructions on the container label to at least one prescribed medication and in 70% of cases this non-adherence was intentional. In most cases the patient did not believe that the medication was necessary. In a similar study by Chryssidis *et al.* (1982), in Australia, some patients expressed a "fear of poisoning". In light of the common age-related adverse clinical events (Table 1) such as urinary incontinence with diuretics, falls with hypnotics and constipation, impaction or intestinal obstruction with anticholinergics, tricyclics and antihistamines, these findings are not surprising. Gryfe and Gryfe (1984) note that patients who had age-related difficulties with urination found genitourinary related drug side-effects severe enough to cause them to stop taking the medication. Disturbed sleep and anticholinergic reactions were mentioned by elderly patients as a reason for discontinuing medication or for not following prescribed regimens. It has been suggested that elderly patients, sometimes wisely, reject some of the medications that are prescribed for them - perhaps the incidence of ADRs in the elderly population would dramatically increase if the patients took all the medicines they receive! Although this statement is probably true, the solution is to ensure adherence in patients and reduce dosage or number of drugs prescribed. In this way healthcare providers will obtain more definitive information from patient monitoring of the effectiveness of the medicines the patient is taking.

It is notable that the people who constitute today's elderly population were mostly born in the 1920s and grew up in an era before the widespread availability of drugs for both life-threatening as well as self-limiting conditions. This unfamiliarity with medicines may well be a contributing factor to the suspicions held by this generation with regard to medical treatments. It will be interesting to see if the elderly population of twenty or thirty year's time, born in the 1950s and 1960s exhibit similar sentiments.

NUMBER OF MEDICATIONS AND ADHERENCE

In general, elderly patients take more medication than their younger counterparts. Studies have shown that while persons over 65 years of age represent about 15% of the population in the UK, they receive 39% of the prescription items dispensed (Cartwright, 1990). The mean number of drugs prescribed for an elderly person in the UK is said to be 2–3 in the community (Nolan and O'Malley, 1988), around 5 in hospital (Nolan and O'Malley, 1988) and around 3 in nursing homes (Hatton, 1990; Primrose *et al.*, 1987). Stewart (1990) reported that the average patient in the USA (under 65 years old) receives 4.3 new and refill prescriptions per annum compared with 10.7 for patients over 65 years of age. Within the elderly population the number of non-prescribed drugs also increases with age. In the USA, among patients 65–69 years old, 66% use non-prescribed drugs, while for the above 85–years old, 69.2% use non-prescribed drugs (Gryfe and Gryfe, 1984). Although multiple disease states undoubtedly contribute to the high numbers of drugs prescribed to this section of the community, the problem of a degree of unnecessary and excessive prescribing has been recognised for many years. A study of 200 long-stay psychiatric patients in a London hospital, published in 1976, found that 50% were receiving unnecessary and excessive psychotropic drugs (Fotrell *et al.*, 1976).

In a more recent study examining 416 successive admissions of elderly patients to a teaching hospital in the UK, a total of 175 drugs from 113 admissions were discontinued on or shortly after admission because they were deemed unnecessary. This study also revealed that 48 patients were taking 51 drugs with absolute contraindications (Lindley *et al.*, 1992). The link between numbers of medications and adherence has been frequently highlighted in the literature. For example, in a study in England, by Brooke and Mukherjee (1988) the percentage of elderly patients taking more than 50% of their drug items correctly decreased with an increase in the number of items taken from approximately 60% for up to three drugs down to zero for eight to eleven items (Figure 1). Another study on elderly patients' adherence patterns, after discharge from hospital, revealed a fifteen fold increase in dosage errors when the number of prescribed drugs increased from one to four (Parkin *et al.*, 1976).

In addition, a link between adverse drug reactions and numbers of medications has been highlighted in many studies (Smith *et al.*, 1966; Hurwitz, 1969; Kellaway and McCrae 1973; Nolan and O'Malley, 1989). In most studies the incidence of ADRs increases with the number of drugs taken and in fact this relationship would appear to be exponential rather than linear (Stewart and Cooper, 1994). The association between ADRs and non-adherence has been described earlier.

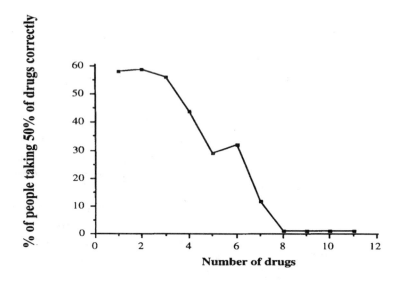

FIGURE 1   The relationship between the percentage of people taking more than 50% of their drug items correctly and the number of drugs taken (after Brook and Mukherjee, 1988).

REGIMEN COMPLEXITY AND ADHERENCE

The greater the complexity of drug dosage regimens the more likely the patient is to make administration errors. This has been clearly demonstrated by Pullar *et al.* in their study (not restricted to elderly patients) published in 1988. They compared adherence to low dose phenobarbitone tablets (phenobarbitone used as a marker of adherence rather than for pharmacological activity) prescribed to be taken as a daily, twice daily or three times a day dosage in a group of 179 patients, with Non Insulin Dependent Diabetes, randomly allocated to one of the three dosing groups. The mean ages of patients in the three groups were 64.9, 63.5 and 63.6 years respectively. Analysis of blood levels of phenobarbitone suggested similar adherence with once and twice daily dosing, with both being better than three times a day regimens (Pullar *et al.*, 1988). In a more recent longitudinal cross-sectional survey of 157 elderly patients (aged 70 years or over) in Amsterdam, 22% of prescribed drugs were not used as directed. Drug regimens of twice daily and more than twice daily had odds ratios (95% confidence intervals) of 4.5 (1.2–12) and 4.2 (1.7–11) respectively for non-adherence (measured via interviews and pharmacy records) compared to once daily regimens (Lau *et al.,* 1996). In this study, drug regimens of twice a day or more were therefore four times more likely to lead to non-adherence than once daily regimens in the population studied.

TYPE OF MEDICATION AND ADHERENCE

The type of medication prescribed also influences adherence patterns. For example, one study has shown that cardiac and anti-diabetic drugs have the highest adherence rates (80–90%). Antihypertensives and diuretics came next (60–70%), with relatively low adherence rates for drugs such as sedatives, hypnotics, analgesics and antacids (40–50%) (Macdonald and Macdonald, 1982). Cooper *et al.* (1982), found a rate of 60% non-adherence with musculoskeletal drugs, 35% with antibiotics, and 18% with gastro-intestinal drugs.

A recent multivariate analytical study on self-reported medication non-adherence among a population of 512 elderly patients (aged 65 or over) in Northern Ireland confirmed variations in adherence with different pharmacological drug classes. For example, patients who were prescribed benzodiazepines were significantly more likely to report non-adherence while those prescribed diuretics were significantly less likely to report non-adherence to medication regimens. Interestingly, this study also implicated an increased usage of non-prescription medications with non-adherence to prescribed treatment regimens (McElnay *et al.*, 1996b). These findings are discussed in more detail in the section describing modelling of adherence behaviour.

EFFECT OF PATIENT KNOWLEDGE OF DRUG PURPOSE AND DISEASE STATE ON ADHERENCE

The influence of patient knowledge about disease and treatments on adherence in the elderly is conflicting. German *et al.* (1982) found that although knowledge of disease processes and medication purpose were significantly lower for elderly patients, adherence was similar in both young and old patients. Hussey (1994), examined medication knowledge and adherence among the elderly by using a colour-coded method, which was designed to tailor the medication regimen to the person's daily schedule. In this latter study, a control group received verbal teaching only, whereas the intervention group received verbal teaching and the colour-coded medication schedule. Although knowledge increased significantly in both groups, adherence to the medication schedule increased only in the intervention group. These results suggest that knowledge of the medication regimen does not guarantee adherence. The fact that elderly patients have less knowledge, but adhere as readily as younger patients, suggests that many elderly patients take their medication without understanding the reason why (Smith and Andrews, 1983).

TYPES OF PACKAGING/CONTAINERS AND ADHERENCE

There is a diminution of tactile sensations resulting in difficulty with fine muscle control in tasks requiring eye-hand co-ordination in elderly people. Patient adherence may be adversely affected, for example, by elderly patients with diabetes attempting to manipulate an insulin syringe, or by the difficulty with fractional dosage (less than one tablet as a single dose) when a elderly patient with arthritic hands is unable to split tablets (Gryfe and Gryfe, 1984).

Elderly patients are aware of problems associated with their medication containers, but are unaware of the methods available to overcome the difficulty in opening and closing them. Robbins and Jahingen (1984) in their study of the push down and turn type of child-resistant container, observed that one in four of the patients (average age 86 years) were unable to open the container. In a further elderly patient study conducted by Murray *et al.* (1993), 31 elderly (over 60 years) outpatients (each taking three or more prescribed medications) were randomly assigned to one of three groups. Group one (n=12) had no change in dosing or packing of their medicines (control), group two (n=10) had a change in their dosing regimens to twice a day but the medication packaging remained unchanged, while group three (n=9) had a change in their dose to twice daily as well as a change in the medication packaging to unit-dose packaging (each dose individually sealed in a single unit). Adherence was significantly better in group three than in the other two groups (which were not significantly different from each other) indicating the importance of the type of packaging in adherence among elderly people. More recently, Nikolaus *et al.* (1996) in a study on 119 elderly patients in hospital and at home found that 10.1% failed to open at least one of their medication containers.

THE EFFECT OF VISUAL ACUITY ON ADHERENCE

The lens of the eye tends to yellow with age. This can lead to problems with glare and differentiating between blue and green becomes more difficult (Hurd and Blevins, 1984). This may result in difficulties in distinguishing between medicines of similar appearance. Problems in reading container labels undoubtedly also influences adherence. In one study, 60% of elderly patients were found to have problems reading medication labels (Zuccollo and Liddel, 1985).

COPING MECHANISMS AND THEIR EFFECT ON ADHERENCE

It is important to note that ageing encompasses much more than simply a set of biological changes and although these changes play an important role in adherence to medications, they are not the only factors. The elderly, as pointed out by Kane *et al.* (1994), rather than being viewed as victims, should be looked upon as survivors. In the face of loss and limitation most elderly patients develop coping mechanisms. Often these adaptive techniques for coping with disability and disease play an important role in adherence to medical treatment. For example, a patient with hearing impairment may talk a great deal to hide the problem and therefore may not receive adequate information on their medication. Patients may simply deny or ignore the fact that they have a particular disease and therefore do not take their medication because they believe that they do not need it. This latter type of coping strategy has been implicated in intentional non-adherence.

Another coping mechanism may involve the cost of drugs. Clinical experience in the USA, suggests that elderly patients on limited incomes sometimes make strategic decisions about which medications they can afford and which ones they cannot (Salzmann, 1995). For example, in the survey conducted by Col *et al.* (1990) referred to earlier in this chapter, cost was the reason given for non-adherence by 10% of patients. In addition, patients who were not covered by medical insurance were more likely to be non-adherent in their study.

MODELLING OF ADHERENCE TO MEDICAL TREATMENT

How the many factors, known to influence adherence in elderly people, work in combination to influence adherence in a given individual is, as yet, not clear. Many models and theories have been proposed and research is ongoing in this area. A number of researchers have attempted to produce regression models for patient adherence to medical treatment for all ages of patients. Most of these have involved linear regression. For example, incorporation of the Theory of Reasoned Action (Ajzen and Fishbein, 1980) into the Health Belief Model (Rosenstock, 1966) (one of the first models used to explain adherence) only accounted for 29% of the variance in adherence between individual patients (Ried and Christensen, 1988). In this latter study the Health Belief Model only accounted for 10% of the variability. Other models incorporating perceived strengths of the Health Belief Model together with a spectrum of other approaches such as the Health Decision Model (Eraker *et al.*, 1984), Health Locus of Control models (Nagy and Wolf, 1984) and Rotter's Social Learning Theory (Schlenk and Hart, 1984) have produced inconsistent results.

Coons *et al.* (1994), developed a logistic regression model for self-reported non-adherence (defined as taking medications more or less often than prescribed in the month preceding the interview) from data obtained in 785 patients aged over 55 years of whom 165 reported non-adherence. They found non-adherence to be significantly associated ($p < 0.05$) with higher socio-economic status, greater numbers of medications and higher psychological stress. The types of medications taken by the patients were not entered into the model and no information on the sensitivity or specificity of the model was reported.

In a similar cross-sectional study by Lau *et al.* (1996) on 157 community-dwelling elderly patients (aged 70 years or over), non-adherence (defined as not using drugs according to the prescribed instructions) was found to be related to the knowledge of the purpose of a drug, the complexity of the drug regimen and the type of prescriber (specialist versus general practitioner). When the knowledge of the purpose of a drug decreased, non-adherence increased. The authors pointed out that they were unsure if the lack of knowledge led to poorer adherence or if non-adherence led to less knowledge of drug purpose. There was also an increased risk of non-adherence with a dosage regimen involving drug administration of two or more times a day, as discussed previously. Finally, adherence was found to be much higher when the drug was prescribed by a specialist compared to a general practitioner. This study did not confirm the association of non-adherence with increased numbers of drugs and again the types of medications were not investigated. No information on the sensitivity or specificity of the model was given (Lau *et al.*, 1996).

Recently, a logistic regression model for self-reported non-adherence (taking less or more than the prescribed amount of medication) to medication treatment in 512 elderly patients (aged 65 years or more) in Northern Ireland, had an overall predictive accuracy of 81% (McElnay *et al.*, 1996b). Five variables were shown to significantly influence self-reported non-adherence to prescribed medications in the population studied. Elderly patients who took two or more non-prescription drugs (odds ratio, OR = 3.2), or who were prescribed bronchodilators (OR = 2.4), benzodiazepines (OR=2.8) or who took their medications independently (OR = 2.6) were significantly more likely to report non-adherence than their counterparts. Conversely, elderly patients who were prescribed diuretics (OR = 2.9) were significantly more likely to report-adherence to their medication regimens. The most strongly associated risk factor for self-reported non-adherence in the model was taking more than one non-prescribed medication. Patients with this risk factor were over 3.2 times more likely to report non-adherence than patients who took one or no non-prescription drugs. A further recent study carried out on self-medication habits of elderly people in Northern Ireland revealed that almost one quarter of those interviewed (n= 515) were already taking a prescribed medication for which the non-prescribed drug was requested (McElnay and

McCallion, 1996). The authors suggested that these patients may have been taking a non-prescribed drug in preference to their prescribed medications which could be indicative of dissatisfaction with the expected outcome of prescribed medicines. In fact, the self-medication study indicated that one third of elderly patients who took both prescribed and non-prescription medicines to treat the same conditions stated that they did so to supplement therapy. A further one quarter of these patients stated that they self-treated because they considered their prescribed therapy to be ineffective (McElnay and McCallion, 1996).

The model described above indicated that elderly patients who took diuretics were almost three times more likely to report good adherence compared to elderly patients who did not take diuretics . These results add weight to the findings of the SHEP (Systolic Hypertension in the Elderly Program) pilot study which provided evidence, based on two objective measures of adherence, namely pill-counts and urine tests, as well as self-reported data, that high levels of adherence occur with antihypertensive treatments among the elderly (Black *et al.*, 1987). On the other hand, patients who were prescribed bronchodilators were shown to be 2.4 times more likely to report non-adherence than patients who did not. These findings are in agreement with the results of others (Rand and Wise, 1994; Horn *et al.*, 1990; Tettersell, 1993). Adverse effects of benzodiazepines in the elderly have been documented frequently in the literature, for example, studies have shown that elderly people are more sensitive to the sedative effects of diazepam after short-term administration than younger adults (Montamat *et al.*, 1989). The benzodiazepines, particularly those with longer half-lives, have been implicated as one of the drug classes associated with falls leading to hip fracture in elderly patients (Gales and Menard, 1995; Cummings *et al.*, 1995). Excessive drowsiness, confusion and ataxia, are the most commonly reported adverse drug reactions to the longer acting benzodiazepines such as flurazepam (Gurwitz and Avorn, 1991). Such adverse effects are likely to decrease adherence to medication regimens.

The model described was much more successful at predicting self-reported adherence (specificity = 89%) than non-adherence (sensitivity = 33%) to treatment in the elderly. This may well be a reflection of the problems associated with the use of interviews as a technique to assess adherence since, although self-reporting is the simplest indirect method, it is adversely affected by favourable bias (patients say that they are adherent when they are not) and forgetfulness on the part of the patient. Although our understanding of adherence to treatment in the elderly continues to improve, a strong model to predict those patients who will be non-adherent still does not exist. This may be due in part to the wide variety of techniques employed to assess adherence, discussed in detail by Myers and Midence, Chapter 1. Each method has specific limitations, and none is totally reliable.

METHODS TO IMPROVE MEDICATION ADHERENCE IN ELDERLY PATIENTS

In the absence of an accurate predictor of non-adherent patients, all (elderly) patients should be considered to be potential non-adherers to medical treatment. The many risk factors highlighted in the previous sections should be addressed when formulating a strategy to optimise adherence.

Simplification of Dosage Regimen

Where possible we should aim for a reduction in the numbers of drugs prescribed and a simplification of the treatment regimen. As a result of a study, not restricted to elderly patients, in which adherence was shown to improve when regimens were decreased from three times a day to once daily, it was suggested that: "probably the simplest and single most important action that health-care providers can take to improve compliance (adherence) is to select medications that permit the lowest daily dose frequency possible" (Eisen *et al.*, 1990). Where a regimen cannot be simplified by a reduction in the frequency of dosing, it may be possible to introduce modification by "prioritising" it, for example, by emphasising the necessity of adherence to particularly critical aspects of treatment; or by minimising the effects of forgetfulness and inconvenience by matching the regimen to regular activities carried out by the patient; or by implementing the regimen gradually, breaking the treatment plan into less complex stages that can be introduced sequentially (Eraker *et al.*, 1984). For patients with chronic conditions, such as diabetes, Eraker *et al.* (1984) suggest that the perception of short-term therapy can be achieved by arranging follow-up visits with the patient in quick succession when progress is apparent. This provides the patient with a sense of the importance of the treatment and a feeling of accomplishment. The availability of slow release or combination dosage forms may help in regimen simplification.

Dosage Forms

Slow release dosage forms are available for many short half-life drugs (drugs which remain in the blood at high enough concentrations to exert a therapeutic effect for only a short time). This permits less frequent administration and therefore aids adherence, for example, many types of slow-release forms of calcium channel blockers are now available. Alternatively a combination dosage form such as a non-steroidal anti-inflammatory and gastroprotective agent can be used to decrease the number of formulations to be administered daily. Such approaches are particularly pertinent to the elderly in order to decrease regimen complexity.

Drug-Forgiveness

The term drug-forgiveness has been recently introduced to apply to "...drugs in the same pharmacological class which may differ in their ability to maintain pharmacological and/or therapeutic action in the face of omitted doses" (Urquhart, 1994). Research into the level of "forgiveness" of individual drugs is fairly new (Meredith and Elliott, 1994) but consideration of this phenomenon may prove useful in the treatment of patients who have a poor record of adherence to medication regimens, particularly where forgetfulness is a problem.

Oral Communication and Counselling

Salzmann (1995) suggests that methods to improve adherence with medical treatments should begin by examining communication between the elderly patient and their physician since good communication should help the patient understand their illness, the importance of their medications, potential drug interactions and the limitations of a particular treatment. This equally applies to other health-care professions. Several studies have looked at the effect of counselling on adherence. While many of these studies indicate that one-to-one counselling appears to improve adherence in all age-groups (Hussar, 1985; Hecht, 1974; Nessman *et al.*, 1980; Zismer *et al.*, 1982), not all research supports these findings. It has been shown, for example, in elderly patients, while knowledge of treatments may improve with verbal communication, adherence does not necessarily improve (Hussey, 1994). This has been discussed in more detail in a previous section.

Written Communication

Health-care providers should consider the possibility that some elderly patients may have a limited attention span and only hear parts of an oral conversation (Salzmann, 1995). The coping strategies discussed earlier may also play a role here. It is therefore important to back up all oral communications with clear written instructions. The use of written instructions and charts, in addition to verbal information, has been shown to be helpful (Lamy *et al.*, 1992; Coe *et al.*, 1984) in improving adherence. Vague instructions such as "take as directed" or instructions printed in small fonts have been shown to be associated with non-adherence in the elderly (Lamy *et al.*, 1992; Zuccollo and Liddel, 1985). Misinterpretation of written instructions have, however, been highlighted. For example, Eraker *et al.* (1984) noted that in one study, the direction "Every six hours" was interpreted correctly by only 36% of patients (over a range of age-groups) studied. One report published more recently involved an elderly patient (68 year old male) who was prescribed dihydrocodeine (a narcotic analgesic) with the labelled instruction "ONE TO BE TAKEN, 6 to 8 hourly". The patient took one tablet every ten minutes, and two hours later, having taken twelve tablets, was admitted to the casualty department of a local hospital (Anon, 1993). The need to use clear instructions is highlighted by this example. In another study it was shown that patients often misinterpreted common medical words (Gibbs *et al.*, 1987). The extent of misinterpretation is depicted in figure 2. In a meta-analysis of articles

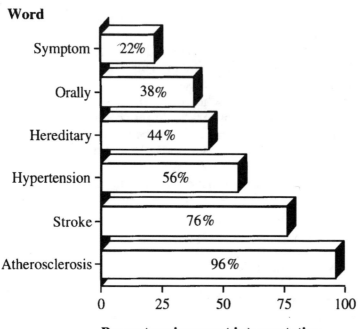

Word

Percentage incorrect interpretation

FIGURE 2   Misunderstanding of common medical words (adapted from Gibbs *et al.*, 1987)

written between 1961 and 1984 on intervention strategies, not restricted to elderly people, written interventions were shown to produce an increase in knowledge and a decrease in dosing errors (Mullen *et al.*, 1985). The meta-analysis also revealed that patient information leaflets (PILs) exert only a limited effect on increasing knowledge or decreasing medication errors. Recent research has indicated that many PILs and patient brochures are not written in language easily understood by the lay-person (Gibbs *et al.*, 1987; Bradley *et al.*, 1994). For a review on written information see Raynor, Chapter 4.

Adherence Packs and Aids

An adherence package has been defined as a pre-packaged unit that provides the patient with one treatment cycle of their medication in a ready-to-use package. In the UK, increasingly tablets and capsules are being packaged in calendar blister packs. While these have been shown to be beneficial in younger age-groups, elderly people, particularly those with manual dexterity problems, may have difficulty opening blister packs and this fact should be borne in mind.

Several additional medication adherence devices have been developed to aid patients in self-administration by organising the dosage regimens and enabling the patient to monitor administration. They have been shown to significantly improve adherence to medication treatments in elderly patients particularly where forgetfulness is a problem or where patients are confused by complex regimens (Martin and Mead, 1982; Wong and Norman, 1987; Ware and Holford, 1991). Two of the most popular and commonly used aids for oral medications are the Medi-dose® and Dosett® systems which both consist of twenty-eight compartments – four compartments for different time-periods (e.g. morning, noon, evening and bed-time) for each day of the week (Rivers, 1992). Many other devices, such as the Prescript TimeCap® (a container cap with a modified alarm clock), are also commercially available. Such devices can be set for the day and hour when the medicine is to be taken, including several dosing times during the day. An audio signal bleeps to alert the patient when the preset time is reached and once the dose is removed from the container the device is reset automatically for the next preset time. A survey of all community pharmacists (n=520) in Northern Ireland, conducted by McElnay and Thompson in 1992, showed that the majority (93.9%) of respondents (n=346) would be willing to identify non-adherent elderly patients who regularly attended their pharmacy and to dispense their medications into a adherence system. Of the respondents, however, 36.1% indicated that they would only be willing to provide this service if they were paid for doing so. The length of time taken to dispense medications into a range of adherence aids was highlighted as a potential drawback of providing such a service with mean times to fill various adherence aids with a week's supply of drugs from a standard three item prescription ranging from 1 minute 45 seconds for the Dosett® up to 9 minutes 59 seconds for the Supercel® pouch card (a system designed by hospital pharmacists in Salford, UK).

Accurate administration of eye-drops is particularly important when treating glaucoma, a not uncommon condition in elderly patients. A number of devices such as Auto-Drop®, Easidrop® and Opticare® are available to help with aiming the drop. The

Opticare® devise also aids squeezing the eye-drop bottle (Rivers, 1992). A range of other devices are available for use with inhalers, where co-ordination of firing the dose and inhaling can be particularly problematic in elderly patients.

Combination of Approaches

Probably the best way to improve adherence in elderly patients is to use a combination of the techniques discussed. One study looked at the effectiveness of verbal instructions alone, verbal plus written instructions, verbal plus a medication reminder calendar and verbal plus a medication reminder package, in a group of ambulatory elderly (aged over 60 years) cardiovascular patients using one or more medications. The intervention that combined oral instructions plus the medication reminder package was superior to controls in improving self-reported adherence (Ascione and Shimp, 1984). In a more recent study on 88 elderly patients discharged to their own homes, a hospital based multi-faceted self-medication programme was shown to significantly improve adherence to treatments as well as improve knowledge of drug purpose in the intervention group, assessed ten days after discharge. The self-medication programme involved rationalisation of their medications, an assessment of patients understanding of their medications, their ability to read labels, their ability to open containers, plus a reminder chart, completed by a pharmacist, who also discussed medicines with each patient during their hospital stay. The intervention (self-medication programme) patients were then given increased responsibility for taking their own medicines while in hospital (Lowe *et al.*, 1995).

The pharmaceutical industry has applied this "combination" approach to packaging. In the USA in 1988, a then unique type of packaging called a "MACPAC" was released. This pack consisted of blister packaging plus reminder aids plus an information leaflet. The MACPAC box contained seven blister-pack cards each containing four daily doses of Macrodantin (nitrofurantoin). The doses were labelled "breakfast", "lunch", "dinner" and "bedtime" to help patients to remember to take the medication at the correct time and to see if they had missed a dose. A reminder card (reminding the patient of the importance of completing the course) was placed between the third and fourth medication cards and the pack also

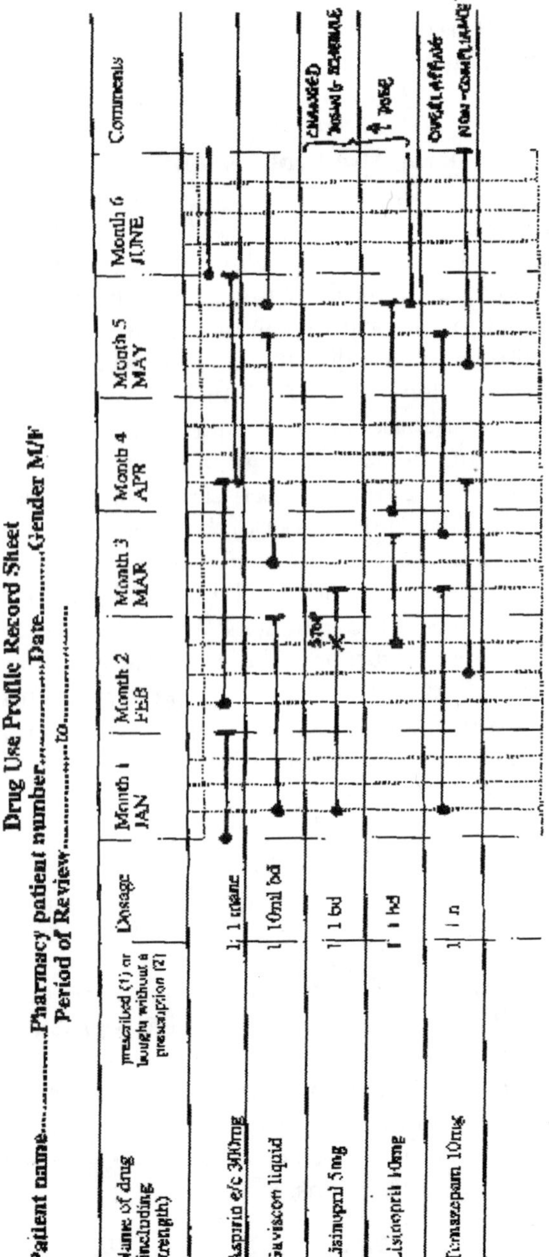

Initially developed by Professor A. G. Forsius, Department of Pharmacy, University of Utrecht and further refined by Dr J.W.F. van Mil, Working Group on Social Pharmacy and Epidemiology, University of Groningen.

FIGURE 3 Example of drug use profile chart

contained an information booklet on urinary tract infections. Today, several other products, particularly those for hormone replacement therapy, have adopted a similar approach.

Monitoring Drug Use-Drug Use Profiles (DUPs)

In many instances the pharmacist, with the aid of patient medication records (PMRs), is the member of the health-care team ideally placed to monitor adherence to medical treatments. A drug use profile (DUP) is a graphic, chronological review of drug use which can be used to help simplify and rationalise therapies as well as indicate if there are adherence problems (Figure 3). In constructing the DUP, drugs are arranged into therapeutic classes for an individual patient. Taking each drug in turn, the starting point of the medicine (date of dispensing) is marked on the record sheet with a dot. The projected end date (based on the dose and number of days treatment supplied) is marked with a vertical dash. The distance between the dot and the dash is completed with a horizontal line. This procedure is carried out for all the drugs in the patient's PMR to produce a profile similar to that shown in Figure 3. The resulting pictorial view of the person's medication profile can highlight problems with adherence as shown in Figure 3 i.e. gaps between "dashes" and "dots" (possible under-adherence) or overlap of horizontal lines (possible over-adherence).

CONCLUSIONS

Much has yet to be done to aid understanding and improve adherence to medical treatments. While non-adherence is a problem common to all age-groups, it is particularly important in elderly people because they are more likely than younger people to suffer adverse consequences from non-adherence. Improvements in adherence among the elderly population may be achieved by health-care workers addressing the following questions:-

- does the patient really need all the drugs prescribed?
- is the patient impaired mentally, physically or financially?

- could the patients regimen be simplified e.g. by the use of slow-release or combination formulations of prescribed drugs?
- could the doses be adjusted to align administration with regular daily activities of the patient?
- if the patient is prescribed a benzodiazepine, is it one with a shorter half-life?
- does the patient know the names and purpose of the drugs they are prescribed?
- does the patient fully understand the dosing regimen for each of their medications?
- can the patient differentiate between their different medications?
- can the patient read (and understand) the label and any additional written information?
- can the patient open their containers easily?
- has the patient complained of any problems which could be drug-induced?
- does the patient live alone?
- does the patient get help when taking their medicines?
- would a medication aid be of benefit?
- does the patient take non-prescription medications?
- are any non-prescription medicines taken by the patient for the same condition for which a medication has been prescribed?
- will the patient be monitored by a member of the health-care team?

Co-operation between different members of the health-care team will be required to ensure that all these issues are properly addressed. Such a comprehensive approach is likely to have a major input on this ubiquitous problem in the case of elderly patients.

REFERENCES

Ajzen, I. and Fishbein, M.. (1980) *Understanding attitudes and predicting social behaviour.* Englewood Cliffs N.J. : Prentice Hall.

Anon. (1993) Misunderstanding leads to overdose. *The Pharmaceutical Journal* **250**, 338.

Ascione, F.J. and Shimp, L.A.(1984) The effectiveness of four education strategies in the elderly. *Drug Intelligence and Clinical Pharmacy* **18,** 926–931.

Barber, H.E., Hawksworth, G.M., Petrie, J.C., Rigby, J.W., Robb, O.J. and Scott, A.K. (1980) Pharmacokinetics of atenolol and propranolol in young and elderly subjects. *Proceedings of the BPS* **10– 12th Sept,,** 118–119.

Belmin, J., Levy, B.I. and Michel, J.B. (1994) Changes in the renin-angiotensin aldosterone axis in later life. *Drugs and Aging* **5** , 391–400.

Bender, A.D. (1965) The effect of increasing age on the distribution of peripheral blood flow in man. *Journal of the American Geriatrics Society* **13,** 1045–1046.

Black, D.M., Brand, R.J., Greenlick, M., Hughes, G. And Smith, J. (1987) Compliance to treatment for hypertension in elderly patients: the SHEP pilot study *Journal of Gerontology* **42,** 552– 557.

Bradley, B.M., Singleton, M. And Li Wan Po, A. (1994) Readability of patient information leaflets on over-the-counter (OTC) medications. *Journal of Clinical Pharmacy and Therapeutics* **19,** 7–15.

Brooke, A. and Mukherjee, S.K. (1988) Drug treatment in the elderly in South Nottinghamshire. a community audit. *The British Journal of Clinical Practice* **42,** 17–20.

Caranasos, G.J., Stewart, R.B. and Cluff, L.E. (1974) Drug induced illness leading to hospitalisation. *Journal of the American Medical Association* **228,** 713–717.

Cartwright, A. (1990) Medicine taking by people aged 65 or more. *British Medical Bulletin* **46,** 63–76.

Chryssidis, E., Frewin, T.A., Frewin, D.B. and Howard, A.F. (1982) Drug compliance in the elderly. *Australian Journal of Hospital Pharmacy* **12,** 8–10.

Coe, R.M., Prendergast, C.G., and Psathas, G. (1984) Strategies for obtaining compliance with medication regimens. *Journal of the American Geriatrics Society* **32,** 589–594.

Col, N., Fanale, J.E. and Kronholm, P. (1990) The role of medication noncompliance and adverse drug reactions in hospitalisations of the elderly. *Archives of Internal Medicine* **150,** 841–845.

Conn, V., Taylor, S., Faan, R.N. and Miller, R. (1994) Cognitive impairment and medication adherence. *Journal of Gerontological Nursing* **20,** 41–47.

Coons, S.J., Sheahan, S.L., Martin, M.S., Hendricks, J., Robbins, C.A. and Johnson, J.A. (1994) Predictors of medication noncompliance in a sample of older adults. *Clinical Therapeutics* **16**, 110–117.

Cooper, J.K., Love, D.W. and Raffoul, P.R. (1982) Intentional prescription nonadherence (noncompliance) by the elderly. *Journal of the American Geriatric Society* **30**, 329–333.

Cummings, S.R., Nevitt , M.C., Browner, W.S., Stone, K., Fox, K.M., Ensrud, K.E., Cauley, J., Black, D. and Vogt, T.M. (1995) Risk factors for hip fracture in white women. *New England Journal of Medicine* **332**, 767–773.

Cunningham, G., Dodd, T.R.P., McMurdo, M.E.T., Richards, R.M.E. and Grant, D.J. (1994) Drug related hospital admissions of elderly patients. *Age and Ageing (Suppl. 2)* **23**, 6.

Cusack, B., Kelly, J., O'Malley, K., Noel, J., Lavan, J., and Horgan, J. (1979) Digoxin in the elderly: Pharmacokinetic consequences of old age. *Clinical Pharmacology and Therapeutics* **25**, 772–776.

Davies, D.F. and Shock, N.W. (1950) Age changes in the glomerular filtration rate, effective renal plasma flow, and tubular excretory capacity in adult males *Journal of Clinical Investigation* **29**, 496–507.

Eisen, S.A., Miller, D.K., Woodward, R.S., Spitznagel, E. and Przybeck, T.R. (1990) The effect of prescribed daily dose frequency on patient medication compliance. *Archives of Internal Medicine* **150**, 1881–1884.

Eraker, S.A., Kirscht, J.P. and Becker, M.H. (1984) Understanding and improving patient compliance. *Annals of Internal Medicine* **100**, 258–268.

Farinati, F., Formentini, S., Della Libera, G., Valiante, F., Fanton, M.C., Mario, F., Vianello, F., Pilotto, A. and Naccarato, R. (1993) Changes in parietal and mucous cell mass in the gastric mucosa of normal subjects with age, amorphometric study. *Gerontology* **39**, 146–151.

Fotrell, E., Sheikh, M. and Kothari, R. (1976) Long-stay patients with long-stay drugs: a case for review, a cause for concern. *Lancet* **i**, 81.

Gales, B.J. and Menard, S.M. (1995) Relationship between the administration of selected medications and falls in hospitalised elderly patients. *The Annals of Pharmacotherapy* **29**, 354–357.

German, P.S., Klein, L.E. and Mcphee, S.J. (1982) Knowledge of and compliance with drug regimens in the elderly. *Journal of the American Geriatrics Society* **30**, 568–571.

Gibbs, R.D., Gibbs, P.H. and Henrich, J. (1987) Patient understanding of commonly used medical vocabulary. *Journal of Family Practice* **25**, 176–178.

Greenblatt, D.J. (1979) Reduced serum albumin concentration in the elderly: a report from the Boston Collaborative Drug Surveillance Program. *Journal of the American Geriatrics Society* **23**, 20–23.

Gryfe, C.I. and Gryfe, B.M. (1984) Drug therapy of the aged: the problem of compliance and the roles of physicians and pharmacists. *Journal of the American Geriatrics Society* **32**, 301–307.

Grymonpre, R.E., Mitenko, P.A., Sitar, D.S., Aoki, F.Y. and Montgomery, P.R. (1988) Drug-associated hospital admissions in older medical patients. *Journal of the American Geriatrics Society* **36**, 1092–1098.

Gunashera, J.B.L., Lee, D.R., Jones, L., Maskrey, C.G. and Jackson, S.H.D. (1996) Does serum albumin fall with increasing age in the absence of disease? *Age and ageing (suppl. 1)* **25**, 29.

Gurwitz, J.H. and Avorn, J. (1991) The ambiguous relation between aging and adverse drug reactions. *Annals of Internal Medicine* **114**, 956–966.

Hatton, P. (1990) "Primum non nocere" – an analysis of drugs prescribed to elderly patients in private nursing homes registered with Harrogate Health Authority. *Care of the Elderly* **2**, 166–169.

Hecht, A.B. (1974) Improving medication compliance by teaching outpatients. *Nursing Forum* **13**, 112–129.

Horn C.R., Clark, T.J.H. and Cochrane, G.M. (1990) Compliance with inhaled therapy and morbidity from asthma. *Respiratory Medicine* **84**, 67–70.

Hurd, P.D. and Blevins, J. (1984) Aging and the color of pills. *New England Journal of Medicine* **310**, 202.

Hurwitz, N. (1969) Predisposing factors in adverse reactions to drugs. *British Medical Journal* **1**, 536–539.

Hussar, D.A. (1985) Improving patient compliance – the role of the pharmacist. In *Improving medication compliance: proceedings of a symposium in Washington D.C., November 1, 1984* Virginia: National Pharmaceutical Council.

Hussey, L.C. (1994) Minimizing effects of low literacy on medication knowledge and compliance among the elderly. *Clinical Nursing Research* **3**, 132–145.

Iber, F.L., Murphy, P.A. and Connor, E.S. (1994) Age-related change in the gastrointestinal system effect on drug therapy. *Drugs and Aging* **5**, 34–48.

Jackson, A.E., Hall, J. and Chadha, D. (1992) Elderly patients and their drugs. avoiding hospital admissions *The Pharmaceutical Journal (suppl.)* **249**, R25.

Kane, R.L., Ouslander, J.G. and Abrass, I.B. (1994) *Essentials of clinical geriatrics. Third Edition.* New York: McGraw-Hill.

Kellaway, G.S.M. and McCrae, E. (1973) Intensive monitoring for adverse drug effects in patients discharged from acute medical wards. *New Zealand Medical Journal* **78**, 525–528.

Key data [UK Social and Economic statistics] Central Statistics Office, 1995/96. Alison Button (ed.) London: HMSO.

Lamy, P.P., Salzmann, C. and Nevis-Olesen, J. (1992). Drug prescribing patterns risks, and compliance guidelines. In C. Salzmann (ed) *Clinical geriatric psychopharmacology. Second edition.* Baltimore: Williams and Wilkins Publishers.

Lau, H.S., Beuning, K.S., Postma-Lim, E., Klein-Beernink, L., de Boer, A. and Porsius, A.J. (1996) Non-compliance in elderly people: evaluation of risk factors by longitudinal data analysis. *Pharmacy World and Science* **18**, 63–68.

Levy, M., Kewitz, H., Altwein, W., Hillebrand, J. and Eliakim, M. (1980) Hospital admissions due to adverse drug reactions: a comparative study from Jerusalem and Berlin. *European Journal of Clinical Pharmacology* **17**, 25–31.

Lindley, C.M., Tully, M.P., Paramsothy, V. and Tallis, R.C. (1992) Inappropriate medication is a major cause of adverse drug reactions in elderly patients. *Age and Ageing* **21**, 294–300.

Lowe, C.J., Raynor, D.K., Courtney, E.A., Purvis, J. and Teale, C. (1995) Effects of a self medication programme on knowledge of drugs and compliance with treatments in elderly patients. *British Medical Journal* **310**, 1229–1231.

Macdonald, E.T. and Macdonald, J.B. (1982). *Disease management in the elderly. Volume 1. Drug treatment in the elderly.* New York: John Wiley and Sons.

Martin, D.C. and Mead, K. (1982) Reducing medication errors in a geriatric population. *Journal of the American Geriatrics Society* **4**, 258–260.

Meredith, P.A. and Elliott, H.L. (1994) Therapeutic coverage: reducing the risks of partial compliance *British Journal of Clinical Practice* **73**, 13–17.

Miller, J.H., McDonald, R.K. and Shock, N.W. (1952) Age change in the maximal rate of renal tubular reabsorption of glucose. *Journal of Gerontology* **1**, 196–200.

Miller, R.A. (1994). "The biology of aging and longevity". In W.L. Hazzard, E.L. Bierman, J.P. Blass, W.H. Ettinger, J.B. Halter, R. Andres (eds) *Principles of geriatric medicine and gerontology. Third edition.* New York: McGraw-Hill.

Miller, R.R. (1974) Hospital admission due to adverse drug reactions. A report from the Boston Collaborative Drug Surveillance Program. *Archives of Internal Medicine* **134**, 219–223.

McElnay, J.C. and McCallion C.R. (1996) Non-prescription drug use by elderly patients. *The International Journal of Pharmacy Practice* **4**, 6–11.

McElnay, J.C. and Thompson, J. (1992) Dispensing of medicines in compliance packs. *International Pharmacy Journal* **6**, 10–15.

McElnay, J.C., McCallion, C.R., Al-Deagi, F. and Scott, M.G. (1997) Development of a risk model for adverse drug events in the elderly *Clinical Drug Investigation* **13**, 47–55.

McElnay J.C., McCallion, C.R., Al-Deagi, F. and Scott, M.G. (1996b) Self-reported medication non-compliance in the elderly. *Unpublished observations.*

McKenny, J.M. and Harrison, W.L. (1976) Drug-related hospital admissions. *American Society of Hospital Pharmacists* **33**, 792–795.

Montamat, S.C., Cusack, B.J. and Vestal, R.E. (1989) Management of drug therapy in the elderly. *New England Journal of Medicine* **73**, 303–309.

Mullen, P.D., Green, L.W. and Persinger, G.S. (1985) Clinical trials of patient education for chronic conditions: a comparative meta-analysis of intervention types. *Preventive Medicine* **14**, 753–781.

Murray, M.D., Birt, J.A., Manatunga, A.K. and Damell, J.C. (1993) Medication compliance in elderly outpatients using twice-daily and unit-of-use packaging. *Annals of Pharmacotherapy* **27**, 616–621.

Nagy, V.T. and Wolfe, G.R. (1984) Cognitive predictors of compliance in chronic disease patients. *Medical Care* **22,** 912–921.

Nessman, D.G., Carnahan, J.E. and Nugent, C.A. (1980) Increasing compliance: patient-operated hypertension groups. *Archives of Internal Medicine* **140,** 1427–1430.

Nicolson, A., Gladman, C.W., Smith, C.W., Bendall, M.J. and Arie T. (1994) Multicentre survey of adverse drug reactions in elderly people admitted to hospital. *Age and Ageing (Suppl 2)* **23,** 40.

Nikolaus, T., Kruse, W., Bach, M., Spechtleible, N., Oster, P. and Schlierf, G. (1996) Elderly patients' problems with medications – an in-hospital and follow-up study. *European Journal of Clinical Pharmacology* **49,** 255–259.

Nolan, L. and O'Malley, K. (1988) Prescribing for the elderly. Part II. Prescribing patterns:differences due to age. *Journal of the American Geriatric Society* **36,** 245–254.

Nolan, L. and O'Malley, K. (1989) Adverse drug reactions in the elderly. *British Journal of Hospital Medicine* **41,** 447–456.

Norell, S.E. (1985) Memory and medication compliance. *Journal of Clinical and Hospital Pharmacy* **10,** 107–109.

O'Malley, K., Crooks, J., Duke, E. and Stevenson, I.H. (1971) Effect of age and sex on human drug metabolism. *British Medical Journal* **3,** 607–609.

Parker, B.M., Cusack, B.J. and Vestal, R. (1995) Pharmacokinetic optimisation of drug therapy in elderly patients. *Drugs and Aging* **7,** 10–18.

Parkin, D.M., Henney, C.R., Quirk, J. and Crooks, J. (1976) Deviation from prescribed drug treatment after discharge. *British Medical Journal* **2,** 686–688.

Popplewell, P.Y. and Henschke, P.J. (1982) Acute admissions to a geriatric assessment unit. *Medical Journal of Australia* **1,** 343–344.

Primrose, W.R., Capewell, A.E., Simpson, G.K. and Smith, R.G. (1987) Prescribing patterns observed in registered nursing homes and long-stay geriatric wards. *Age and Ageing* **16,** 25–28.

Pullar, T., Birtwell, A.J., Wiles, P.G., Hay, A. and Feely, M.P. (1988) Use of a pharmacologic indicator to compare compliance with tablets prescribed to be taken once, twice, or three times daily. *Clinical Pharmacology and Therapeutics* **44,** 540–545.

Rand, C.S. and Wise, R.A. (1994) Measuring adherence to asthma medication regimens. *American Journal of Respiratory Critical Care Medicine* **149,** S69–S76.

Ried, L.D. and Christensen, D.B. (1988) A psychosocial perspective in the explanation of patients drug-taking behavior. *Social Science and Medicine* **27**, 277–285.

Rivers, P.H. (1992) Compliance aids – do they work? *Drugs and Aging* **2**, 103–111.

Robbins, L.J. and Jahingen, D.W. (1984) Child resistant packaging and the geriatric patient. *Journal of the American Geriatrics Society* **32**, 450–452.

Rosenstock, I.M. (1966) Why people use health services. *Milbank Memorial Fund Quarterly* **44**, 94–127.

Salzmann, C. (1995) Medication compliance in the elderly. *Journal of Clinical Psychiatry (Suppl. 1)* **56**, 18–22.

Schlenk, E.A. and Hart, L.K. (1984) Relationship between health locus of control, health value, and social support and compliance of persons with diabetes mellitus. *Diabetes Care* **7**, 566–574.

Smith, J.W., Seidel, L.G. and Cluff, L.E. (1966) Studies on the epidemiology of adverse drug reaction. *Annals of Internal Medicine* **65**, 629–640.

Smith, P. and Andrews, J. (1983) Drug compliance not so bad, knowledge not so good, the elderly after hospital discharge. *Age and Ageing* **12**, 336–342.

Smuker, W.D. and Kontak, J.R. (1990) Adverse drug reactions causing hospital admission in an elderly population: experience with a decision algorithm. *Journal of the American Board of Family Practice* **3**, 105–109.

Stewart, R.B. and Cooper, J.W. (1994) Polypharmacy in the aged – practical solutions. *Drugs and Aging* **4**, 449–61.

Stewart, R.B. (1990) Polypharmacy in the elderly: a fait accompli? *The Annals of Pharmacotherapy* **24**, 321–323.

Tessier, E.G. (1993). Practical drug use in the elderly: pharmacokinetic and pharmacodynamic considerations. In J.D. McCue, E.G. Tessier, P. Gaziano, P. Lamhut (eds) *Geriatric drug handbook for long-term care.* London: Williams and Wilkins Press.

Tettersell, M.J. (1993) Asthma patients' knowledge in relation to compliance with drug therapy. *Journal of Advanced Nursing* **18**, 103–113.

Urquhart, J. (1994) Role of patient compliance in clinical pharmacokinetics. a review of recent research. *Clinical Pharmacokinetics* **27**, 205–215.

Vestal, R.E., Norris, A.H., Tobin, J.D., Cohen, B.H., Schock, N.W. and Andres, R. (1975) Antipyrine metabolism in man: influence of age, alcohol, caffeine, and smoking. *Clinical Pharmacology and Therapeutics* **18**, 425–432.

Wallace, S., Whiting, B. and Runcie, J. (1976) Factors affecting drug binding in plasma of elderly patients. *British Journal of Clinical Pharmacology* **3**, 327–330.

Ware, G.J. and Holford, N.H.G. (1991) Unit dose calendar packaging and elderly patient compliance. *New Zealand Medical Journal* **104**, 495–497.

Warren, P.M. (1978) Age changes in small intestine mucosa. *The Lancet* **II**, 849.

Williamson, J. and Chopin, J.M. (1980) Adverse reactions to prescribed drugs in the elderly: a multicentre investigation. *Age and Ageing* **9**, 73–80.

Woodhouse, K.W. and James, O.F. (1990) Hepatic drug metabolism and ageing. *British Medical Bulletin* **46**, 25–35.

Wong, B.S.M. and Norman, D.C. (1987) Evaluation of a novel medication aid, the calender blister-pak, and its effect on drug compliance in a geriatric outpatient clinic. *Journal of the American Geriatric Society* **35**, 21–26.

Zismer, D.K., Gillum, R.F., Johnson, C.A., Becerra, J. and Johnson, T.H. (1982) Improving hypertension control in a private medical practice. *Archives of Internal Medicine* **142**, 297–299.

Zuccollo, G. and Liddel, H. (1985) The elderly and the medication label: doing it better. *Age and Ageing* **14**, 371–376..

10

Adherence in Ethnic Minorities : The Case of South Asians in Britain

Mary Sissons Joshi

BACKGROUND

Health care professionals have traditionally regarded non-adherence with medical advice as a major factor in the explanation of poor outcomes. Non-adherence can be defined narrowly as failing to take prescriptions in accordance with instruction (in respect of quantity, frequency and timing) and missing follow-up appointments; more broadly as not adopting recommended changes in behaviour; and even more broadly to include not seeking medical advice at all. The phenomenon of non-adherence occurs in patients of all social classes, ethnic groups, and health care delivery systems (Hays and DiMatteo, 1987), and regardless of symptom severity or medical assessment of disease severity (Haynes, 1979). Despite the ubiquity of non-adherence, it is nevertheless worth considering whether there are any categories of patients whose adherence rates are different from those of other groups, or for whom the sources of non-adherence vary. Interest in this topic has been shown by researchers desiring a better understanding of the topic of adherence and by practitioners who aim to encourage greater adherence from those with low rates so that such patients may better benefit from what the health system has to offer.

Ethnicity in the UK

The 1991 Census of Population indicates that ethnic minority members constitute 5.5% of the population of Great Britain (Owen, 1996). Issues concerning categorisation of respondents into ethnic groups are discussed elsewhere (e.g. Bulmer, 1996; Dale and Marsh, 1993; Peach, 1996; Sillitoe and White, 1992). The *Health of the Nation* Government strategy document (Department of Health, 1993) set targets for the improvement of health and pointed to the need to ensure that all members of the community share in the improvements. Ethnic minority groups are mentioned as being likely to have specific needs. If all are to have an equal chance of adhering to medical advice, it will be worth considering whether members of minority groups are likely to have particular difficulties in accessing services and/or following advice. Difficulties would arise if, for example, patients lacked knowledge of services, were unfamiliar with either the English language or with the rules and rituals of the medical encounter in the UK, or if medical advice clashed with culturally specific beliefs and practices. However, since health behaviour can only be understood with reference to other beliefs and behaviours (Fabrega, 1974; Kleinman, 1980; Landrine and Klonoff, 1992) and to the wider socio-economic and political context (Townsend, Davidson and Whitehead, 1988), it would be incorrect to study adherence and ethnicity as if ethnic minority members constituted one undifferentiated group. While ethnic minority members may share, to a greater or lesser extent, the psychological experience of being "different" from the dominant culture and the unpleasantness of being the subject of interpersonal prejudice and institutional discrimination, a great many social, economic and cultural factors also differentiate between ethnic groups.

South Asians in the UK

In its review of ethnicity and adherence to medical regime, this chapter, for a number of reasons, will focus on South Asians (i.e. Indians, Pakistanis and Bangladeshis) in Britain. The largest ethnic minority identified in the 1991 Census comprised those who identified themselves as Indian, constituting 1.5% of the total population. Those identifying themselves as Pakistani and Bangladeshi constitute

0.87% and 0.30% of the total population respectively (Office of Population Censuses and Surveys, OPCS, 1993). The generic term South Asian is commonly used to encompass all three groups (Mason, 1995; Smaje, 1995) and this composite grouping accounts for 2.7% of the total population and 49.2% of the ethnic minority population. Within the medical field, more research appears to have been conducted on disease epidemiology and service-use among South Asians than among other ethnic groups, such as Afro-Caribbeans. One explanation for this bias is that prior to recent regular ethnic monitoring within the health service, ethnicity was not transparent in patient records – except amongst South Asians where surname is a good indicator of religious background and thereby, to a certain extent, of ethnicity. Low rates of inter-ethnic marriage (Berrington, 1996) further add to the reliability of surname as an ethnic indicator for South Asians. Additionally, it is suggested by Mason (1995) that research focuses disproportionately on "high-status areas of medical practice" so that coronary heart disease (amongst South Asians) has had a significantly higher public profile than hypertension (amongst Afro-Caribbeans).

Care must be exercised in the use of the category South Asian since it is a term which originates outside the group to which it refers, and may be criticised as reflecting the tendency of the majority population to "conceptualise themselves as individuals, while outsiders are seen as members of a group" (Mason, 1995). It is important to note that ethnic identity may or may not indicate other categories and identities. Ethnic grouping is not indicative of country of birth – for example amongst the Indian group, 41.2% were born in the UK, 36.8% in India, and 16.9% in East Africa (Robinson, 1996). Further, while the Islamic religion characterises the majority of those of Pakistani and Bangladeshi descent, the term Indian encompasses those of Hindu, Muslim, Sikh, Parsi, Jewish and Christian faith, and more besides. Language transcends national and religious boundaries – for example Urdu and Punjabi may be spoken by those from Pakistan and India, and Gujarati may be spoken by Muslims from East Africa and Hindus from India. Ethnic identification is contextual – while a person may be willing to allocate him or herself to a general label such as Indian, self-perception may, depending on situation, be in terms of a narrower linguistic or regional grouping (Ballard, 1994).

Demographically speaking, the 1991 Census and numerous social science enquiries have made it clear that the Indian, Pakistani and

Bangladeshi ethnic groups can be contrasted with each other in terms of age structure, patterns of migration to UK, geographical distribution within UK, initial and subsequent employment, and housing (Ballard, 1996; Eade, Vamplew and Peach, 1996; Robinson, 1996). For example, while all three groups have a younger age structure than the white majority, Indians have an older age structure than the Bangladeshis and Pakistanis (Mason, 1995). Amongst the Indians, 11.4% of employed males are in professional occupations, in comparison to 6.7% of Whites, 5.9% of Pakistanis and 5.2% of Bangladeshis; Pakistanis and Bangladeshis have a "concentration in manual employment and very high unemployment rates" (29% and 32% respectively) (Peach, 1996). Further, the Indian group should not be considered as a unitary group for it comprises people from various countries practising a variety of religions and speaking a variety of languages with, as Robinson (1984; 1996) has noted, a diversity of trajectory after arrival.

Notwithstanding the diversity both among and between component groups, this chapter will review literature pertaining to South Asians in Britain. The argument in favour of reviewing material on these three ethnic categories (i.e. Indian, Pakistani and Bangladeshi) is that, as outlined above, religious and cultural/regional identity may cut across ethnic identity; and that experience of discrimination and exclusion may similarly shape the experiences of all three groups (and sub-groups) such that to be South Asian becomes an identity in certain circumstances. It has also been argued by some that there are important commonalities of belief amongst South Asians in the sub-continent (Hofstede, 1980; Kakar, 1978; 1982) and abroad (Roland, 1988; Clarke, Peach and Vertovec, 1990).

MEDICAL DIVERSITY AND THE SEEKING OF ADVICE

In order to follow medical advice, one must first seek it. A tendency for observers to see South Asians as members of an exotic "other" culture can result in notions of competing ideology and alternative medical systems as explanations for poor adherence. Some research has supported this viewpoint. For example, focusing on Muslim Mirpuris from Pakistan living in Bradford, West Yorkshire, Aslam and Healy (1983) describe an "alternative" health service and suggest that belief in "traditional" concepts can interfere with adherence to physicians' advice. In a small-scale study of Bangladeshi women's antenatal interactions in Oxford, Miller (1995) emphasises the competing influence of the "all-embracing" Muslim faith. However, in a consideration of ethnographic data, it is important to remember that alternative beliefs are not found exclusively in minority cultures but are common amongst the majority white population as Helman's (1978) work on doctor-patient discourse and lay beliefs about colds and fevers has amply demonstrated.

While certain specific lay beliefs may indeed be in contradiction to those of orthodox medicine, the systems themselves are not necessarily viewed as alternatives by the consumers. Western medicine has a long and complex history in India (Arnold, 1993) and current research on consultation patterns in the subcontinent reveals that patients do not choose *between* systems but consult *several* or more systems – often simultaneously (Madan, 1969; Minocha, 1980; Nichter, 1980). In Hunte and Sultana's (1992) study of health-seeking behaviour in a rural area in North West Pakistan, parents sought on average 3.9 treatments for a child's illness, ranging from home-based remedies to over-the-counter pharmaceutics and from visits to religious healers to consultation with hospital physicians. Within Britain, on a negative note, Aslam, Davis and Healy (1979) have warned of the widespread use and the potential toxicity of Asian medications. In contrast, is Bhopal's (1986) study of the health beliefs and practices of 65 Punjabis (of Muslim, Sikh and Hindu religion) in Glasgow, Scotland. Knowledge of Asian traditional remedies was high, particularly amongst older respondents, but their use was not extensive. Bhopal (1986) concluded that traditional Asian medicine did not pose a health threat, respect for Western medicine was widespread, and that in the community he studied "general practice consultation rates were unaffected by knowledge or utilization of Asian health remedies". Consultation rates with Asian healers were low, except on trips back to India. Research in London with Gujarati patients with diabetes indicated awareness of Ayurvedic theory (i.e. the traditional Hindu system of medicine) and the medicinal properties of various foods and herbs, but suggests little risk of conflict between Ayurvedic and Western medicine in daily practice (Khajuria and Thomas, 1992). In a household survey in the West Midlands, Johnson, Cross and Cardew (1983) found that "the majority of Asians felt that scientific medicine was preferable to traditional remedies".

Many studies in fact report that Asian patients have an above average rate of consultation with their general practitioners (GPs; Wright, 1983; Sutcliffe, 1985; Donaldson, 1986; Gillam *et al.*, 1989). However, in Heatley and Yip's (1991) study, where Asian patients were matched with non-Asian patients by age, gender and address, there was no significant difference between the groups in general practice consultation rates. Also see Gillam *et al.* (1989) and Smaje (1995) for discussion of the problems of disentangling attitude factors from medical need in the interpretation of consultation rates). Interestingly, in Pakistan, Hunte and Sultana (1992) note that it is not the consultation of different systems of medicine which is likely to lead to medical problems, but the practice of consulting more than one cosmopolitan practitioner in quick succession. This habit when combined with the over-prescription of drugs by practitioners (Greenhalgh, 1987) and augmented by the patient's traditional practice of mixing ingredients in home-based medicines, can result in a hazardous mixing of medicinal substances. But as Ahmad (1992) has noted, the self-modification of drug regime either through multiple consultation or the sharing of medicine with family members is likely to be a characteristic of patients from a wide variety of social and cultural backgrounds, particularly in the face of increasing prescription costs.

Material in the above paragraphs demonstrates that it would be inaccurate to depict South Asians in Britain as being opposed to Western medicine or to be, in any general sense, underusing the service. Balarajan and Raleigh (1995) warn against complacency in the face of equal use of service, pointing out that since minority ethnic people are more prone to certain chronic disease of middle age (e.g. diabetes in the case of South Asians), *higher* rates of hospital-based care should be expected. Furthermore, Gillam *et al.* (1989) indicate that it may be unwise to make any general statements about service use. Their study investigated general practice consultation in terms of patient ethnicity, age and condition, and found differences which could in part be interpreted in terms of morbidity but also in terms of patient attitude. Thus, Asian patients with respiratory disease were found to consult more frequently than other patients with the same disease, and the authors suggest that this "may reflect understandable anxiety over respiratory symptoms in communities originating from countries where respiratory infections, particularly tuberculosis, remains a common cause of death" .

Certain other services, including health-related services, appear to be under-used in absolute terms. Elderly South Asians make low use of domiciliary and other social services (Blakemore and Boneham, 1994). Atkin *et al.*'s study (1989) revealed low knowledge about a range of domiciliary services but also an interest in using the services once they had been described.

Services have to be culturally sensitive if they are actually to be acceptable. Neither service managers nor ground staff, if they are of white ethnicity, are likely to be fully aware of Hindu and Muslim cultural practices surrounding eating, bathing and other domestic behaviours. The matching of client with care worker which is advised by many authors (e.g. Poonia and Ward, 1990) will only be feasible in areas of ethnic concentration, and in any event should not be thought of as a complete solution. Ahmad *et al.*'s (1991) study found that "Asian-qualified doctors held less favourable attitudes towards Asian patients than other doctors". Various factors have been proposed to explain why non-Asian *and* Asian GPs report their consultations with Asian patients as less satisfying. These include characteristics of the patients, social class differences between doctors and patients, and the notion of Asian doctors internalising racial stereotypes common in the wider society (Ahmad *et al.*, 1991; Smaje, 1995). Further, gender matching between health professional and patient may be as important as linguistic or cultural matching, especially for Muslim women (see Rudat, 1994).

DOCTOR-PATIENT RELATIONSHIPS

Use of service will relate to experience within it, and the doctor-patient relationship has been identified as a key factor in explaining variation in patient adherence (DiMatteo and DiNicola, 1982; Taylor, 1995; see Noble, Chapter 3 for a discussion of doctor-patient communication). The quality of the communication between doctor and patient can be considered from both the informational and affective viewpoints (DiNicola and DiMatteo, 1984). Patients cannot follow instructions if they have not understood them in the first place, and clearly anyone who is not fluent in the language of the encounter will be placed at a severe disadvantage. Since detailed medical instructions may be given in written form, as well as orally, literacy in the relevant language will also be required (Ley, 1988). Bhatt (1992) has suggested that in the absence of full literacy, audio-visual health education material will be more effective and acceptable in some South Asian communities.

English fluency has been identified as a problem for Pakistani Mirpuris in Bradford (Ahmad, Kernohan and Baker, 1989) and Bangladeshi Sylhetis in Tower Hamlets, London (Jones, 1987). In the East Midlands town of Leicester, English language was not seen to be a problem for the majority of South Asians (Rashid and Jagger, 1992). However, also in Leicester, in a sample of 726 South Asians over 65 years, Donaldson (1986) noted that only 2% of women and 37% of men reported an ability to speak English. Further, amongst those who could speak English, explaining a problem to a doctor was judged, by the respondents themselves, to be the most difficult of six suggested social situations. Telephoning to rearrange an outpatient appointment was also held to be difficult and likely to require an interpreter.

Use of vocabulary and its relationship to the presentation of symptoms has long been noted as a factor likely to impede communication and distort diagnosis in a medical encounter (Zborowski, 1952; Zola, 1966). Many authors have warned practitioners of the need to be aware of cultural differences in the presentation of psychiatric symptoms by Asian patients (Rack, 1982; Kleinman, 1987) but similar issues need to be considered in general medicine. For example, Homans (1980) found that "pregnant Asian women tended to say *I feel weak* rather than *I think I am pregnant* at their initial GP visit". However, as Smaje (1995) has commented, no generalisations can be made about English language use and fluency and the South Asian population given the diversity of that population with respect to age, education and recency of migration. Furthermore, while language currently may be a severe problem for some groups, as outlined above, this will diminish as South Asian British children progress through the school system. Indeed it is worth noting that, in Britain, Indian school pupils are currently "achieving levels of success consistently in excess of their white counterparts in some (but not all) urban areas" (Gillborn and Gipps, 1996).

Communication between doctor and patient is eased by more than vocabulary. Argyle's (1972) social skill model has demonstrated that successful communication arises from each participant sharing an understanding of the meaning of non-verbal and extra-linguistic signals. Gumperz, Jupp and Roberts (1979) have shown how South Asian-English speakers can sound unintentionally hostile due to a different pattern of emphasis and tone from that used by English-English speakers. Such mismatches open the door to cultural misunderstanding and may go part of the way to explaining why some studies have found negative attitudes to Asian patients amongst GPs (Wright, 1983; Ahmad *et al.*, 1991). Heatley and Yip (1991) have suggested that GPs' perceptions of Asian patients as over-consulting relates to language and cultural barriers, and to Asians frequently presenting out of hours, "hence appearing to represent a disproportionately large share of the workload". Such an observation is concordant with the psychological phenomenon of illusory correlation – i.e. the cognitive tendency for two behaviours or categories which are unusual to be regarded as causally connected by the perceiver (Hamilton and Gifford, 1976).

There is evidence to suggest that South Asian patients are the recipients of much direct emotionally-toned prejudice in their encounters with doctors and ancillary staff. Bowler (1993) interviewed midwives about their attitudes towards and beliefs about their South Asian patients, most of whom were recent migrants from rural areas in Pakistan or Bangladesh. The Asian women's lack of English led to the midwives characterising them as "unresponsive, rude and unintelligent". Maternity patients interviewed by Bowler (1993) were aware, for example, that they were being judged as unintelligent, but were unable to challenge this or other views about them through lack of language and lack of knowledge of the appropriate cultural script (Garfinkel, 1967; Goffman, 1969). Non-colloquial use of English by the patients (as in the frequent use of the imperative, and the lack of use of "please" and "thank you") distanced them from the midwives, as did the midwives' use of culturally specific euphemisms for parts of the body. Midwives were hostile when Asian women failed to conform to "the prevailing (Western) model of motherhood", preferring for example to bottle-feed rather than breastfeed, but the midwives made no mention, however, of their Asian patients' positive behaviours, such as not smoking. Social psychological studies have frequently demonstrated how stereotypes not only fail to alter in the light of incoming contradictory evidence but affect perception itself so that the "same" action is construed differently depending on the identity of the performer (Duncan, 1976). It is clear that the medical encounter is rife with prejudicial possibilities, particularly in view of the inherently unequal status positions of patient and practitioner.

In their focus on the interpersonal aspect of doctor-patient relations, social scientists must be careful not to overlook the resource context in which patients seek and are given care. Studies in the USA have suggested that treatment offered can vary with ethnicity. For example, Peterson *et al.* (1994) showed that following myocardial infarction, black people were significantly less likely to receive various treatments, after controlling for age, severity of infarction and hospital characteristics. In the UK, Shaukat, de Bono and Cruickshank (1993) controlled for age, gender and extent of coronary disease, and found that Indian patients experienced greater delays in being referred to a regional specialist centre than did white patients. Smaje (1995) notes the sparsity the literature on the topic of ethnic differences and the quality of care, and also rightly points to the difficulties in disentangling demand side from referral bias factors. However, in their review of the USA data, Ford and Cooper (1995) suspect that subtle personal factors, including physician bias in referral, may be important. In the context of this chapter's focus on adherence, it is important also to register Ford and Cooper's (1995) comment that "unfriendly contacts with the medical system" may have led to a distrust of the system and affected black patients' acceptance of referrals.

ATTITUDES, KNOWLEDGE, AND PREVENTIVE HEALTH BEHAVIOUR

Adherence to medical advice can be considered as an example of health behaviour. Thus, the usual models which have been applied to the understanding of health behaviour can be applied to adherence – viz. the health belief model (HBM, Rosenstock, 1966, Becker, 1974) and the theory of reasoned action (TRA, Fishbein and Ajzen, 1975), with its revision in the form of the theory of planned behaviour (TPB, Ajzen, 1988). This chapter will not attempt to review these models in full but, citing examples from the area of preventive health, will use a selection of the models' key theoretical concepts to further understanding of the relationship between ethnicity and adherence. For a description of the models, see Horne and Weinman, Chapter 2.

Knowledge and attitude are key determinants of health behaviour for both the HBM and the TPB. Some health promoting behaviours are imposed by law – such as wearing of car seatbelts, but for voluntary behaviours, a person must both desire health and place it at a high priority if he or she is to engage in the appropriate behaviours. While it is clear from the high consultation rates described above that South Asians in the UK have a desire for health, there may be specific areas in which lack of knowledge limits the use of certain services. In order to engage in preventive health behaviour one must know of the disease in question, know of the preventive behaviour, and believe in the efficacy of the recommended health action.

Immunisation

Much research has focused on the uptake of childhood immunisation. Measures have included whether a full course was taken, and also whether the course was taken at the recommended time. Baker, Bandaranayake and Schweiger (1984) studied the uptake of DPT (diptheria, pertussis/whooping cough, tetanus), poliomyelitis, measles and BCG (tuberculosis) immunisations in Bradford. The Indian group had the best rate of immunisation in terms of proportion of children immunised and age at immunisation. The Pakistani group had good uptake proportionately, but a delay in timing at the early months. The Bangladeshi group had lower rates and did not differ from the "British" group. The authors speculate that delayed take-up may relate to frequent changes of address, perception of the child as being in poor health on the scheduled day, and/or poor understanding/motivation. In a London study, recent immigration was given as a reason by parents of Bangladeshi children (aged 4.5 to 6 years) who had had no immunisations (Bedford, Masters and Kurtz, 1992). In a study of Punjabis in Glasgow, where Asian and European children were matched for gender and post-code, Bhopal and Samim (1988) found that Sikhs had the highest immunisation rates for DPT, measles and polio, and Muslims and Hindus had higher uptakes of pertussis/whooping cough vaccination but were similar to controls for the other immunisations. The authors invoke a variety of cultural factors to explain these high rates including fear of infectious disease resulting from experiences in the Indian subcontinent, faith in injections, and practical support from the extended family which gives mothers time to attend the relevant clinics. Bhopal and Samim (1988) also make the intriguing suggestion that due to a poorer grasp of English, some Asian parents may be unaware of the adverse media publicity which has surrounded the pertussis/whooping cough vaccine, noting that "paradoxically, in this instance language and cultural barriers may be aiding, not hindering, health care".

Screening

Cervical cancer is one of the cancers which the *Health of the Nation* strategy targets for reduction by the year 2000 (Department of Health, 1993). Noting the high incidence of cervical cancer in some Asian countries, Balarajan and Raleigh (1995) call for more studies of rates among Asian women in the UK. Uptake of cervical smear screening has generally been found to be low (Firdous and Bhopal, 1989). In a Leicester study, McAvoy and Raza (1988) attribute low uptake to women's lack of specific knowledge about the test rather than to attitude factors such as dislike of internal examination or to normative factors such as husband's disapproval. More recently, in Oldham, Greater Manchester, Bradley and Friedman (1993) found cervical smear uptake, at 61%, to be equal in Asian (Pakistani) and non-Asian women aged 50–64 years. Naish, Brown and Denton (1994) studied attitudes to cervical screening using a small number of focus groups drawn from Bengali and Punjabi women living in East London. Attitudes to cervical screening were generally positive among the women, most of whom had had their first smear taken at a postnatal examination, but many women were not aware that such screening had to be repeated at regular intervals. The women made practical suggestions for the improvement of uptake such as the provision of childcare facilities in surgeries so that children did not have to be present for the examination.

It is important to note that low uptake rates across a community may not necessarily be indicative of low knowledge or negative attitude, since demographic characteristics may structure a community's response to a screening programme. For example, in a questionnaire study of attitudes to cervical screening in the outer London district of Ealing, Doyle (1991) suggests that the greater rate of mobility within the UK of Asians will result in call/recall letters failing to reach their addressees. In an intervention study of breast screening amongst 247 Pakistani and Bangladeshi women aged 50–64 years, Hoare *et al.*(1994) found that of the 102 women who could not be contacted, 26 were visiting Asia. Since visits to Asia can be for substantial periods, such women are likely to be inaccessible to a screening programme.

PERCEIVED VULNERABILITY

The extent to which patients and potential patients perceive themselves to be vulnerable to various diseases is a well established factor in the prediction of health behaviour among those researchers who use the HBM, and it is important to examine adherence and ethnicity from this point of view.

Sickle/Beta Thalassaemia

Certain diseases are inherited and vary in their prevalence between ethnic groups – for example, cystic fibrosis is more common among North European populations (Smaje, 1995). Sickle/beta thalassaemia is found disproportionately among people originating from South Asia, Southern Europe and the Middle East (Anionwu, 1993; Smaje, 1995). One in twenty people of South Asian descent carry the trait and when both partners carry the trait each child has a one in four chance of being affected (Anionwu, 1993; Mason, 1995). Studies by Darr (1990) of Pakistanis from Mirpur resident in UK and by Jani *et al.* (1992) of a Gujarati community in North London suggest that there is insufficient awareness of the disease, its inherited nature and the possibility of testing adults and unborn babies with respect to carrier and disease status. Richards and Ponder (1996) note that lay understanding of genetics is generally very limited in the UK, but additionally raise the possibility that South Asians may have culturally specific reasons to be ill at ease with certain ideas which are likely to form part of genetic counselling and inheritance. Richards and Ponder (1996) suggest that lay understanding of heredity is grounded in kinship structures which is further sustained by everyday social activities. Within English culture, kinship is broadly speaking bilateral with an equal role given to both sides of the family (Strathern, 1992). Genetic counsellors need to be aware that Hindu, Sikh and Muslim cultures draw fine and differentiating distinctions between the paternal and maternal side of the family, and that these representations may affect lay ideas about genetics and the inheritance of disease. Risk perception is affected not only by the dissemination of medical knowledge but also by a variety of cognitive biases, such as the availability heuristic (Tversky and Kahneman, 1973), whereby people may reject pure probability statements in favour of more immediately available knowledge such as, in the case of an inherited disorder, the very many healthy children within the family.

Malaria

Malaria is the single most important disease hazard facing travellers to most tropical countries (Hall,1989). Behrens (1993) has reported that people from ethnic minorities visiting relatives abroad are three times more likely to return to the UK with malaria than are tourists. While this higher risk may in part relate to geographical area visited and length of stay abroad, there is some suggestion in the literature that ethnic minority travellers are less likely to take chemoprophylaxis than business or tourist travellers (Bradley and Warhurst, 1993). Joshi and Khan (1995) interviewed 200 South Asians, resident in Britain, about their knowledge and attitudes towards malaria and their use of preventive measures on trips to the subcontinent or East Africa during the preceding three years. Forty eight per cent of the sample embarked upon taking malaria tablets, but only 6% took them for the recommended four weeks after returning to the UK. Adherence did not relate to socio-economic status, age or gender. The most frequently mentioned reason for not taking tablets, given by 47% of non-adherers, was a belief in immunity thought to have arisen from periods of time (for instance as a child) spent in malarious zones or, in some cases, from "ethnicity" itself. Recent health propaganda has attempted to disabuse lay people of the immunity belief since current medical thinking indicates that if a person has developed immunity in a tropical country, it will wear off during the first year of stay in the UK. Nineteen per cent of non-adherers rated the risk of malaria as low or zero in their locale – often seeing malaria as a problem of "other" poorer communities, but not their own. Reluctance to take medication over a long period was expressed by 10% of non-adherers not so much because of the specific side-effects associated with malaria prophylactic drugs, but more because the notion of long-term medication conflicted with ideas about the healthiness of the body in its "natural" unmedicated state.

Joshi and Khan's (1995) study illustrates another aspect of medication behaviour. Social psychologists such as Tajfel (1981) have frequently noted that individuals claim and demonstrate their social identities in a variety of ways – choice of dress, language, accent and so on. While being interviewed about adherence to anti-malaria prophylaxis, some South Asian respondents indicated their dislike of taking malaria tablets on "home" visits since the very taking of such medication marked their status as an outsider and someone who no longer belonged. The study indicates that the imagery of a disease, such as malaria, and of its attendant medication will vary according to cultural identity. Similarly, in a questionnaire study of beliefs about medication among students at a university in the south of England, Horne (1997) found that Asians believed more strongly than Europeans that medicines in general are harmful.

Coronary heart disease

Epidemiologists differentiate between relative and absolute risk (Rose, 1992) and the study of perceived vulnerability would be incomplete if it focused only on conditions where South Asian groups may be at higher risk than other groups but nevertheless at low absolute risk. Concentrating on diseases such as maternal and child death, sickle/beta thalassaemia, rickets, malaria and tuberculosis, further "exoticises" and "pathologises" ethnic minority members especially if life-styles are seen as causal agents (Hopkins, 1993; Sheldon and Parker, 1992). (See Gabe and Thorogood, (1986) and Morgan and Watkins (1988) for relevant research on prescribed drug use in Afro-Caribbean and white patients in the UK).

A ranking of the common causes of death shows that the health problems of ethnic minorities are in fact broadly similar to those of the general population (Bhopal, 1991) with circulatory diseases, cancer and respiratory diseases being the major killers (Smaje, 1995). Lay perceptions of the risk factors associated with coronary heart disease, a common cause of death, are similar in South Asian and non-Asian groups in the UK (Davison, Davey Smith and Frankel, 1991; Lambert and Sevak, 1996). Stress, heredity, smoking and diet are amongst the causal agents invoked by both groups, and health promotion messages are sometimes rejected when they are disconfirmed by contradictory examples encountered in daily life.

The perception of vulnerability to coronary heart disease requires study since it is well established that the South Asian population in UK is not only at absolute risk of coronary heart disease, but is also at greater relative risk than the indigenous population. McKeigue and Chaturvedi (1996) state that "across all age groups, the rates are 40% higher in South Asians, and for deaths before the age of 40 years there is a two fold excess of deaths in South Asian men. At later ages, South Asian women are especially affected". Preliminary work investigating attitudes to diet and coronary heart disease in London and Leicester (Thomas, Joshi, and Lamb, 1996) suggests that many South Asians are aware that, *as a group*, they are at higher risk of coronary heart disease than the indigenous population but nevertheless think that, *as individuals*, they are not at risk. Such perceptions, in line with the well-known phenomenon of unrealistic optimism (Weinstein, 1980), may well deter individuals from responding to health messages.

NORMATIVE FACTORS

Health decisions are socially and inter-personally located (Kippax and Crawford, 1993), and the TRA/TPB draws attention to the influence which family and friends can have over an individual's health care decisions. Due to a juxtaposition of financial constraints and ideological shifts in health service management in the UK, patients are discharged from hospital care earlier than in the past while still needing to follow complex treatment regimes. The influence of family and friends is likely to be greater in the domestic than in the hospital setting. Further, the home management of chronic conditions can have a bearing on patients' lives and the lives of those with whom they interact. Fishbein and Ajzen (1975) primarily conceptualise the influence of significant others upon individuals as an interpersonal matter, but there are grounds for suggesting that culture may partly determine the extent of normative influence.

Diabetes

Non-insulin dependent diabetes mellitus is a disease for which South Asians have high levels of absolute and relative risk. It is estimated to be about five times higher in South Asians than in Europeans; and in the UK "by the age of 55 years about 20% of South Asian men and women are diabetic" (McKeigue and Chaturvedi, 1996). The successful management of diabetes not only involves patients in regular and frequent assessments of bodily state through precise measurement but also in dietary change which many patients find oppressive and difficult. See Warren and Hixenbaugh, Chapter 16 for a discussion of adults with diabetes. Low rates of adherence to the diabetic regime are common for patients in general (Shillitoe and Miles, 1989) and some research suggests that dietary adherence is particularly difficult for South Asian patients. Commenting on an adherence survey by Samanta *et al.* (1987), Burden (1993) writes that "the results were frankly shocking: sugar was taken freely by many people, and there were high fat and calorie intakes".

Part of the blame for low adherence is laid at the door of poorly translated health messages (where, for example, sugar could be taken to refer to only white sugar) and inappropriate dietary listings which concentrated on Western rather than South Asian food items (see also Khajuria and Thomas, 1992). Furthermore, simplistic medical prescription for South Asian patients to avoid certain high fat/high sugar foods is culturally problematic when such items are of crucial social and symbolic importance. Hindus with diabetes interviewed in Bombay (Joshi, 1995) and Muslims with diabetes interviewed in East London (Kelleher and Islam, 1996) reported explicit pressure from friends and relations to eat medically unsuitable food on social and ceremonial occasions. As members of a culture which, in certain settings, values conformity and deference rather more than individuality and difference (Roland, 1988; Sinha and Tripathi, 1994), South Asian patients may take the views of family members into consideration to a much greater extent than do Western patients. Moreover, some South Asian women live in

family power-structures where their immediate interests are sub-
jugated to those of their husbands and older family members (Agarwal, 1994).

The self in relation to other

In the subjective norm component of the TRA/TPB model, the
participant's perception of the views of significant others is explicitly
mediated by the separate factor of his/her motivation to adhere to
the expectations of those significant others. Thus it is inherent in the
model that the individual is free, theoretically at least, *not* to adhere
to the advice of significant others. Such a model is concordant with
the Western philosophical tradition which places the individual cen-
tre-stage, clearly delineated from context. Thus, the TRA/TPB model
poses a picture of a bounded individual evaluating the views of
others as conceptually distinct from his or her own views. In many
other cultures, including South Asian cultures, the self is construed
more socially (Geertz, 1975; Shweder and Bourne, 1982), and more
importance is given to individuals' roles than to their personalities.
These considerations affect the way in which individuals construe
themselves and their needs (Roland, 1988), and Markus and
Kitayama (1991) argue that in non-Western cultures "it is the *other*
or the *self-in-relation-to-other* that is focal in individual experience".
As a result of boundary differences such as these, the conceptual
separation of self from other in the TRA/TPB model is culturally
unsuited to describing the psychology of South Asian patients.

Empirically, it is important for Western health care workers to
recognise that South Asian patients may not simply be behaviourally
responsive to family pressure but, due to an inter-dependent view of
self, may not conceptually isolate their needs as patients from their
needs to fulfil other more social roles. For example, in the case of the
Hindus with diabetes interviewed by Joshi (1995), patients felt
obliged to be good guests and eat unsuitable food not just in order
to please others but from an internally motivated desire, in the words
of one respondent, not to appear "as a separate person". Such a
statement raises conceptual problems for Ajzen and Madden's (1986)
TPB model in which perceived behavioural control (i.e. the extent to
which a person feels capable of performing a given action) is added
as a further component to the TRA model and seen as quite distinct

from the normative component. Perceived behavioural control has been assumed to encompass feelings of self-efficacy as well as the more concrete skills relevant to the action in question. However in a cultural context in which pressures of a moral or social kind are felt to be overwhelming, or have even been internalised, perceived behavioural control cannot usefully be distinguished from normative influence as is usual in the TPB model.

IN CONCLUSION

The literature on health attitudes and behaviour among South Asians in Britain is full of contradictory imagery. The community is depicted as knowing little of the concept of screening, and yet on the Indian subcontinent, the determination of foetal gender by amniocentesis is well-known to the point of abuse (Pandya, 1988). The culture is characterised as retrograde with respect to the seclusion of women and yet the support of the extended family system is seen to be beneficial. Overcrowding is used as an indicator of poverty and thereby implicated in poor health, but it has also been noted that the cultural practice of parental-infant bed sharing may limit the occurrence of sudden infant death syndrome (Farooqi, 1994). Sub-groups of the community are described in terms of "good" and "bad" health practices. For example, alcohol and cigarette consumption is low in Pakistani and Indian females (Ahmad, Kernohan and Baker, 1988) but the habit of betel nut chewing has been implicated in the excess cases of oral cancer found amongst South Asians (Donaldson and Clayton, 1984). Any attempts to generalise about health in general or adherence are further complicated by the confounding of ethnicity with class (Navarro, 1990; LaVeist, 1996). Poor adherence may be as much, if not more, related to structural than to attitude barriers.

Within an ethnic group, adherence in one health area may not predict adherence in another (Langlie, 1977), and it will be clear from the material reviewed in this chapter that the study of adherence in one ethnic minority will not necessarily throw light on adherence in any other group. What then can be learnt of *general* interest from the study of adherence in a *particular* ethnic group ? Two very pertinent points are raised in Anderson's (1986) study of the health ideology of Chinese immigrants to Canada. Firstly, cultural factors may affect health priority setting in a subtle manner. In an ethnographic study of families caring for a chronically ill child at home, Anderson (1986) found that Anglo-Canadian families strove to normalise the experiences of the child whereas immigrant Chinese families gave priority to fostering the "happiness" and "contentment" of the child. It is argued that in these two ideologies adherence to treatment is structured differently. The Anglo-Canadian families saw treatment as a way of achieving normalisation rather than "going down hill" whereas there was a tendency for the Chinese families to desist from rehabilitative procedures if any discomfort was shown by the child. Secondly, Anderson (1986) noted that ethnic differences amounted to a lack of reciprocity between practitioners and families. Practitioners *instructed* families without due recognition of "the network of cultural and social meanings in which the experience and management of illness is grounded". The danger in any doctor-patient encounter is that practitioners will see non-adherence as a "problem" to be corrected with even more rigorous instruction. But a sensitive study of ethnicity and adherence provides the very important service of reminding us of Zola's (1981) advice that we should "no longer speak of *medication compliance* but rather of *therapeutic alliance* ".

REFERENCES

Ahmad, W.I.U. (1992) The maligned healer: the 'hakim' and western medicine. *New Community* **18**, 521–536.

Ahmad, W.I.U., Baker, M. and Kernohan, E. (1991) General practitioners' perceptions of Asian and non-Asian patients. *Family Practice – An International Journal* **8**, 52–56.

Ahmad, W.I.U., Kernohan, E.E.M. and Baker, M.R. (1988) Alcohol and cigarette consumption among white and Asian general practice patients. *Health Education Journal* **47**, 128–129.

Ahmad, W.I.U., Kernohan, E. and Baker, M. (1989) Patients' choice of general practitioner: influence of patients' fluency in English and the ethnicity and sex of the doctor. *Journal of the Royal College of General Practitioners* **39**, 153–155.

Agarwal, B. (1994) *A field of one's own.* Cambridge: Cambridge University Press.

Ajzen, I. (1988) *Attitudes, personality, and behavior.* Chicago: Dorsey Press.

Ajzen, I. and Madden, T. (1986) Prediction of goal-directed behaviour: attitudes, intentions, and perceived behavioral control. *Journal of Experimental Social Psychology* **22**, 453–474.

Anderson, J. (1986) Ethnicity and illness experience: ideological structures and the health care delivery system. *Social Science and Medicine* **22**, 1277–1283.

Anionwu, E. (1993) Sickle cell and thalassaemia: community and official responses. In W.I.U. Ahmad (ed.) *'Race' and health in contemporary Britain.* Buckingham: Open University Press.

Argyle, M. (1972) *The psychology of interpersonal behaviour, 2nd edition.* Harmondsworth: Penguin.

Arnold, D. (1993) *Colonizing the body : state medicine and epidemic disease in nineteenth century India.* Berkeley: University of California Press.

Aslam, M., Davis, S.S. and Healy, M.A. (1979) Heavy metals in some Asian medicines and cosmetics. *Public Health London* **93**, 274–284.

Aslam, M. and Healy, M.A. (1983) Asian medicine. *Update* **27**, 1043–1048.

Atkin, K., Cameron, F., Badger, F. and Evers, H. (1989) Asian elders' knowledge and future use of community social and health services. *New Community* **15**, 439–445.

Baker, M.R., Bandaranayake, R. and Schweiger, M.S. (1984) Differences in rate of immunisation among ethnic groups. *British Medical Journal* **288**, 1075–1078.

Balarajan, R. and Raleigh, V.S. (1995) *Ethnicity and health in England.* London: HMSO.

Ballard, R. (1994) Introduction: the emergence of Desh Pardesh. In Desh Pardesh (ed.) *The South Asian presence in Britain.* London; Hurst and Co.

Ballard, R. (1996) The Pakistanis: stability and introspection. In C. Peach (ed.) *Ethnicity in the 1991 Census. Volume 2. The ethnic minority populations of Great Britain.* London: HMSO.

Becker, M.H. (1974) The health belief model and sick role behavior. *Health Education Monographs* **2**, 409–419.

Bedford, H.E., Masters, J.I. and Kurtz, Z (1992) Immunisation status in inner London primary schools. *Archives of Disease in Childhood* **67**, 1288–1291.

Behrens, R. (1993) Prevention of malaria. *The Practitioner* **237**, 714–716.

Berrington, A. (1996) Marriage patterns and inter-ethnic unions. In D. Coleman and J. Salt (eds.) *Ethnicity in the 1991 census. Volume 1. Demographic characteristics of the ethnic minority populations.* London: HMSO.

Bhatt, A. (1992) *Evaluation of Amar Dil: a video for South Asians.* Centre for Mass Communication Research, University of Leicester.

Bhopal, R.S. (1986) The inter-relationship of folk, traditional and western medicine within an Asian community in Britain. *Social Science and Medicine* **22**, 99–105.

Bhopal, R.S. (1991) Health education and ethnic minorities. *British Medical Journal* **302**, 1338.

Bhopal, R.S. and Samim, A.K. (1988) Immunisation uptake of Glasgow Asian children: paradoxical benefit of communication barriers? *Community Medicine* **10**, 215–220.

Blakemore, K. and Boneham, M. (1994) *Age, race and ethnicity.* Buckingham: Open University Press.

Bradley, S. and Friedman, E. (1993) Cervical cytology screening: a comparison of uptake among 'Asian' and 'non-Asian' women in Oldham. *Journal of Public Health Medicine* **15**, 46–51.

Bradley, D.J. and Warhurst D.C. (1993) Malaria imported into the United Kingdom during 1991. *Communicable Disease Report* **3**, R25–R28.

Bowler, I. (1993) 'They're not the same as us:' midwives' stereotypes of South Asian descent maternity patients. *Sociology of Health and Illness* **15**, 157–178.

Bulmer, M. (1996) The ethnic group question in the 1991 Census of population. In D. Coleman and J. Salt (eds.) *Ethnicity in the 1991 census. Volume 1. Demographic characteristics of the ethnic minority populations.* London: HMSO.

Burden, A. (1993) Diabetes: impact upon black and ethnic minority people. In A. Hopkins and V. Bahl (eds.) *Access to health care for people from black and ethnic minorities.* London: Royal College of Physicians.

Clarke, C., Peach, C. and Vertovec, S. (1990) *South Asians overseas: migration and ethnicity.* Cambridge: Cambridge University Press.

Dale, A. and Marsh, C. (eds.) (1993) *The 1991 census users' guide.* London: HMSO.

Darr, A.R. (1990) The Social implications of Thalassaemia among Muslims of Pakistani origin in England-family experience and service delivery. *Unpublished PhD Thesis.* University of London.

Davison, C., Davey Smith, G. and Frankel, S. (1991) Lay epidemiology and the prevention paradox: the implications of coronary candidacy for health education. *Sociology of Health and Illness* **13**, 1–19.

Department of Health (1993*)* *The health of the nation : a strategy for health in England.* London: HMSO.

DiMatteo, M.R. and DiNicola, D.D. (1982) *Achieving patient compliance.* Elmsord, NY; Pergamon.

DiNicola D.D. and DiMatteo M.R. (1984) Practitioners, patients, and compliance with medical regimens: A social psychological perspective. In A. Baum, S.E. Taylor and J.E. Singer (eds.) *Handbook of psychology and health. Volume 4.* Hillsdale: Lawrence Erlbaum.

Donaldson, L. (1986) Health and social status of elderly Asians: a community survey. *British Medical Journal* **293**, 1079–1082.

Donaldson, L.J. and Clayton, D.G. (1984) Occurrence of cancer in Asians and non-Asians. *Journal of Epidemiology and Community Health* **38**, 203–207.

Doyle, Y. (1991) A survey of the cervical screening service in a London district, including reasons for non-attendance, ethnic responses and views on the quality of service. *Social Science and Medicine* **32**, 953–957.

Duncan, B.L. (1976) Differential social perception and the attribution of intergroup violence: testing the lower limits of stereotyping Blacks. *Journal of Personality and Social Psychology* **34**, 590–8.

Eade, J., Vamplew, T. and Peach,C. (1996) The Bangladeshis: the encapsulated community. In C. Peach (ed.) *Ethnicity in the 1991 Census. Volume 2. The ethnic minority populations of Great Britain.* London: HMSO.

Fabrega, H. (1974) *Disease and social behavior: an interdisciplinary perspective.* Cambridge, MA: MIT Press.

Farooqi, S. (1994) Ethnic differences in infant care practices and in the incidence of sudden infant death syndrome in Birmingham. *Early Human Development* **38**, 209–213.

Firdous, R. and Bhopal, R.S. (1989) Reproductive health of Asian women: a comparative study with hospital and community perspectives. *Public Health* **103**, 307–315.

Fishbein, M. and Ajzen, I. (1975) *Belief, attitude, intention and behavior*. Reading, Mass: Addison-Wesley.

Ford, E.S. and Cooper, R.S. (1995) Implications of race/ethnicity for health and health care use. *Health Services Research* **30**, 237–252.

Gabe, J. and Thorogood, N. (1986) Prescribed drug use and the management of everyday life: the experiences of black and white working-class women. *Sociological Review* **34**, 7337–7772.

Garfinkel, H. (1967) *Studies in ethnomethodology*. Englewood Cliffs, NY: Prentice-Hall.

Geertz, C. (1975) On the nature of anthropological understanding. *American Scientist* **63**, 47–53.

Gillam, S.J., Jarman, B., White, P. and Law, R. (1989) Ethnic differences in consultation rates in urban general practice. *British Medical Journal* **299**, 953–957.

Gillborn, D. and Gipps, C. (1996) *Recent research on the achievements of ethnic minority pupils*. Ofsted Reviews of Research, London: HMSO.

Goffman, E. (1969) The insanity of place. *Psychiatry* **32**, 357–387.

Greenhalgh, T. (1987) Drug prescription and self-medication in India: an exploratory survey. *Social Science and Medicine* **25**, 307–318.

Gumperz, J.J., Jupp, T.C. and Roberts, C. (1979) *Crosstalk: an introduction to cross-cultural communication. New edition, 1990.* London: BBC TV Continuing Education and Training Department.

Hall, A. (1989) Malaria. In R. Dawood (ed.) *Travellers' health*. Oxford: Oxford University Press.

Hamilton, D.L. and Gifford, R.K. (1976) Illusory correlations in interpersonal perception: a cognitive basis of stereotypic judgments. *Journal of Experimental Social Psychology* **12**, 392–407.

Haynes, R.B. (1979) Introduction. In R.B. Haynes, D.W. Taylor and D.L. Sackett (eds.) *Compliance in health care*. Baltimore: Johns Hopkins University Press.

Hays R.D. and DiMatteo M.R. (1987) Key issues and suggestions for patient compliance assessment: sources of information, focus of measures, and nature of response options, *Journal of Compliance in Health Care* **2**, 37–53.

Heatley, P.T. and Yip, R.Y.W. (1991) Analysis of general practice consultation rates among Asian patients. *British Journal of General Practice* **41**, 476.

Helman, C.G. (1978) 'Feed a cold, starve a fever': folk models of infection in an English suburban community, and their relation to medical treatment. *Culture, Medicine and Psychiatry* **2**, 107–137.

Hoare, T., Thomas, C., Biggs, A., Booth, M., Bradley, S. and Friedman E. (1994) Can the uptake of breast screening by Asian women be increased? A randomized controlled trial of a linkworker intervention. Journal of Public Health Medicine **16**, 179–185.

Hofstede, G. (1980) *Culture's consequences.* Beverly Hills, CA: Sage.

Homans, H. (1980) Pregnant in Britain: a sociological approach to Asian and British women's experiences, *Unpublished PhD Thesis.* University of Warwick.

Hopkins, A. (1993) Envoi. In A. Hopkins and V. Bahl (eds.) *Access to health care for people from black and ethnic minorities.* London: Royal College of Physicians London.

Horne, R. (1997) *Unpublished Ph.D. thesis.* Department of Pharmacy, University of Brighton.

Hunte, P.A. and Sultana, F. (1992) Health-seeking behavior and the meaning of medications in Balochistan, Pakistan. *Social Science and Medicine* **34**, 1385–1397.

Jani, B., Mistry, H., Patel, N., Anionwu, E. and Pembrey, M. (1992) A study of beta thalassaemia in the Gujarati community of north London. *Paediatric Reviews and Communication* **6**, 191–192.

Janz, N.K. and Becker M.H. (1984) The health belief model: a decade later. *Health Education Quarterly* **11**, 1–47.

Johnson, M.R.D., Cross, M. and Cardew, S.A. (1983) Inner-city residents, ethnic minorities and primary health care. *Postgraduate Medical Journal* **59**, 664–667.

Jones, V.M. (1987) Current infant weaning practices within the Bangladeshi community in the London borough of Tower Hamlets. *Human Nutrition: Applied Nutrition* **41a**, 349–352.

Joshi, M.S. (1995) Lay explanations of the causes of diabetes in India and the UK. In Markova and R.M. Farr (eds.) *Representations of health, illness and handicap.* Chur, Switzerland: Harwood Academic Publishers.

Joshi, M.S. and Khan, S. (1995) The use of malaria prophylaxis amongst South Asians resident in the UK. *Proceedings of the British Psychological Society* **4**, 38.

Kakar, S. (1978) *The inner world : a psycho-analytic study of childhood and society in India.* Delhi: Oxford University Press.

Kakar, S. (1982) *Mystics, shamans and doctors*. Delhi : Oxford University Press.

Kelleher, D. and Islam, S. (1996) 'How should I live?' Bangladeshi people and non-insulin-dependent diabetes. In D. Kelleher and S. Hillier (eds) *Researching cultural differences in health*. London: Routledge.

Khajuria, S. and Thomas, J. (1992) Traditional Indian beliefs about dietary management of diabetes – an exploratory study of the implications for the management of Gujarati diabetics in Britain. *Journal of Human Nutrition and Dietetics* **5**, 311–321.

Kippax, S. and Crawford, J. (1993) Flaws in the Theory of Reasoned Action. In D.J. Terry, C. Gallois and M. McCamish (eds.) *The theory of reasoned action: its application to Aids-preventive behaviour*. Oxford: Pergamon.

Kleinman, A. (1980) *Patients and healers in the context of culture*. Berkeley: University of California Press.

Kleinman, A. (1987) Culture and clinical reality: commentary on culture-bound syndromes and international disease classifications. *Culture, Medicine and Psychiatry* **11**, 49–52.

Lambert, H. and Sevak, L. (1996) Is 'cultural difference ' a useful concept?: perceptions of health and the sources of ill health among Londoners of South Asian origin. In D. Kelleher and S. Hillier (eds.) *Researching cultural differences in health*. London: Routledge.

Landrine, H. and Klonoff E.A. (1992) Culture and health-related schemas: a review and proposal for interdisciplinary integration. *Health Psychology* **11**, 267–276.

Langlie, J.K. (1977) Social networks, health beliefs, and preventive health behavior. *Journal of Health and Social Behavior* **18**, 244–260.

LaVeist, T.A. (1996) Why we should continue to study race .. but do a better job : an essay on race, racism and health. *Ethnicity and Disease* **6**, 21–29.

Ley, P. (1988) *Communicating with patients*. London: Chapman and Hall.

Madan, T.N. (1969) Who chooses modern medicine and why? *Economic and Political Weekly* **4**, 1475–1484.

Markus, H.R. and Kitayama, S. (1991) Culture and the self: implications for cognition, emotion, and motivation. *Psychological Review* **98**, 224–253.

Mason, D. (1995) *Race and ethnicity in modern Britain*. Oxford: Oxford University Press.

McAvoy, B.R. and Raza, R. (1988) Asian women: (i) contraceptive knowledge, attitudes and usage; (ii) contraceptive services and cervical cytology. *Health Trends* **20**, 11–17.

McKeigue, P. and Chaturvedi, N. (1996) Epidemiology and control of cardiovascular disease in South Asians and Afro-Caribbeans. In *Ethnicity and health: reviews of literature and guidance for purchasers in the areas of cardiovascular disease, mental health and haemoglobinopathies*. York: NHS Centre for Reviews and Dissemination, University of York.

Miller, T. (1995) Shifting boundaries: exploring the influence of cultural traditions and religious beliefs of Bangladeshi women on antenatal interactions. *Women's Studies International Forum* **18**, 299–309.

Minocha, A.A. (1980) Medical pluralism and health services in India. *Social Science and Medicine* **14B**, 217–223.

Morgan, M. and Watkins, C.J. (1988) Managing hypertension: beliefs and responses to medication among cultural groups. *Sociology of Health and Illness* **10**, 561–578.

Naish, J., Brown, J. and Denton, B. (1994) Intercultural consultations: investigation of factors that deter non-English speaking women from attending their general practitioners for cervical screening. *British Medical Journal* **309**, 1126–8.

Navarro, V. (1990) Race or class versus race and class: mortality differentials in the United States. *The Lancet* **336**, 1238–1240.

Nichter, M. (1980) The layperson's perceptions of medicine as perspective into the utilization of multiple therapy systems in the Indian context. *Social Science and Medicine* **14B**, 225–233.

Office of Population Censuses and Surveys /General Register Office for Scotland (1993) *1991 census, ethnic group and country of birth, Great Britain. Two volumes*. London: HMSO.

Owen, D. (1996) Size, structure and growth of the ethnic minority populations. In D. Coleman and J. Salt *Ethnicity in the 1991 census. Volume 1. Demographic characteristics of the ethnic minority populations*. London: HMSO.

Pandya, S.K. (1988) Yearning for baby boys. *British Medical Journal* **296**, 1312.

Peach, C. (1996) Introduction. In C. Peach (ed.) *Ethnicity in the 1991 Census. Volume 2. The ethnic minority populations of Great Britain.* London: HMSO.

Peterson, E., Wright, S., Daley, J. and Thibault, G. (1994) Racial variation in cardiac procedure use and survival following acute myocardial infarction in the Department of Veterans' Affairs. *Journal of the American Medical Association* **271,** 1755–1180.

Poonia, K. and Ward, L. (1990) Fair share of (the) care? *Community Care* **796,** 16–18.

Rack, P. (1982) *Race, culture, and mental disorder.* London: Tavistock.

Rashid, A. and Jagger, C. (1992) Attitudes to and perceived use of health care services among Asian and non-Asian patients in Leicester. *British Journal of General Practice* **42,** 197–201.

Richards, M. and Ponder, M. *(1996)* Lay understanding of genetics: A test of a hypothesis. *Journal of Medical Genetics* **33,** 1032–1036 .

Robinson, V. (1984) Asians in Britain: a study in encapsulation and marginality. In C. Clarke, D Ley and C Peach (eds.) *Geography and ethnic pluralism.* London: Allen and Unwin.

Robinson, V. (1996) The Indians: onward and upward. In C. Peach (ed.) *Ethnicity in the 1991 Census. Volume 2. The ethnic minority populations of Great Britain.* London: HMSO.

Roland, A. (1988*) In search of self in India and Japan: towards a cross-cultural psychology.* Princeton: Princeton University Press.

Rose, G. (1992) *The strategy of preventive medicine.* Oxford: Oxford University Press.

Rosenstock, I.M. (1966) *Why people use health services.* Millbank Memorial Fund.

Rudat, K. (1994) *Black and minority ethnic groups in Britain: health and lifestyles.* London: Health Education Authority.

Samanta, A., Campbell, J.E., Spalding, D.L., Panja, K.K., Neogi, S.K. and Burden, A.C. (1987) Dietary habits of Asian diabetics in a general practice clinic. *Human Nutrition: Applied Nutrition* **47a,** 160–163.

Shaukat, N., de Bono, D.P. and Cruickshank, J.K. (1993) Clinical features, risk factors, and referral delay in British patients of Indian and European origin with angina matched for age and extent of coronary atheroma. *British Medical Journal* **307,** 717–718.

Sheldon, T.A. and Parker, H. (1992) Race and ethnicity in health research. *Journal of Public Health Medicine* **14,** 104–110.

Shillitoe, R.W. and Miles, D.W. (1989) Diabetes mellitus. In A.K. Browne (ed) *Health psychology: processes and applications.* London: Chapman and Hall.

Shweder, R.A. and Bourne, E.J. (1982) Does the concept of the person vary cross-culturally? In. A.J. Marsella and G. White (eds) *Cultural conceptions of mental health and therapy.* Dordrecht: Reidel.

Sillitoe, K. and White, P.H. (1992) Ethnic group and the British census: the search for a question. *Journal of the Royal Statistical Society, Series A* **55**, 141–63.

Sinha, D. and Tripathi, R.C. (1994) Individualism in a collectivist culture. In U. Kim, H.C. Triandis, C. Kagitcibasi, S-C Choi and G. Yoon (eds.) *Individualism and collectivism: theory, method, and applications.* Thousand Oaks: Sage.

Smaje, C. (1995) *Health, 'race' and ethnicity.* London: King's Fund Institute.

Strathern, M. (1992) *After nature: English kinship in the late twentieth century.* Cambridge: Cambridge University Press.

Sutcliffe, R.I. (1985) A comparison of contacts with Asian and British patients: implications of primary care in Asians. In *Trainee projects: occasional paper 29.* London: Royal College of General Practitioners.

Tajfel, H. (1981) *Human groups and social categories.* Cambridge: Cambridge University Press.

Taylor, S.E. (1995) *Health psychology.* New York: McGraw Hill.

Thomas, J., Joshi, M.S. and Lamb, R. (1997) *Diet, attitudes to diet and coronary heart disease among South Asians in the UK.* Report to the Health Education Authority.

Townsend, P., Davidson, N. and Whitehead, M. (1988) *The black report/the health divide.* London: Penguin.

Tversky, A. and Kahneman, D. (1973) Availability: a heuristic for judging frequency and probability. *Cognitive Psychology* **5**, 207–32.

Weinstein, N.D. (1980) Unrealistic optimism about life events. *Journal of Personality and Social Psychology* **39**, 806–820 ..

Wright, C. (1983) Language and communication problems in an Asian community, *Journal of the Royal College of General Practitioners* **33**, 101–104.

Zborowski, M. (1952) Cultural components in responses to pain. *Journal of Social Issues* **8**, 16–30.

Zola, I.K. (1966) Culture and symptoms: an analysis of patients' presenting complaints. *American Sociological Review* **31,** 615–630.

Zola, I.K. (1981) Structural constraints in the doctor-patient relationship: The case of non-compliance. In L. Eisenberg and A. Kleinman (eds.) *The Relevance of Social Science for Medicine.* Dordrecht, Holland: D. Reidel.

Acknowledgments

I would like to thank Bradford Health Libraries and Information Services, Share (King's Fund Institute) and Anne Lee for help in conducting a literature search.

Adherence to different treatments

11

Adherence to Medication: A Review of Existing Research

Robert Horne

The prescription of medication is one of the most common medical interventions and the appropriate use of medicines is a key aspect to the self-management of most chronic illnesses. However, many patients fail to do this and low rates of adherence to medication are seen as problematic in many chronic diseases including asthma (Yeung *et al.*, 1994), diabetes (Glasgow, McCaul and Scafer, 1986), heart disease (Horwitz *et al.*, 1990; Monane *et al.*, 1994), cancer (Lilley-man and Lennard, 1996) and kidney disease (Cleary *et al.*, 1995). The incidence of reported medication non-adherence varies greatly from 4–92% across studies, converging at 30–50% in chronic illness (Haynes *et al.*, 1979; Meichenbaum and Turk, 1987). The reasons for such a wide variation are complex and relate to discrepancies in the definition and measurement of adherence across studies, which are discussed by Myers and Midence in Chapter 1. This chapter will provide an overview of existing research relating to medication adherence and outline some of the implications for practice.

TYPES OF ADHERENCE RESEARCH

Over the last 25 years or so a plethora of research studies have been conducted in an attempt to identify the determinants of adherence and to develop effective interventions to enhance adherence. This research has been characterised by three broad approaches.

Atheoretical approaches

A review of the literature indicates that much of the early research and a portion of more recent research is atheoretical in its approach. Such research is a pragmatic attempt to identify the causes of non-adherent behaviour or to evaluate interventions to change such behaviour. The philosophical starting point for much of this research appears to be the notion that non-adherence is a trait characteristic which may be linked to certain socio-demographic or dispositional features of the patient.

The communication model

This approach focuses on the role of communication and the nature of interactions between patients and health professionals (HPs). Although this research does not appear to be explicitly theory driven, it draws on an implicit theory that the quality of the patient's interaction with the HP is of prime importance. This approach, which is typified by the work of Ley (1982; 1988), stems from the observation that patients either misunderstand or forget treatment instructions or they may lack motivation to take the treatment, because they are dissatisfied with some aspect of the doctor-patient relationship. (For a discussion of doctor-patient communication see Noble, Chapter 3).

The social cognition models and self-regulatory theory

This approach focuses on patients' beliefs and the sociocultural context in which they occur. It draws on a range of theoretical models, commonly referred to as *social cognition models* (SCMs), which attempt to explain health-related behaviours in relation to specific cognitions (Conner and Norman, 1996; Stroebe and Stroebe, 1995). These include expectancy-value models such as the Health Belief Model (HBM; e.g. Rosenstock, 1974), the Theory of Reasoned

Action (TRA; Ajzen and Fishbein, 1980) and its revision the Theory of Planned Behaviour (TPB; Ajzen, 1985) in which the decision whether or not to follow treatment advice is based on the patient's expectations of what the treatment will achieve and the value which they place upon it. In contrast, Leventhal's self-regulatory theory or model (SRM; Leventhal, Meyer and Nerenz, 1980) views adherence as the product of a dynamic interaction between patients experience of and beliefs about the illness, their emotional reaction to it and their appraisal of the impact of adherence/non-adherence on their well-being. (For a description of this model see Chapter 2).

Each of the above approaches has been applied to two key questions "what are the determinants of adherence?" and "how can adherence be enhanced?" This chapter summarises the contribution of this research to our understanding of medication adherence.

THE DETERMINANTS OF NON-ADHERENCE: ATHEORETICAL APPROACHES

The issue of patient non-adherence came to prominence with the publication of the classic reviews of Sackett and Haynes (Haynes, Taylor and Sackett, 1979; Sackett and Haynes, 1976). These reviews summarised a large body of research which attempted to identify the determinants of adherence. Much of this early work was either a search for demographic factors and personality traits which "caused" non-adherence, or for the particular characteristics of the disease or treatment which acted as barriers to following the treatment instructions.

In an early systematic review of 185 studies, (Sackett and Haynes, 1976), no clear relationship emerged between race, gender, educational experience, intelligence, marital status, occupational status, income and ethnic or cultural background and adherence behaviours. The only consistent finding was that non-adherence was associated with extremes of age (see Bryon, Chapter 7 and McKelnay and McCallion, Chapter 9). Meichenbaum and Turk (1987) suggest that this may be because the very young are more averse to bad tasting medicine and the very old are more susceptible to forgetfulness or self-neglect. However, recent research suggests that younger patients may be less adherent (Bosley, Fosbury and Cochrane, 1995; Daniels, Rene and Daniels, 1994; DiMatteo *et al.*, 1993; Frazier, Davis Ali and Dahl, 1994; Lorenc and Branthwaite, 1993; Sherbourne *et al.*, 1992). There is little evidence that adherence behaviours can be explained in terms of trait personality characteristics (Becker, 1979; Bosley *et al.*, 1995; McKim, Stones, Kozma, 1990).

A socio-demographic/dispositional approach to the adherence problem has fundamental limitations. Even if stable associations exist, they would serve to identify certain "at risk" groups but could do little to indicate the type or content of interventions to enhance adherence. Furthermore, socio-demographic characteristics and personality traits are not generally amenable to change and therefore, present few opportunities for interventions. In practice, the idea that stable socio-demographic or dispositional character-istics are the sole determinants of adherence is discredited by evi-dence that an individual's levels of adherence may vary over time and between different aspects of the treatment regimen (Cleary *et al.*, 1995; Hilbrands, Hoitsma and Koene, 1995; Kruse and Weber, 1990; Rudd *et al.*, 1989). Thus, searching for the stable characteristics which make up the "noncompliant patient" is fruitless as a person may comply with some aspects of their treatment but not others. This limitation also applies to the search for disease and treatment char-acteristics as antecedents of adherence, since there are wide varia-tions in adherence between and within patients with the same disease and treatment (e.g. Cleary *et al.*, 1995; Horwitz *et al.*, 1990; Lilleyman and Lennard, 1996).

Failure to recognise these limitations leads to mistaken assump-tions about how the problem of low adherence may be resolved. For example, the observed correlation between regimen complexity and non-adherence (Sackett and Haynes, 1976), seems to have led to the assumption in some quarters that simply reducing the dose fre-quency is enough to prevent non-adherence as evidenced in the marketing of "once daily" pharmaceuticals. However, there is little evidence to support the efficacy of this single strategy in enhancing adherence to medication (Haynes *et al.*, 1979; Myers and Branthwaite, 1992).

The fallacy of "once daily dose" as a panacea for non-adherence is illustrated by a recent prospective study (Myers and Branthwaite, 1992) in which 89 depressed out-patients were randomly allocated to one of three, therapeutically equivalent, daily dosage schedules of the same antidepressant medication (amitripyline and mianserin). Group A received their medication at night, Group B received their medication in three divided doses and Group C were allowed a free choice between regimen A or B. Adherence rates did not differ according to whether the regimen was prescribed once or three times a day. However, patients who chose a three times a day regimen were significantly more adherent than those who were randomly allocated to this regimen. This and other recent studies reinforce the view that if frequency of dosing is a barrier for a particular individual reducing the number of daily doses can facilitate adherence. However, the *routine* choice of once daily regimens is unjustified (Cramer *et al.*, 1989; Eisen *et al.*, 1990). Complexity *per se* is not the key issue but how well the treatment fits in with the individual patient's routine (Cockburn, *et al.*, 1987; Meichenbaum and Turk, 1987).

One of the key findings to emerge from Meichenbaum and Turk's (1987) extensive review of the adherence literature was that stable characteristics such as the nature of the disease and treatment or socio-demographic variables influence the adherence behaviour of some patients more than others. This has led to a greater emphasis on understanding the interaction of the individual with the disease and treatment, rather than identifying the socio-demographic features which characterise the "non-compliant patient". An early example of a more patient-focused approach is research linking patients' knowledge to adherence as discussed below.

MEDICATION KNOWLEDGE AND ADHERENCE

Many patients lack basic knowledge about their medication (al Mahdy and Seymour, 1990; Cartwright, 1994; Eagleton, Walker and Barber, 1993). However, the relationship between a patient's knowledge of their medication regimen and their adherence to it is by no means simple or clear-cut. In his classic, systematic review of the adherence literature, Haynes (1976) concluded that, although 12 studies had demonstrated a positive association between knowledge and adherence, there were at least twice as many studies, which were more methodologically sound, that had failed to demonstrate a link. Studies conducted since then generally reinforce the view that associations between knowledge and adherence are at best small and inconsistent (Eagleton *et al.*, 1993; Lee, Wing and Wong, 1992) In addition, enhancing knowledge does not necessarily improve adherence (George, Waters and Nicholas, 1983; Haynes *et al.*, 1978).

One problem with this approach is that many of the studies linking knowledge and adherence have used cross-sectional designs. This means that it is difficult to assign causality. Are patients less adherent because they lack knowledge or are non-adherent patients less interested in their treatment and so do not seek out information? Another reason for inconsistencies in association between knowledge and adherence is that medication knowledge is not a unitary concept, but rather comprises different knowledge components. This is illustrated by Ascione, Kirscht and Shimp (1986) in a study of 187 ambulatory cardiovascular patients. The authors found wide intra and inter-patient variations in level of knowledge about three aspects of medication. Patients knew most about the purpose of the medication and how to take it. Fewer patients knew what to do if they missed a dose and only a small minority could identify the common side-effects associated with their treatment. Thus, the observed inconsistencies in the relationship between medication knowledge and adherence may be partially explained by variations in the way in which medication knowledge is conceptualised and measured.

Although a basic awareness of how and when to take medication is an essential pre-requisite for adherence (Raynor, Booth and Blenkinsopp, 1993), we should not assume that all we need do to prevent non-adherence is to give patients clear information about how to use their treatment. Adherence research which focuses only on patients' knowledge of the regimen fails to take account of the fact that non-adherence may arise from an active decision on the part of the patient and may not simply be due to a lack of competence or lack of knowledge about how to use the medication (Cooper, Love and Raffoul, 1982). A further point is that there is variation between individuals in the desire for information (Weinman, 1990). Recognition that many patients make decisions about whether or not to take the treatment as instructed underpins the "communication approach" to adherence research (Ley, 1988). This approach suggests that adherence depends on the patient receiving and understanding the necessary information and being able to remember it accurately. It also suggests that patients who are more satisfied with their care will be more likely to adhere to the treatment regimen. Addressing these issues extends the scope of adherence research to include the role of the physician (DiMatteo and DiNicola, 1982) and HP-Patient interactions (Ley, 1988).

HEALTH PRACTITIONER-PATIENT INTERACTIONS AS DETERMINANTS OF ADHERENCE: THE COMMUNICATION APPROACH

Patients do not always understand prescription instructions (Sarriff *et al.*, 1992) and often forget considerable portions of what HPs tell them (Ley and Llewellyn, 1995; Weinman, 1987). It is well recognised that many patients have a poor understanding of terminology which is often used by doctors in communicating details about illness (Boyle, 1970; Weinman, 1987) and medication (Sarriff *et al.*, 1992). Consequently, many patients have a poor understanding of the details of their medication regimen (Cleary *et al.*, 1995; Eagleton *et al.*, 1993; Lee *et al.*, 1992).

There is increasing interest in the role of patient satisfaction as a mediator between information provision, recall and adherence. A number of surveys suggest that many patients are dissatisfied with aspects of consultations with HPs and the amount of information offered to them about their illness and treatment (Cartwright, 1967; Hall, Rotter and Katz, 1988; Ley, 1982; Gibbs and George, 1990). In a national UK survey of patients' satisfaction with medicines information received, over 70% of respondents wanted more information than they were given (Gibbs and George, 1990). Dissatisfaction with attributes of the practitioner or the amount of information and explanation provided may act as a barrier to adherence by making the patient less motivated towards treatment (Hall *et al.*, 1988).

More recent studies have attempted to relate patient satisfaction to the degree to which patient expectations about specific aspects of the consultation were fulfilled (Lassen, 1991; Williams *et al.*, 1995). In a study involving 504 patients of 25 General Practitioners in 10 London practices, patient expectations were determined in terms of needs, requests and desires prior to seeing the doctor. The fulfilment of these expectations was assessed using validated questionnaires.

Patients were generally much more eager to obtain an "explanation of their problem" than they were to obtain "support" or "tests and diagnosis" and the degree to which their expectations were met was predictive of satisfaction with the encounter (Williams *et al.*, 1995).

Further insight into the importance of addressing patients needs for clear explanations of their illness and treatment is provided by the Medical Outcomes Study, a large study of how patients fare with health care in the USA (e.g. Stewart and Ware, 1992). One aim of this study was to examine the influence of physician's characteristics on patient adherence to a range of treatments. In a cohort of over 8,000 patients, reported medication adherence at 2 years was related to (a) reported medication adherence at baseline and (b) the tendency of the physician to report that they saw a greater number of patients per week, and arranged a specific follow up appointment. It is interesting that socio-demographic characteristics of patients and doctors had no influence on adherence and that adherence to one aspect of the treatment (e.g. medication) did not predict adherence to any other (e.g. diet, exercise). The authors hypothesise that adherence was stimulated by scheduling frequent follow-up visits in which the patients' experience with medication could be monitored.

Another aspect of patient satisfaction in relation to medication use is the extent to which the patient's desire to be involved in the decision to prescribe is fulfilled. More studies are needed to establish whether the patients' degree of perceived empowerment within the prescribing decision is correlated with adherence (McCrea *et al.*, 1993).

At this stage it is worth pausing to consider studies evaluating interventions to enhance medication. This is an appropriate stage to review these studies since the majority are based upon the atheoretical or communication approaches described above.

INTERVENTIONS TO ENHANCE MEDICATION ADHERENCE

On reviewing the adherence interventions literature it quickly becomes apparent that although one finds particular interventions which appear to have improved adherence in specific situations, no single intervention seems to stand out as being consistently effective. In a recent systematic review of this literature, Haynes, McKibbon and Kanani (1996) commented that the majority of interventions are limited in scope and that most of the strategies evaluated using rigorous controlled clinical trial methodologies were "not very effective, despite the amount of effort and resources they consumed".

The discovery of a single intervention which is effective in all situations is something of an "adherence Holy Grail" but the fact that it has not yet been found should not surprise us. The search seems to rest on an implicit assumption that adherence is a unitary phenomenon. However, adherence is clearly multifactorial with a large range of determinants. One reason why the success of adherence interventions does not seem to be generalisable is that adherence behaviours are not generalisable. It is likely that the salience of particular determinants will vary between individuals and in the same individual across treatments and over time. A further complication is that non-adherent behaviour may be the intentional result of an active decision by the patient (Cooper *et al.*, 1982). Thus, an intervention which is effective in some situations (e.g. reminding the patient who forgets) may be ineffective in another (e.g. if the patient avoids taking the medication because of unpleasant side-effects).

The multifactorial nature of adherence and the fact that non-adherence is often volitional has led to a shift in the conceptualisation of adherence and a change in the focus of research. Adherence is best thought of as a *state*, rather than a *trait* characteristic (Horne, 1993). Individual patients may adhere to some aspects of their treatment and not others and adherence rates may vary over time. Interventions designed to make the patient more effective at following the prescribed instructions are unlikely to work if the patient has decided not to take a particular medication or if taking it is perceived as unimportant. Consequently, the emphasis of adherence research over the last decade or so has moved away from attempts to identify stable trait factors which characterise the non-adherent patient to achieving a greater understanding of how and why patients decide to take some treatments and not others (Horne, 1993). Much of this research is informed by psychological theories which conceptualise behaviour as the product of cognitions which occur within a social framework. This approach is informed by a recognition that "what a person thinks influences what they do" and has led to a large number of psychologically-based research studies which seek to explain variations in adherence by understanding how people make adherence-related decisions. This research has drawn on two broad theoretical approaches. Social cognition models (SCMs) and Leventhal's self-regulatory theory or model (SRM) These theoretical approaches are described in more detail in Chapter 2.

BELIEFS AS PREDICTORS OF MEDICATION ADHERENCE

Social Cognition Models

SCMs have been used in a number of studies of medication adherence. The most commonly used models in this respect are the HBM and the TRA and its revision the TPB. These models have been applied singly or in combination to medication adherence in a range of illness groups including: hypertension (Nelson *et al.*, 1978; Inui, Yourtee and Wiliamson, 1976; Taylor, 1979; Ried *et al.*, 1985; Miller *et al.*, 1992), renal disease (Hartman and Becker, 1978; Cummings *et al.*, 1981), psychiatric illnesses (Budd, Hughes and Smith, 1996; Cochran and Gitlin, 1988; Pan and Tantam, 1989; Kelly *et al.*, 1987), diabetes (Brownlee-Duffeck *et al.*, 1987) and the treatment of urinary tract infections (Ried and Christensen, 1988)

So what do the SCMs contribute to our understanding of medication adherence? Methodological limitations and inconsistencies in the way in which models have been operationalised and applied in studies of medication taking prevent us from drawing firm conclusions. Common flaws in existing studies include the use of cross-sectional designs to test a predictive model (e.g. Cochran and Gitlin, 1988; Cummings *et al.*, 1981; Hartman and Becker, 1978) and lack of explanation of how constructs were operationalised and validated (e.g. Cummings *et al.*, 1981; Nelson *et al.*, 1978; Taylor, 1979). Marteau (1995) has suggested that the presence of methodological limitations such as these may mean that the models have not been fully evaluated.

Despite its limitations, existing SCM-based research indicates that medication non-adherence may arise from a rational decision on the part of the patient and identifies some of the cognitions which are salient to these decisions. Although there is some variation in the specific type of beliefs which are associated with adherence across studies, the findings show that certain cognitive variables included in the HBM and TPB appear to be prerequisites of adherence in certain situations. For example, beliefs that failure to take the treatment could result in adverse consequences and that one is personally susceptible to these effects tends to be associated with higher adherence rates (Cummings *et al.*, 1981; Kelly *et al.*, 1987; Nelson *et al.*, 1978; Taylor, 1979). Additionally, adherence decisions may be influenced by a cost-benefit analysis in which the *benefits* of treatment are weighted against the perceived *barriers* (Brownlee-Duffeck *et al.*, 1987; Cummings *et al.*, 1981; Nelson *et al.*, 1978; Taylor, 1979). Other studies, based on the TRA/TPB have shown that the perceived views of significant others such as family, friends and doctors (*normative beliefs*) may also influence adherence (Cochran and Gitlin, 1988; Ried and Christensen, 1988; Ried *et al.*, 1985). Several studies have demonstrated the value of interventions based on the HBM in facilitating health-related behaviours, such as attending for medical check-ups (Haefner and Kirscht, 1970), or using emergency care facilities in an acute asthma attack (Jones, Jones and Katz, 1987). However, few studies have applied this model to interventions to enhance medication adherence.

Thus, applied to medication-related behaviours, SCMs have identified cognitions which are germane to decisions about whether or not to take medication. In doing so they help to reframe adherence issues. Within a social cognition framework, medication taking can be seen as a volitional act which is, to some extent, the result of a rational decision by the patient. This contrasts with other adherence research paradigms which, broadly speaking, tend to conceptualise non-adherence as a function of patient incompetence and clinicians' failure to enhance it, or as an unavoidable consequence of certain trait characteristics. Although limited in scope, SCM-related adherence research has opened the door to a broader conception of adherence which recognises that medication adherence may reflect patients *beliefs* as well as their ability to comprehend, remember and follow instructions.

Leventhal's Self-Regulatory Model

The potential utility of the SRM as a theoretical framework for understanding adherence is described in Chapter 2. One of the advantages of this model is that it conceptualises the relationship between beliefs as a dynamic interaction rather than a static one-off decision. It differs from the SCMs in that it includes a feedback loop in the form of an appraisal stage (Leventhal Zimmerman and Gutmann, 1984). Patients evaluate the effect of taking or not taking their medication and adjust their behaviour or beliefs accordingly. The model also acknowledges that illness beliefs, the selection of coping procedures (such as taking medication) and the subjective appraisal of the outcome of coping are all influenced by social and cultural factors and by personality traits (Leventhal *et al.*, 1992). The complexity of the framework contributes to its validity as an explanatory model of adherence, but also makes it difficult to operationalise in its entirety within the constraints of research studies. A further impairment to the empirical testing of the model is that, although the relevant components of the cognitive representation of illness are clearly specified, there was until recently no standard method for operationalising the representations construct. Consequently, there has been little uniformity across studies. This problem has recently been addressed by the development of the Illness Perception Questionnaire (IPQ), a validated method for the quantitative assessment of the 5 components of illness representation (Weinman *et al.*, 1996)

In the absence of a full validation of the SRM as a whole, one is left to judge the merits of the self-regulatory approach on the basis of studies which have empirically evaluated certain key tenants of the model. Some of these studies provide indirect support for a self-regulatory approach, whereas others have specifically used the model to conceptualise their research question.

The importance of symptom perception in influencing illness representations and behaviour was reinforced by a study of patients with diabetes who used perceived symptoms to indicate their blood glucose levels and to guide self-treatment (Gonder-Frederick and Cox, 1991). However, patient's beliefs about their symptoms, and estimations of their own blood glucose levels were often erroneous and resulted in poor diabetic control. Further evidence of the importance of illness representations was obtained by Meyer and colleagues who noted a clear relationship between illness representations and behaviour in their study of patients with hypertension (Meyer, Leventhal and Gutmann 1985). Patients who believed that their hypertension was an acute condition were more likely to drop out of treatment than those who believed it to be a chronic condition. This study also showed that patients' representations of the illness often conflicted with the medical view and provided an insight into the effects of this mismatch. In a group of 50 patients who had continued in treatment, 80% agreed with the statement that " people cannot tell when their blood pressure is up". However, 92% believed that they could tell when their own blood pressure was raised by monitoring symptoms such as tiredness, headache and stress. Patients who believed that their anti-hypertensive medication improved symptoms were more likely to take it. A striking example of this was provided by 5 out of 17 patients who believed that their medication affected symptoms. These patients took their anti-hypertensive medication only when they judged their blood pressure to be raised. The patients had understood and accepted the abstract medical view of hypertension as an asymptomatic condition but their concrete experience of symptoms caused them to hold contrasting beliefs and to behave according to these.

BELIEFS ABOUT MEDICATION AS PREDICTORS OF ADHERENCE

A number of qualitative studies, which have been conducted independently of the SRM, have shown that people hold complex beliefs about medication and suggested that these might influence adherence (Arluke, 1980; Britten, 1994; Conrad, 1985; Donovan and Blake, 1992; Fallsberg, 1991; Morgan and Watkins, 1988). This research is summarised in recent reviews (Blaxter and Britten, 1997; Horne, 1997a). The representations of medicines, identified in these studies, appear to be common across several illness and cultural groups. However, a systematic comparison of findings is hampered by the fact that the few studies which have quantitatively assessed medication beliefs have used different questionnaires or have investigated medication beliefs in the broader context of views about the practice of medicine (Echabe, Guillen and Ozamiz, 1992; Marteau, 1990). Furthermore, some studies have assessed peoples' ideas about medicines in general, whereas others have focused on specific medication prescribed for a particular illness.

   Although it identifies particular beliefs, this research tells us little about the prevalence of these beliefs. We do not know the proportion of people who hold them or how strongly they are held.

Furthermore, we know little about how medication beliefs are cognitively organised. For example, we do not know whether individual beliefs can be grouped together into core themes or components in the same way that illness beliefs are structured around five components (Leventhal and Nerenz, 1985). A key question here is the extent to which patients beliefs about medicines in *general* are differentiated from their beliefs about *specific* medicines prescribed for their illness. Finally, if medication beliefs appear to be related to adherence then there is a need to identify some of the salient factors which determine these beliefs.

These questions have recently been addressed using quantitative methodologies in a sample of over 500 patients suffering from a range of chronic illnesses (Horne, 1997a; 1997b). This research indicates that four "core-themes" or factors underlie commonly held beliefs about medicines. Core beliefs about prescribed medication are its perceived necessity for maintaining health (*Specific-Necessity*) and concerns based on beliefs about the potential for dependence or harmful long-term effects and that medication taking is disruptive (*Specific-Concerns*). Beliefs about medicines in general were also grouped around two themes. The first relates to the intrinsic properties of medicines and the extent to which they are harmful, addictive, poisons which should ·be taken regularly for long periods of time (*General-Harm*). The second theme deals with views about whether medicines are overused by doctors (*General-Overuse*). These themes form the basis for a new questionnaire-based method for assessing cognitive representations of medication: the Beliefs about Medicines Questionnaire (BMQ: Horne, Weinman and Hankins, 1997) .

Correlations between specific medication beliefs, suggested that, for a third of the total chronic illness sample, strong beliefs in necessity coincided with strong concerns. These patients seemed to have a rather complex view of their prescribed medication in which high benefit was balanced by high cost. An analysis of the interaction between medication beliefs and reported adherence behaviours revealed an interesting pattern of results. In all but one of the diagnostic groups studied (psychiatric outpatients), beliefs about prescribed medication were correlated with reported adherence to medication. Multiple linear regression showed that age and medication·beliefs accounted for 27% of the variance in reported medication adherence, with beliefs about prescribed medication contributing 13% to the total variance explained. It is interesting that people's views about the specific medication regimen prescribed for them were much more strongly related to adherence reports than were more general views about medicines as a whole. Moreover, the interplay between concerns and necessity beliefs implied a risk-benefit analysis and subsequent attempts to moderate the perceived potential for harm by taking less. Patients with stronger concerns based on beliefs about the potential for long-term effects and dependence reported lower adherence rates, whilst those with stronger beliefs in the necessity of their medication reported greater adherence to the medication regimen (Horne, 1997a; 1997b).

Further analysis of a sample of 47 patients receiving hospital haemodialysis suggested that the association between treatment beliefs and adherence behaviour was highly specific. Beliefs about separate aspects of the treatment (medication vs. diet) were related to adherence in a meaningful and discriminating way. For example, concerns about prescribed medication were associated with lower rates of self-reported medication adherence but not with lower adherence to fluid and dietary restrictions. Similarly, patients who believed that their fluid and dietary restrictions were too strict were less likely to adhere to them. Furthermore, the observation that adherence to medication was not correlated with adherence to fluid/diet restrictions provided additional evidence that patients may adhere to some aspects of their treatment but not others (Horne, 1997a; 1997b).

The differential effect of medication and illness beliefs has also been explored on two types of adherence behaviour (Horne, 1997a; 1997b). Data from a sample of asthma clinic patients (n=78) showed that the five components of illness representation identified by Leventhal and colleagues (Leventhal, 1985; Leventhal and Diefenbach, 1991; Leventhal *et al.*, 1992) and beliefs about prescribed medication were related to reported adherence in a way which was consistent with self-regulatory theory (Horne, 1997b). Both medication and illness representations were associated with passive non-adherence (PnA) as indicated by the reported frequency of forgetting to take medication. The pattern of correlation between illness and medication beliefs and PnA suggested that these beliefs contributed to the patient's perceptions of the *salience* of their medication which was in turn related to how often they forgot to take it. Patients who believed that their asthma would last a long time and have severe personal consequences also had stronger beliefs in the necessity of their prescribed medication and reported lower rates of PnA. In contrast, reported frequency of active non-adherence (AnA), indicated by reported frequency of deliberately altering the dose of medication, was predicted by *Specific-Concerns* about the asthma medication. In this case, taking less medication could be seen as a coping procedure by which the patient attempts to lessen the risk of dependence and long-term effects by taking less. Medication representations may have a more direct effect on adherence than illness beliefs, suggesting that the explanatory power of the SRM may be enhanced by inclusion of treatment beliefs (Horne, 1997a).

The fact that patients concerns about prescribed medication may be based on mistaken beliefs about the potential for dependence and long-term adverse effects, suggests that Specific-Concerns may be a marker for inadequate communication about medication between HP and patient (Horne, 1997b).

SUMMARY, CONCLUSIONS AND FUTURE DIRECTIONS

Early research into medication adherence attempted to identify the features of a disease or treatment which acted as barriers to adherence. It searched for demographic factors and personality traits which distinguished "the noncompliant patient". The limitations of this research are highlighted by findings that adherence rates often vary between treatments and over time within the same individuals. Most patients are non-adherent some of the time.

A more rewarding avenue of research focused on the identification and removal of barriers to adherence to individual treatment modalities which suggests that improving communication with clear, easily remembered instructions and tailoring the regimen to fit in with the patient's lifestyle enhances adherence in some situations. An interesting aspect of this work was the inclusion of patients' satisfaction with practitioner-patient interactions as a possible determinant of medication adherence. This acknowledges the role of motivation and sees that non-adherence may not just be the unintentional consequence of incompetence or lack of knowledge on the part of the patient. The recognition that what a patient thinks influences what they do stimulated more psychologically-based research into medication adherence.

Psychological research guided by SCMs has identified certain cognitions which underpin adherence decisions. However, some of these approaches are limited by a tendency to conceptualise adherence as the result of a "one-off" rational decision. The SRM conceptualises adherence as a dynamic interaction between the patients beliefs about the identity (including symptom experience), cause, consequences, time-line and potential for control or cure of their illness and their subjective evaluation of the effects of medication upon their illness, with particular emphasis on symptom experience.

An interesting recent development has been a focus on patients' beliefs about medication. This research suggests that patients form coherent beliefs about specific aspects of their treatment which seem to influence adherence. Preliminary findings suggest that, for a significant number of patients with common chronic illnesses, failure to take medication as instructed may be the result of rational but mistaken beliefs about the medication.

However, these findings should be interpreted with caution. The data were obtained from cross-sectional studies in which adherence was assessed by self-report. Further studies are now needed to confirm the causal relationships between medication beliefs and adherence using prospective longitudinal designs in which a range of adherence measures are used. Additionally, there is a need to clarify the dynamic interaction between patients' representations of illness and treatment and their adherence to treatment over time. It is suggested that beliefs about general and specific medication will influence treatment preferences and initial orientation to prescribed medication. However, continued adherence will be determined by a dynamic interplay between abstract beliefs and concerns about medication and the degree to which the patient's concrete experience of symptoms is influenced by the medication.

To date, few intervention studies have been conducted to evaluate whether adherence can be enhanced by changing beliefs which are associated with non-adherence. Allaying concerns about prescribed medication may be best achieved by a more open dialogue between patient and prescriber in which patients are encouraged to express their views about medication and to feedback on its perceived effects and several strategies for achieving this have been suggested (Horne, 1993). Research is needed to quantify the benefits and costs of these and other approaches. Fallowfield (1992), has pointed out that although, eliciting patients' views takes time and skill, good communication does not necessarily increase consultation times. Economic evaluations of strategies to facilitate adherence should include an assessment of the projected cost of non-adherence.

Over the last 25 years research has shown adherence to be a multi-factorial phenomena. Non-adherence may be the intentional result of a rational decision based on personal beliefs about the illness and treatment as well as the unintentional consequences of lack of ability to manage the medication regimen. Recent research calls for a patient-centred approach to the adherence issue which focuses on the patient's own ideas about the illness and treatment and the degree of concordance between the perceptions of patient and HP (Marinker, 1997; Royal Pharmaceutical Society of Great Britain, 1997).

REFERENCES

al Mahdy, H. and Seymour, D.G. (1990) How much can elderly patients tell us about their medications? *Postgraduate Medical Journal* **66,** 116–121.

Arluke, A. (1980) Judging drugs: patients' conceptions of therapeutic efficacy in the treatment of arthritis. *Human Organisation* **39,** 84–88.

Ascione, F.J., Kirscht, J.P. and Shimp, L.A. (1986) An assessment of different components of patient medication knowledge. *Medical Care* **24,** 1018–1028.

Ajzen, I. (1985) From intentions to actions: a theory of planned behaviour. In J Kuhl and J. Beckmann (eds.) *Action-Control: from cognition to behaviour.* Heidelberg: Springer-Verlag.

Ajzen, I. and Fishbein, M. (1980) *Understanding attitudes and predicting social behaviour,* Englewood Cliffs, NJ: Prentice-Hall .

Becker, M.H. (1979) Understanding patient compliance: the contributions of attitudes and other psychosocial factors. In S.J. Cohen (ed.) *New directions in patient compliance.* Toronto: Lexington.

Blaxter, M. and Britten, N. (1997) *Lay beliefs about drugs and medicines and the implications for community pharmacy.* Manchester, UK: Pharmacy Practice Research Resource Centre, University of Manchester.

Booth, C.S., Safer, M.A. and Leventhal, H. (1986) Use of physician services following participation in a cardiac screening program. *Public Health Reports* **101**, 315–319.

Bosley, C.M., Fosbury, J.A. and Cochrane, G.M. (1995) The psychological factors associated with poor compliance with treatment in asthma. *European Respiratory Journal* **8**, 899–904.

Boyle, C.M. (1970) Differences in patients' and doctors' interpretations of some common medical terms. *British Medical Journal* **2**, 286–289.

Britten, N. (1994) Patients' ideas about medicines: a qualitative study in a general practice population. *British Journal of General Practice* **44**, 465–468.

Brownlee-Duffeck, M., Peterson, L., Simonds, J.F., Goldstein, D., Kilo, C. and Hoette, S. (1987) The role of health beliefs in the regimen adherence and metabolic control of adolescents and adults with diabetes mellitus. *Journal of Consulting and Clinical Psychology* **55**, 139–144.

Budd, R.J., Hughes, I.C.T. and Smith, J.A. (1996) Health beliefs and compliance with antipsychotic medication. *British Journal of Clinical Psychology* **35**, 393–397.

Cartwright, A. (1967) *Patients and their doctors*. London: Routledge and Kegan Paul.

Cartwright, A. (1994) The experience of patients and general practitioners. *Journal of the Royal Society of Medicine (Supplement 23)* **87**, 8–10.

Cleary, D.J., Matzke, G.R., Alexander, A.C. and Joy, M.S. (1995) Medication knowledge and compliance among patients receiving long-term dialysis. *American Journal of Health-System Pharmacy* **52**, 1895–1900.

Cochran, S.D. and Gitlin, M.J. (1988) Attitudinal correlates of lithium compliance in bipolar affective disorders. *The Journal of Nervous and Mental Disease* **176**, 457–464.

Cockburn, J., Gibberd, R.W., Reid, A. and Sanson-Fisher, R.W. (1987) Determinants of non-compliance with short term antibiotic regimens. *British Medical Journal* **295**, 814–818.

Conner, M. and Norman, P. (1996) *Predicting health behaviour: research and practice with social cognition models*. Buckingham: Open University Press.

Conrad, P. (1985) The meaning of medications: another look at compliance. *Social Science and Medicine* **20**, 29–37.

Cooper, J.K., Love, D.W. and Raffoul, P.R. (1982) Intentional prescription non-adherence (non-compliance) by the elderly. *Journal of the American Geriatrics Society* **30**, 329–333.

Cramer, J.A., Mattson, R.H., Prevey, M.L., Scheyer, R.D. and Ouellette, V.L. (1989) How often is medication taken as prescribed: a novel assessment technique. *Journal of the American Medical Association* **261**, 3273–3277.

Cummings, K.M., Becker, M.H., Kirscht, J.P. and Levin, N.W. (1981) Intervention strategies to improve compliance with medical regimens by ambulatory haemodialysis patients. *Journal of Behavioural Medicine* **4**, 111–127.

Daniels, D.E., Rene, A.A. and Daniels, V.R. (1994) Race: an explanation of patient compliance – fact or fiction? *Journal of the National Medical Association* **86**, 20–25.

Diefenbach, M., Leventhal, H. and Leventhal, E., 1996. The Sensitive Soma Scale. *Personal communication.*

DiMatteo, M.R., Sherbourne, C.D., Hays, R.D., Ordway, L., Kravitz, R.L., McGlynn, E.A., Kaplan, S. and Rogers, W.H. (1993) Physicians' characteristics influence patients' adherence to medical treatment: results from the Medical Outcomes Study. *Health Psychology* **12**, 93–102.

DiMatteo, M.R. and DiNicola, D.D. (1982) *Achieving patient compliance: the psychology of the medical practitioner's role*, New York: Pergamon Press.

Donovan, J.L. and Blake, D.R. (1992) Patient non-compliance: deviance or reasoned decision making? *Social Science and Medicine* **34**, 507–513.

Eagleton, J.M., Walker, F.S. and Barber, N.D. (1993) An investigation into patient compliance with hospital discharge medication in a local population. *International Journal of Pharmacy Practice* **July,** 107–109.

Echabe, A.E., Guillen, C.S. and Ozamiz, J.A. (1992) Representations of health illness and medicines: coping strategies and health promoting behaviour. *British Journal of Clinical Psychology* **31**, 339–349.

Eisen, S.A., Miller, D.K., Woodward, R.S., Spitznagel, E. and Przybeck, T.R. (1990) The effect of prescribed daily dose frequency on patient medication compliance. *Archives of Internal Medicine* **150**, 1881–1884.

Fallowfield, L. (1992) The ideal consultation, *British Journal of Hospital Medicine.* **47,** 364–367.

Fallsberg, M. (1991) *Reflections on medicines and medication: a qualitative analysis among people on long-term drug regimens.* Linkoping, Sweden: Linkoping University.

Frazier, P.A., Davis Ali, S.H. and Dahl, K.E. (1994) Correlates of noncompliance among renal transplant recipients. *Clinics in Transplantation* **8,** 550–557.

George, C.F., Waters, W.E. and Nicholas, J.A. (1983) Prescription information leaflets: a pilot study in general practice *British Medical Journal* **287,** 1193–1196.

Gibbs, S.W. and George, W.E. (1990) Communicating information to patients about medicine. Prescription information leaflets: a national survey. *Journal of the Royal Society of Medicine* **83,** 292–297.

Glasgow, R.E., McCaul, K.D. and Scafer, L.C. (1986) Barriers to adherence among persons with insulin-dependent diabetes. *Journal of Behavioural Medicine* **9,** 65–77.

Gonder-Frederick, L.A. and Cox, D.J. (1991) Symptom perception, symptom beliefs and blood glucose discrimination in the self-treatment of insulin dependent diabetes. In J.A. Skelton and R.T. Croyle (eds.) *Mental representation in health and illness.* New York: Springer-Verlag.

Haefner, D.P. and Kirscht, J.P. (1970) Motivational and behavioural effects of modifying health beliefs. *Public Health Reports* **85,** 478–484.

Hall, J.A., Roter, D.L. and Katz, L.R. (1988) Meta-analysis of provider behaviour in medical encounters. *Medical Care* **26,** 657–675.

Hartman, P.E. and Becker, M.H. (1978) Non-compliance with prescribed regimen among chronic hemodialysis patients. *Dialysis and Transplantation* **7,** 978–985.

Haynes, R.B. (1976) A critical review of the 'determinants' of patient compliance with therapeutic regimens. In D.L. Sackett and R.B. Haynes (eds.) *compliance with therapeutic regimens.* London: John Hopkins University Press.

Haynes, R.B., Sackett, D.L., Gibson, E.S., Taylor, D.W., Roberts, R.S. and Johnson, A.L. (1978) Patient compliance with antihypertensive regimens. *Patient Counselling and Health Education* **1,** 18–21.

Haynes, R.B., Taylor, D.W. and Sackett, D.L. (1979) *Compliance in health care.* Baltimore: John Hopkins University Press.

Haynes, R.B., McKibbon, K.A. and Kanani, R. (1996) Systematic review of randomised clinical trials of interventions to assist patients to follow prescriptions for medications. *Lancet* **348**, 383–386.

Hilbrands, L.B., Hoitsma, A.J. and Koene, R.A. (1995) Medication compliance after renal transplantation. *Transplantation* **60**, 914–920.

Horne, R. (1993) One to be taken as directed: reflections on non-adherence (noncompliance). *Journal of Social and Administrative Pharmacy* **10**, 150–156.

Horne, R. (1997a) Representations of medication and treatment: advances in theory and measurement. In K.J. Petrie and J. Weinman (eds.) *Perceptions of health and illness: current research and applications*. London: Harwood Academic.

Horne, R (1997b) The nature, determinants and effects of medication beliefs in chronic illness. *Unpublished PhD thesis*. University of London.

Horne, R., Weinman, J. and Hankins, M. (1997) The Beliefs about Medicines. Questionnaire (BMQ): a new method for assessing cognitive representations of medication. *Unpublished manuscript.*

Horwitz, R.I., Viscoli, C.M., Berkman, L., Donaldson, R.M., Horwitz, S.M., Murray, C.J., Ranshoff, D.F. and Sindelar, J. (1990) Treatment adherence and risk of death after a myocardial infarction. *Lancet* **336**, 542–545.

Inui, T.S., Yourtee and Williamson, J.W. (1976) Improved outcomes in hypertension after physicians tutorials. *Annals of Internal Medicine* **84**, 646–651.

Jones, P.K., Jones, S.L. and Katz, J. (1987) Improving compliance for asthma patients visiting the emergency department using a health belief model intervention. *Journal of Asthma* **24**, 199–206.

Kelly, G.R., Mamon, J.A. and Scott, J.E. (1987) Utility of the health belief model in examining medication compliance among psychiatric outpatients. *Social Science and Medicine* **25**, 1205–1211.

Kruse, W. and Weber, E. (1990) Dynamics of drug regimen compliance–its assessment by microprocessor-based monitoring. *European Journal of Clinical Pharmacology* **38**, 561–565.

Lassen, L.C. (1991) Connections between the quality of consultations and patient compliance in general practice. *Family Practice* **8**, 154–160.

Lee, S., Wing, Y.K. and Wong, K.C. (1992) Knowledge and compliance towards lithium therapy among Chinese psychiatric patients in Hong Kong. *Australian and New Zealand Journal of Psychiatry* **26**, 444–449.

Leventhal, E.A., Leventhal, H., Schaefer, P. and Easterling, D. (1993b) Conservation of energy, uncertainty reduction, and swift utilisation of medical care among the elderly. *Journals of Gerontology* **48**, 78–86.

Leventhal, H., Zimmerman, R. and Gutmann, M. (1984) Compliance: a self-regulation perspective. In D Gentry (ed.) *Handbook of behavioural medicine.* New York: Pergamon Press.

Leventhal, H. (1985) The role of theory in the study of adherence to treatment and doctor-patient interactions. *Medical Care* **23**, 556–563.

Leventhal, H., Diefenbach, M. and Leventhal, E.A. (1992) Illness cognitions: using common-sense to understand treatment adherence and affect cognition interactions. *Cognitive Therapy and Research* **16**, 143–163.

Leventhal, H. and Diefenback, M. (1991) The Active Side of Illness Cognition. In J.A. Skelton and R.T. Croyle (eds.) *Mental representation in health and illness.* New York: Springer Verlag.

Leventhal, H. and Nerenz, D. (1985) The assessment of illness cognition. In P. Karoly (ed.) *Measurement strategies in health psychology.* New York: Wiley and Sons.

Leventhal, H. and Cameron, L. (1987) Behavioral theories and the problem of compliance. *Patient Education and Counseling* **10**, 117–138.

Leventhal, H., Meyer, D. and Nerenz, D. (1980) The common sense representation of illness danger. In S. Rachman (ed.) *Contributions to medical psychology.* Oxford: Pergamon Press.

Ley, P. (1982) Satisfaction, compliance and communication. *British Journal of Clinical Psychology* **21**, 241–254.

Ley, P. (1988) *Communicating with patients.* London: Crown Helm.

Ley, P. and Llewellyn, S. (1995) Improving patients' understanding, recall, satisfaction and compliance. In A. Broome and S. Llewellyn (eds.) *Health psychology: processes and applications. Second edition.* London: Chapman and Hall.

Lilleyman, J.S. and Lennard, L. (1996) Non-compliance with oral chemotherapy in childhood leaukaemia: an overlooked and costly cause of late relapse. *British Medical Journal* **313**, 1219–1220.

Lorenc, L. and Branthwaite, A. (1993) Are older adults less compliant with prescribed medication than younger adults? *British Journal of Clinical Psychology* **32**, 485–492.

Marinker, M. (1997) From compliance to concordance: achieving shared goals in medicine taking. *British Medical Journal* **314**, 747–748.

Marteau, T.M. (1995) Heath beliefs and attributions. In A. Broome and S. Llewellyn (eds.) *Health psychology: processes and applications. Second edition* London: Chapman and Hall.

Marteau, T.M. (1990) Attitudes to doctors and medicine: the preliminary development of a new scale. *Psychology and Health* **4**, 351–356.

McCrea, J.B., Ranelli, P.L., Boyce, E.G. and Erwin, W.G. (1993) Preliminary study of autonomy as a factor influencing medication taking by elderly patients. *American Journal of Hospital Pharmacy* **50**, 296–298.

McKim, W.A., Stones, M.J. and Kozma, A. (1990) Factors predicting medicine use in institutionalized and non-institutionalized elderly. *Canadian Journal on Ageing* **9**, 23–34.

Meichenbaum, D. and Turk, D.C. (1987) *Facilitating treatment adherence: a practitioner's handbook.* New York: Plenum Press.

Meyer, D., Leventhal, H. and Gutmann, M. (1985) Common-sense models of illness: the example of hypertension. *Health Psychology* **4**, 115–135.

Miller, P., Wikoff, R. and Hiatt, A. (1992) Fishbein's model of reasoned action and compliance behaviour of hypertensive patients. *Nursing Research* **41**, 104–109.

Monane, M., Bohn, R.L., Gurwitz, J.H., Glynn, R.J. and Avorn, J. (1994) Noncompliance with congestive heart failure therapy in the elderly. *Archives of Internal Medicine* **154**, 433–437.

Morgan, M. and Watkins, C.J. (1988) Managing hypertension: beliefs and responses to medication among cultural groups. *Sociology of Health and Illness* **10**, 561–578.

Moss-Morris, R., Petrie, K.J. and Weinman, J. (1996) Functioning in Chronic Fatigue Syndrome: do illness perceptions play a regulatory role? *British Journal of Health Psychology* **1**, 15–25.

Myers, E.D. and Branthwaite, A. (1992) Out-patient compliance with antidepressant medication. *British Journal of Psychiatry* **160**, 83–86.

Nelson, E.C., Stason, W.B., Neutra, R.R., Solomon, H.S. and McArdle, P.J. (1978) Impact of patient perceptions on compliance with treatment for hypertension. *Medical Care* **XVI**, 893–906.

Pan, P. and Tantam, D. (1989) Clinical characteristics, health beliefs and compliance with maintenance treatment: a comparison between regular and irregular attenders at a depot clinic. *Acta Psychiatrica Scandinavica* **79**, 564–570.

Petrie, K.J., Weinman, J., Sharpe, N. and Buckley, J. (1996) Predicting return to work and functioning following myocardial infarction: the role of the patient's view of their illness. *British Medical Journal* **312**, 1191–1194.

Raynor, D.K., Booth, T.G. and Blenkinsopp, A. (1993) Effects of computer generated reminder charts on patients' compliance with drug regimens. *British Medical Journal.* **306**, 1158–1161.

Ried, L.D., Oleen, M.A., Martinson, O.B. and Pluhar, R. (1985) Explaining intention to comply with antihypertensive regimens: the utility of health beliefs and the theory of reasoned action. *Journal of Social and Administrative Pharmacy* **3**, 42–52.

Ried, L.D. and Christensen, D.B. (1988) A psychosocial perspective in the explanation of patients' drug-taking behavior. *Social Science and Medicine* **27**, 277–285.

Royal Pharmaceutical Society of Great Britain (1997) *From compliance to concordance: achieving shared goals in medicine taking.* London.

Rosenstock, I. (1974) The health belief model and preventative health behaviour. *Health Education Monographs* **2**, 354–386.

Rudd, P., Byyny, R.L., Zachary, V., LoVerde, M.E., Titus, C., Mitchell, W.D. and Marshall, D. (1989) The natural history of medication compliance in a drug trial: limitations of pill counts. *Clinical Pharmacology and Therapeutics* **46**, 169–176.

Sackett, D.L. and Haynes, R.B. (1976) *Compliance with therapeutic regimens.* London: John Hopkins University Press.

Safer, M.A., Tharps, Q., J., Jackson, T.C. and Leventhal, H. (1979) Determinants of three stages of delay in seeking medical care at a medical clinic. *Medical Care* **17**, 11–29.

Sarriff, A., Aziz, N.A., Hassan, Y., Ibrahim, P. and Darwis, Y. (1992) A study of patients' self-interpretation of prescription instructions. *Journal of Clinical Pharmacology and Therapeutics* **17**, 125–128.

Sherbourne, C.D., Hays, R.D., Ordway, L., DiMatteo, M.R. and Kravitz, R.L. (1992) Antecedents of adherence to medical recommendations: results from the Medical Outcomes Study. *Journal of Behavioral Medicine* **15**, 447–468.

Smith, R. (1991) *Health Of The Nation: The BMJ View.* London: British Medical Journal.

Stewart, A.L. and Ware, J.E.(1992) *Measuring functioning and wellbeing: the Medical Outcomes Study approach.* Chapel Hill, NC: Duke University Press.

Stroebe, W. and Stroebe, M.S. (1995) *Social psychology and health,* Pacific Grove, CA, US: Brooks/Cole Publishing Co.

Taylor, D.W. (1979) A test of the Health Belief Model in hypertension. In R.B. Haynes, D.L. Sackett and D.W. Taylor (eds.) *Compliance in health care.* Baltimore and London: John Hopkins University Press.

Weinman, J. (1987) *An Outline of Psychology as Applied to Medicine. Second edition.* Bristol: Wright.

Weinman, J. (1990) Providing written information for patients : psychological considerations. *Journal of the Royal Society of Medicine* **83**, 303–305.

Weinman, J., Petrie, K.J., Moss-Morris, R. and Horne, R. (1996) The Illness Perception Questionnaire: a new method for assessing cognitive representations of illness. *Psychology and Health* **11**, 431–445.

Williams, S., Weinman, J., Dale, J. and Newman, S. (1995) Patient expectations; what do primary care patients want from the GP and how far does meeting expectations affect patient satisfaction. *Family Practice* **12**, 193–201.

Yeung, M., O'Connor, S.A., Parry, D.T. and Cochrane, G.M. (1994) Compliance with prescribed drug therapy in asthma. *Respiratory Medicine* **88**, 31–35.

Acknowledgements

The production of this paper was funded by the Department of Health, Pharmacy Enterprise Scheme and I would like to thank Jennette Howe and Peter Wilson for their support. I am also grateful to Professor John Weinman, Unit of Psychology, United Medical School of Guy's and St Thomas, London for helpful comments on an early draft.

12

Adherence to Lipid-Lowering Dietary Advice

Kathryn Nicholson Perry, Lorna Rapoport and Jane Wardle

EATING, HEALTH AND DIET

Messages about the food that we eat are ubiquitous in western society, coming from food manufacturers, public health bodies, or self-appointed health gurus. Messages range from advertising claims, books which offer advice on how to relieve the problems of every-day living through dietary changes, public health campaigns and weight reduction plans, to exotic gourmet cookery programmes. The ubiquity of such messages gives an indication of the central place of food and eating in society: it is not only the means by which we supply ourselves with energy, but is also a vehicle of social interaction, a representation of our cultural heritage, and a source of pleasure. Patterns of eating within cultures develop over thousands of years, and as individuals our eating preferences are shaped and refined from childhood. Diet has also become a major contemporary issue because of its contribution to health. Improved nutrition and food preparation practices have reduced the risk of disease from food-borne pathogens, while developments in nutritional science have led to increased knowledge about the composition of foods and the components of a healthy diet. Relationships between nutrition and disease are well recognised in many areas, such as coronary heart disease, stroke, cancer, diabetes, obesity, dental caries, as well as diseases related to nutritional deficiencies. Against this complex background, dietary advice is offered as a way of preventing the deterioration of health, and in some cases, reversing the course of chronic diseases. The enormous range of possible dietary behaviour changes and the diversity of the groups affected by the need to change their diet, underlines the complexity of the adherence issue. In this chapter we aim to illustrate the ways in which promoting dietary change presents a unique challenge to health professionals (HPs). The chapter draws principally on the literature on adherence to dietary advice in the context of lipid lowering in relation to Coronary Heart Disease (CHD). Raised cholesterol is relevant to a wide range of HPs because of the enormous numbers of people which it affects, and the cost of CHD to the health service and the economy. In the UK Health of the Nation White Paper, reductions in the prevalence of hypercholesterolaemia was identified as critical in reducing the burden of CHD (Department of Health, 1991).

We shall discuss adherence to dietary advice in relation to the different types of interventions and populations affected. We shall also examine the characteristics of interventions and individuals which are associated with better adherence. Finally, we shall summarise the important issues involved in promoting successful dietary change.

INVESTIGATING ADHERENCE TO DIETARY ADVICE

Adherence is a complex concept encompassing both the behavioural goal and the processes and context of that change. The assessment of adherence therefore requires a clear specification of the desired behaviour change, and a valid method of detecting whether the change has taken place (see Myers and Midence, Chapter 1). Dietary interventions prove problematic in both of these respects. The change is often specified in nutritional not behavioural terms – e.g.. reduce energy intake, reduce the percentage of energy as fat, and translating nutritional goals into food choices is far from straightforward. Consequently, it may not be clear what exactly the respondents are adhering to.

It is equally difficult to carry out assessments of the diet to determine whether change has occurred. The most direct measure of adherence depends upon evaluation of the characteristics of the diet which are targeted in the intervention, which can include the types of foods consumed, the amounts of foods consumed, the timing of consumption, or the average nutritional composition of the diet over a specified period –varying from one day to weeks. In free living individuals, assessment will almost certainly depend on the report of the individual, either prospectively or retrospectively, since direct observations are rarely practicable. One alternative, though a very expensive one, is the duplicate portion method, in which all foods consumed are stored in duplicate form for later analysis. The "gold standard" is a seven day record of exact weights of all food consumed, with detailed information on composition of home-made foods (e.g.. it was made up from 5 mls brand A olive oil with 100 grams of potato) and product information on prepared foods. The most inconvenient and intrusive aspect of this is the weighing, so one alternative is an estimated record of portion size –matched either against familiar measures of volume (spoons, cups etc.) or pictorial representations of portions. The record keeping process itself is subject to a wide range of errors, from inaccurate portion information, lapses of memory and conscious or unconscious bias.

If the target behaviour change is defined in terms of specific foods then the food record itself, or an abbreviated form, can be used to generate food consumption frequencies, but if the target is either composition (for example fat intake), or energy intake, then a nutritional analysis may be required. This itself is both imprecise and time consuming. Nutrient composition tables have been prepared for basic foods and the most frequently consumed ready-made foods, and these are available in computerised forms, such as Microdiet (Fletcher, 1993). The type and quantity of the food are taken from the dietary record, but in practice many of the recorded foods will be home made with inadequate specification of constituents, or ready made, but the product information is not in published databases, and in either case portion information is highly imprecise. In addition, such a process requires estimation of the quantities and compositions of foods, and often requires supplementation through contact with food manufacturers to obtain nutritional information on new products. Given the range of possible errors in the process of recording and analysis, it will be readily apparent that dietary composition cannot be estimated very accurately even with co-operative participants.

The development of methods of biochemical validation has helped to overcome errors of systematic bias due either to different methods of dietary assessment or from consistent over-or under-reporting by participants. Independent methods for validating dietary assessments include comparing 24 hour urine nitrogen output with reported protein intake (Isaksson, 1988), doubly-labelled water techniques to validate reported energy intake (Livingstone *et al.*, 1990) and indirect calorimetry and labelling food with 13C-glucose in order to assess adherence from the 13C02 enrichment in expired air (Lyon *et al.*, 1995). The development of intermediate markers, such as cheek cell compositional changes whereby changes in fatty acid composition reflects changes in dietary fatty acid intake, may provide a way forward (Sampigna *et al.*, 1988). All of these methods can be used to assess the correspondence between reports of adherence and the measure in question, but they are not exact reflections of the change. Another important consideration is their expense, both in terms of time and money.

A commonly used alternative to assessing behavioural adherence is to use the level of a clinically relevant outcome as an index of dietary change, for example changes in serum lipid profile or weight. However, this does not necessarily reflect adherence to specialist dietary advice, since the patient may have instituted other measures which are responsible for the changes observed. An individual patient may achieve the outcome without following the prescribed behavioural change, for example reducing weight by eating only one chocolate bar each day. The other problem is that the relationship between dietary change and physiological change is not entirely consistent across individuals. There are known to be biological determinants to responsiveness, such as genetic factors which determine differences in lipid levels, which need to be taken into account when extrapolating adherence from clinical outcomes (Denke, 1995). For example, when a consistent dietary change which was implemented in a closed community of Trappist monks to reduce the saturated fat content of the monks' daily diet, serum cholesterol reductions showed individual variation (Katan *et al.*, 1988). In addition, the longer the time period over which adherence is being monitored, the more the opportunity for other variables to have an effect on outcome.

The problems raised by defining or assessing adherence to dietary advice are augmented by the design of interventions. The goals of interventions are often stated in different ways. Some may advise that an absolute target for a food should be met, such as having less than 10 grams of fat in each meal, while others emphasise changing the overall balance of nutritional intake, for example increasing the ratio of different types of fat in the diet. Comparison of the efficacy of different interventions may be difficult to establish since interventions are frequently labelled in broad terms, such as behavioural techniques. This makes it difficult to compare the components of different interventions and therefore difficult to understand their effect on adherence. The range of different methods of defining dietary adherence complicates the process of comparing characteristics of programmes or individuals which contribute to higher levels of adherence. However, some studies report levels of change which are beneficial to the patients in terms of clinical outcomes, and thus their methods clearly bear closer examination. There is also some consensus concerning the characteristics of successful individuals and the salient components of effective interventions on which to base the construction of future dietary treatments.

PROMOTING HEALTHY DIETS

Nutrient and dietary targets, and recommendations for a healthy diet, have been produced for many years in different forms throughout the world, and notwithstanding the myth that nutritionists cannot agree, there is remarkable consistency between them (Cannon, 1992). There is virtually unanimous agreement in developed countries about the main recommendations, which are: (i) to limit fat and saturated fat intake; (ii) to increase consumption of fruit, vegetables and foods rich in starch and fibre; (iii) to control body weight; (iv) to eat a variety of foods; and (v) to limit intake of sugar, salt and alcohol.

Some of these recommendations are presented in a complex form relating to recommended intake of specific nutrients, while others address quite simple changes. Many attempts have been made to give people a practical message about the recommended balance of foods in the diet to help people understand healthy eating via pictorial representations, for example the "Balance of Good Health" (Health Education Authority, HEA, 1994). The benefit of such pictorial representations is that they communicate that people do not have to give up the foods they most enjoy for the sake of their health. They also emphasises positive actions, such as substitution and balance. In contrast, advice to reduce fat, for example, may communicate as an entirely negative message regarding healthy eating.

At the clinical level, the job of the HP is to provide advice on dietary change in a form which promotes adherence. Economic, social and cultural conditions, as well as food preferences need to be taken into account, which may result in a compromise between what is dietetically desirable and what is acceptable and hence potentially attainable.

There are three target groups for dietary interventions: (i) the general population who eat the usual western diet, which is therefore likely to be too high in energy, fat, sugar and salt, and too low in plant-based foods, (ii) those who are at increased risk of disease because of concurrent illness, raised risk factors, or genetic predisposition and, (iii) those who require treatment due to active disease or as part of secondary rehabilitation. Unlike other aspects of behaviour change, the participants may have eaten entirely "normal" diets, that is, they eat the same kinds of foods, in the same kinds of quantities, as most other people in their community. However, normal diets generally do not concur with healthy eating guidelines. Accordingly, dietary interventions may be designed to improve food choices to meet recommended standards, rather than to bring them into line with those around them.

Dietary intervention may be targeted to the needs of specific individuals, or it may be organised at the community and population level. Over the last decade, there has been an integration of preventive programmes at community and population level aimed at a range of diseases such as obesity, CHD and cancer. This strategy aims to shift behavioural, eating and drinking patterns to improve overall health among large groups of people. A wide range of opportunities for promoting healthy eating have been identified in the UK (Department of Health, 1991) which involve the participation of a broad spectrum of public and commercial organisations. On a community level they involve interventions of varying intensity, from predominantly passive information dissemination in the form of leaflets, posters or advertising, to groups or courses and specialist health events. At the population level they can include strategies such as fortification of certain foods with vitamins and minerals to prevent deficiency, modifying the pricing structure for foods or regulating labelling.

ADHERENCE TO DIETARY INTERVENTIONS IN GENERAL POPULATIONS

In this section we shall examine some examples of adherence to community-wide dietary interventions, which are usually designed to prevent the development of diet-related disorders. Their value is commonly assessed against their impact on health indicators across a wide spectrum of risk factors. There is a need to balance effort and cost against the numbers of people who change their behaviour, and the impact on health (Rose, 1982). Given the large numbers of people usually targeted, good dietary assessment is particularly difficult. We are, therefore, even more reliant on clinical outcomes as a proxy measure of adherence in these cases.

An important consideration in these interventions is the varying levels of both exposure and motivation among such broad populations. The target population may not even see or hear the message or they may be unaware of the relevance of the messages to their personal situations. Lack of perception of susceptibility may also influence the behaviour of significant proportions of the population (Becker, 1974).

Two of the earliest community intervention programmes for CHD were the Stanford Three Community Study (California, USA) and the North Karelia Project (Finland) during the 1970s. The Stanford Three Community Study (Fortmann *et al.*, 1981) was a long running, community-wide, cardiovascular risk reduction programme which aimed to modify diet in the intervention community so as to reduce the intake of dietary cholesterol and fat. The intervention ran for two years using mass media techniques, intensive education and direct clinical interventions with high risk individuals from one of the intervention communities. Adherence to dietary advice was measured using a diet history interview to record usual dietary behaviour at baseline and at the subsequent annual surveys. Significant differences between the intervention and control communities were observed in intake of both dietary cholesterol and dietary saturated fat. Overall, both body weight and plasma cholesterol levels increased over time, but the intervention communities had significantly smaller increases than the control community. These results suggest that the intervention had a modest impact, both in relation to the targeted dietary change and the predicted risk factor change.

In the North Karelia Project, which monitored the effects of a community-wide dietary behaviour change programme over ten years (Puska *et al.*, 1985), a different pattern emerged. The project came about as a result of awareness of and concern about the high morbidity and mortality rates due to CHD in the North Karelia area of Finland. The aim of the study was to encourage positive risk factor changes across the community, in this case smoking, blood pressure and cholesterol levels. The intervention was based on media communication across the whole population, and through the recruitment of opinion leaders, both formally and informally, who disseminated information and influenced others. The emphasis was on improving both knowledge and skills within a environment which supported the changes advocated by the project. The activities of the project included the identification and training of informal opinion leaders in the community, training of key professional groups, and media based education projects. In addition, high risk and clinically ill individuals were more intensively supported, with, for example, secondary prevention programmes for myocardial infarction being offered (Puska *et al.*, 1981). A baseline survey in 1972 revealed high levels of cholesterol and blood pressure. Given the high levels of morbidity and mortality due to CHD in North Karelia, there can be no doubt that the population would have included some individuals with active clinical disease and some with a very high likelihood of developing CHD during the follow-up period (Puska *et al.*, 1985).

Adherence to behavioural dietary changes was monitored with a number of questions on the main survey, for example on fat intake, although few details are given on this. We are therefore largely dependent upon changes in risk factors to obtain some assessment of adherence in this case. Repeat cross-sectional surveys were carried out in North Karelia in 1977 and 1982, and the results showed positive self-reported changes in dietary behaviour. Serum cholesterol levels were significantly reduced in men (4% in the first five years, and a further 3% in the second five years) but smaller changes were not significant, reductions among women. Positive changes in smoking rates and blood pressure were also reported, although again the smoking reduction among women was not significant. Unlike in the Stanford Three Community Study, the reference community in this study also showed general improvements in the risk factors, but they were significantly smaller than those in the treatment communities. The results of this study thus seem promising, with larger than otherwise expected reductions in cholesterol levels across the board. It certainly delivered valuable clinical results overall, with a reduction of CHD mortality among North Karelian men of 24%.

The Stanford Five-City Project, successor to the Stanford Three Community Study, also aimed to reduce CHD modifiable risk factors: plasma cholesterol levels, blood pressure, resting pulse rate, and smoking prevalence. Education campaigns were carried out over 6 years in two intervention communities and they were compared with three control non-intervention communities over the same time period (Farquhar *et al.*, 1990; Fortmann *et al.*, 1993). In this study a wider age range of individuals were used, between 12 and 74 years. A sample of the population, known as the "cohort survey sample", was re-surveyed four times at two yearly intervals, and in addition, four cross-sectional surveys were conducted. Dietary intake was assessed using 24-hour recall interviews and food intake questions which were included in the surveys, although these were reported to correlate poorly with the 24-hour recall interview data (Fortmann *et al.*, 1993). The strategies used to promote the nutritional intervention package included encouraging the setting of general and specific dietary change goals and increasing social support, for example through the "Healthy Living Program" a mass media promotion using self-help materials and newsletters (Fortmann *et al.*, 1993). The aim was to reduce mean plasma cholesterol by 4%, reduce dietary saturated fat intake to less than 10% of calories and dietary cholesterol to less than 250 mg per day (Fortmann *et al.*, 1993). Initially, the intervention focused on raising awareness and knowledge through the mass media and special booklets, in both English and Spanish. In years 3 to 6 of the intervention further educational materials were distributed, including a cookbook of low-fat recipes. Participants were encouraged to set general and specific dietary goals for each year of the intervention. By the end of the fifth year participants had been exposed to a wide range of television and print educational materials. Sixty percent reported seeing at least one public service announcement and 70% recalled at least one or more of the print materials (Fortmann *et al.*, 1993).

The results showed an increase in knowledge of CHD risk factors in all communities, but with significantly greater increases in intervention communities in both the cross-sectional and longitudinal data sets. As assessed by 24-hour recall, dietary cholesterol intake declined significantly over time, but dietary fat intake was unchanged, and there were no significant differences between intervention and control communities in either measure (Fortmann *et al.*, 1993). The findings were consistent across separately analysed high risk groups, in whom one might have expected to see greater changes, and those who smoked or took medications which might cause cholesterol levels to be raised.

Plasma cholesterol levels showed initial reductions in all communities, and significantly greater reductions in the intervention communities at first. However, by the fourth survey significant differences were detected only in the longitudinal sample, which implies that the assessments themselves could have influenced adherence (Farquhar *et al.*, 1990). Changes in body mass index were even more discouraging, and increases in Body Mass Index (BMI) were seen in both data sets, with no consistent differences between intervention and control communities (Farquhar *et al.*, 1990; Taylor *et al.*, 1991).

Overall, the 5 years of intervention appeared to achieve 15% reduction in all cause mortality risk and 16% reduction in CHD risk scores among the cohort participants (Farquhar *et al.*, 1990), which is largely accounted for by the reduction in smoking. Dietary behaviour change was modest at best, as indicated by the food records, and this was supported by the small changes in plasma cholesterol levels and BMI. This major, community-wide initiative clearly had an impact on knowledge, but despite the emphasis on dietary behaviour change the effects on dietary patterns was negligible (Fortmann *et al.*, 1993), which was reflected in the poor outcomes in terms of BMI and plasma cholesterol change.

Following in the footsteps of these early community intervention attempts are a new wave of projects, and one of the most ambitious, nutritionally-based, risk reduction initiatives is the "5 A Day – For Better Health" campaign (Foerster *et al.*, 1995). The programme was specifically directed at cancer risk reduction, although it could be expected to impact on CHD mortality if effective, but the sheer scale of the programme and its attempt to work only at the community level makes it of interest. One of the programmes was carried out in California in 1990–1 by the Nutrition and Cancer Prevention Program. The aim of the initiative was a doubling of fruit and vegetable consumption among the 19 million residents of California to five servings each day. As part of this project a new public health unit was created through which intervention strategies were developed and carried out. The interventions were mainly carried out through mass media public health messages, backed up by point of purchase messages about the need to increase fruit and vegetable consumption. Five campaign waves were conducted through the mass media and participating retailers, and it was estimated that California residents were exposed to more than one hour of health education materials annually during the campaign. There was a good level of commercial support, with up to 1800 supermarkets involved at the peak of the promotion. Unlike the North Karelia Project, for example, there were no additional intervention packages for those identified as being a high risk of cancer or having manifest disease. The outcome of the trial was measured through the 1989 and 1991 California Dietary Practices Surveys (CDPS). The CDPS conducted telephone interviews of approximately 1000 randomly selected adults during each survey.

Following the period of the intervention, changes in awareness, knowledge and belief moved in the direction of the campaign message (Foerster *et al.*, 1995). There were significant increases in the percentage of the total sample who agreed that what people consume affects their chance of getting cancer (from 51% to 65%). There were significant increases in the percentage of the sample who identify fruit and vegetables as linked to cancer prevention (from 24% to 32%), and increases in the proportion who thought they personally should eat more fruit and vegetables (from 52% to 60%).

These changes in cognitive factors are important when self-reported behavioural changes are examined. Among the total sample there was a non-significant increase in the number of portions of fruit and vegetables consumed on the previous day, while among the Hispanic participants, who had shown most increase in thinking that they should eat more fruit and vegetables, there was a significant decline in fruit consumption, which was most marked among the least educated (Foerster *et al.*, 1995). The authors suggest that the overall changes reflected long-term trends for changes in fruit and vegetable consumption in the United States as a whole. The 5 A Day programme demonstrated that resources can be combined across public and commercial organisations in support of health education, but it is disappointing that despite massive effort, the self-reported changes in knowledge and attitude were not translated into meaningful behavioural changes.

On the whole, the results of community intervention studies are mixed. The Stanford Three Community Study and the North Karelia Project suggest that a combination of broad stroke public health and more intensive interventions with clinical populations can result in modest dietary behaviour change. Pure community strategies, however, like the 5 A Day seem to be less effective at producing behaviour change, although changes in knowledge do seem possible. However, the overall conclusion has to be that adherence to public health or community-based dietary advice has been minimal, with the exception of the North Karelia study, despite the huge efforts which were put into all the interventions described. The level of exposure to educational materials achieved by purely community-based interventions may well be too low for complex messages to be conveyed, and the better results in the North Karelia may be due to the high level of public concern about the issue out of which the intervention arose. The findings suggest that both motivation to change and delivery of intervention are implicated in the success, or otherwise, of community-based interventions.

ADHERENCE TO DIET IN HIGHER RISK POPULATIONS

This section will focus on the adherence achieved by high risk groups in dietary intervention trials. One of the most important differences between this group and the interventions targeted at the general public is the likely increased perception of personal susceptibility among this group. Interventions are also more likely to be associated with more rigorous evaluations, resulting in more in-depth attempts at assessing adherence to the prescribed dietary changes. An example of a large scale primary prevention programme among individuals at high risk for CHD is the Multiple Risk Factor Intervention Trial (MRFIT; Neaton, Grimm and Cutler, 1987). MRFIT recruited 12866 high risk participants from an original screening population of 361,662 men aged between 35 and 57 years of age. The participants were free of clinical evidence of coronary heart disease, but were high on some or all of serum cholesterol, smoking and blood pressure. The trial was carried out through 22 clinics in the United States with the men randomised to either usual care (UC) or special intervention (SI) conditions. The participants in the SI group received a treatment programme tailored to their particular risk factors: (i) stepped-care treatment for hypertension; (ii) counselling for smokers; and (iii) dietary advice for lowering cholesterol levels. UC participants were referred back to their local health care providers. All participants were seen annually for a medical examination and assessment of risk status. All the participants were followed for six years.

The SI participants attended a series of ten weekly intervention groups, with a partner or friend, which addressed all three risk factors (Multiple Risk Factor Intervention Trial Research Group, 1982). Participants were subsequently seen every four months or more. They were prescribed an initial, basic eating pattern followed by a maintenance, or progressive eating pattern, once the basic pattern had been established. The dietary goals were to (i) increase polyunsaturated fat consumption to 10% of calories; (ii) decrease saturated fat consumption to less than 10% of calories, subsequently revised to less than 8%; and (iii) decrease dietary cholesterol to less than 300 mg per day, subsequently revised to less than 250. Weight reduction goals were also set for men whose weight was 115% or greater than the desirable weight. Weight reduction interventions involved caloric restriction and exercise.

Dietary changes were monitored in two ways. Firstly, through the use of a specially designed scoring system, called the food record rating, which was kept for three days by each SI participant. In this method, points are allocated for foods eaten based on their saturated fat, cholesterol and polyunsaturated fat content. Secondly, the nutritionists working on the trial undertook an investigation of the suitability of the home and work environment, evidence of deviation from the prescribed eating pattern and level of motivation of each participant (Dolecek *et al.*, 1986). This attempt to measure behavioural adherence is clearly more sophisticated than those used in the community intervention studies.

Overall, the SI participants in MRFIT achieved a reduction of 4% in percentage of energy from saturated fat to 10%, in contrast to the insignificant reduction made by the usual care group, and this translated into a 7.5% reduction in serum cholesterol levels. The most dramatic reductions were achieved between the first screening visit and the first annual review, although these levels were largely maintained for the duration of the trial. Dolecek *et al.* (1986) comment that the reductions achieved were not as large as had been anticipated on the basis of the study design. Two reasons were advanced for this: (i) that participants initially ate a lower-fat diet than the population on which the study had been based; and (ii) that other interventions offered as part of the SI package were affecting the responses. Participants being treated only for raised cholesterol had greater cholesterol reductions than those receiving additional interventions, cholesterol reductions were greater among the non-smoking, non-hypertensive participants.

The Hypertension Prevention Trial (Meinert, Borhani, and Langford, 1989) whilst not offering low fat dietary interventions, is of particular interest as it take into account some adherence issues, for example frequency of lapses. The participants in the study were normotensive individuals, but their blood pressure was slightly raised and they were therefore thought to be at risk of developing hypertension at a future date. The study aimed to achieve changes in dietary consumption of sodium, potassium and calories, and sustain the changes for two years. Eight hundred and forty one men and women were recruited as participants and dietary adherence was assessed throughout the trial by interview and 24 hour food diaries, and validated by urinary sodium and potassium analysis.

Participants were randomised to one of four treatment groups (calorie restriction, sodium restriction, sodium and calorie restriction, and sodium restriction and potassium increase) or a control group. The treatments were offered through group counselling with a nutritionist and behaviourist (Jeffrey *et al.*, 1989). During the initial phase of the treatment, from randomisation to 14 weeks, participants attended 12 group sessions. They received a diet-specific cook book and nutrient content guide. Specific attention was given to motivational factors in the initial phase of the treatment programme. Strategies used included encouraging expression of feelings, emphasising the importance of the research programme, tastings of new foods, encouraging significant others to attend the groups and use of a token reward system. Results were presented separately by gender and weight group (Shah *et al.*, 1990). None of the sub-groups reduced their total daily sodium intake to the target level, and only the normal weight, treatment condition men increased their potassium levels to the target level. However, normal weight treated women were only 1% above the desired level of daily sodium intake. Reducing consumption of sodium from salt, meats and grain products had been specifically targeted. Significant differences between control and treated participants were observed in most food groups, and treated participants consumed approximately one third less sodium than control group participants. Specifically targeted foods in relation to increasing potassium consumption were fruits, vegetables, nut/legumes and salt substitute. All potassium treated participants showed significantly greater consumption of fruit than control participants, but in the other target foods the findings were inconsistent.

The Dietary Alternatives Study (McCann *et al.*, 1990) was similarly directed towards a healthy high risk target population, but it included a focus on predictors of adherence such as social support, self-efficacy and motivation. The study examined adherence to a low-fat, low-cholesterol diet among 531 hypercholesterolaemic or combined hyperlipidaemic men, who were recruited through an aeroplane manufacturer in the USA. The participants and their partners attended eight weekly change classes, run by registered dieticians as part of the company's coronary disease prevention programme. This was followed up with individual and optional group sessions with dieticians and psychologists during the first year of follow-up. The programme was based on techniques derived from behavioural self-management and social-learning theory, for example self-monitoring, goal-setting and inclusion of partners in the treatment programme (McCann *et al.*, 1990). In particular, attention was paid to maintenance of initial changes, through provision of a helpline answered by a dietician, a quarterly newsletter and group maintenance sessions in which adherence difficulties were specifically addressed. Adherence was measured using four day food diaries, which were collected on a monthly basis initially, and subsequently every three or six months.

Data have only been published on 254 men and their spouses, among whom median fat intake reduced from 36% to between 19% and 26% at the end of the active treatment phase. These gains were maintained at two years post-intervention, when the median fat intake was 22–28%. However, data available from other trials, such as changes in cholesterol levels, which were used to validate measures of behavioural dietary adherence were not presented in this study. This and the uncertainty over the fate of the other 277 participants limits the value of these results.

The Women's Health Trial (Henderson *et al.,* 1990; Urban *et al.,* 1992; subsequently known as DIET FIT and Women's Health Initiative) reported initial and long-term adherence to the low-fat diet (fat less than 20% of total calories) prescribed to reduce risk of developing breast cancer. Although not intended to target a population especially at risk of hyperlipidaemia, its advocacy for a low-fat diet makes it relevant. In the initial feasibility study, The Women's Health Trial Vanguard Study (Henderson *et al.,* 1990), the 303 participants were women of 45 to 69 years of age with an increased risk of breast cancer but without any indication of current or past cancer. Recruits were excluded if they were already following a low-fat eating plan or if they would be unavailable for long-term follow-up. It is notable that one additional exclusion criteria was that the dietician involved with the trial suspected that the individual might not adhere to the dietary advice. Sixty percent of participants were randomised to an intervention condition which involved 8 weekly group sessions, followed by 4 bi-weekly meetings, and subsequent monthly meetings. The groups were run by a nutritionist and were reported to be based on nutritional and behavioural principles. Adherence to the diet was monitored using 4 day food diaries at randomisation, after 3 months of intervention and at 6, 12 and 24 months post-intervention. Among the intervention group the percentage of energy from fat fell significantly from 39.1% at baseline to 21.6% at 12 months and 22.6% at 24 months. In contrast, the levels remained steady among the participants in the control group. A significant difference in weight between the intervention and control groups was also observed, with the intervention group losing 1.91 kg compared with a weight loss of 0.08 kg in the control group. Baseline measures of total plasma cholesterol were not obtained for the control group participants. However, among the intervention group, reductions of 13.9 mg/Dl at the 12 month follow-up were observed. These changes demonstrate that dietary advice can achieve significant reductions in dietary fat and total plasma cholesterol. However, it seems likely that it was the highly selected nature of the population, combined with a high risk of a very threatening disease which were primarily responsible for the high degree of adherence, and the remarkable persistence.

Drawing together the results of these intervention studies with higher risk populations, it is important to remain mindful of the role of extraneous variables in the changes achieved. This group are more likely to have a clearer perception of their own vulnerability to the disease in question, which is likely to increase their motivation. They also received more intensive interventions, allowing them the opportunity to discuss and resolve misunderstanding and difficulties with the prescribed dietary changes and to receive feedback on their progress. In addition, their health in general may be subject to more scrutiny with advice being received to tackle other health problems, for example receiving medication for hypertension. The MRFIT study participants without complicating factors were able to reduce their consumption of saturated fat from a low starting point, to an even lower end-point, and the results of the Women's Health Trial showed a similar pattern of results. The male participants in the Dietary Alternatives Study, who had a more elaborate intervention, seemed able to maintain only moderate reductions, and were not able to sustain the most strict diet. The interesting interaction between gender and adherence to the calorie restriction diet in the Hypertension Prevention Trial is a clue perhaps to the need to consider adherence as a situational issue. In general, it seems that among well motivated individuals, with access to intensive professional support, substantial changes in diet type with effects on physiological parameters can be achieved, but no-one has really looked at adherence or its predictors in these studies.

ADHERENCE TO DIET IN CLINICAL POPULATIONS

There is a likelihood that clients from clinical populations, who therefore have frank disease, may be more receptive to action aimed at ameliorating their hyperlipidaemia since they could expect demonstrable benefits. Again, evaluations of adherence are limited by the difficulties of measurement and definition, as previously discussed. Clinical outcomes are all the more important in this area, and invasive methods of monitoring clinical change, such as angiography, are used. As with less invasive measures of clinical outcome used in previous studies of higher risk individuals, these are often used as substitutes for direct measures of adherence to dietary behaviour change.

The highly intensive interventions carried out in the Lifestyle Heart Trial, by Dean Ornish and his colleagues is perhaps the best known dietary intervention study in clinical populations (Ornish *et al.*, 1990). The study prescribed a "lifestyle" programme (including low-fat vegetarian diet, moderate aerobic exercise, stress management training, stopping smoking and group support in the form of twice-weekly discussion groups led by a clinical psychologist) to 22 free-living adults, all of whom had documented coronary artery disease. Quantitative coronary angiography at baseline and after a year assessed the progression or regression of the primary clinical outcome indicator, coronary artery lesions. Adherence to the dietary behaviour changes was checked using a 3-day diet diary at baseline and after one year. Data collected from this source were combined with adherence to other elements of the intervention to produce an overall adherence score, with a score of one indicating 100% adherence to the programme. The diet prescribed was very low in fat, with less than 10% of calories as fat, and severe reductions in consumption of animal products. Additional recommendations, such as sodium restriction for hypertensive participants, were given as necessary. Direct attention to adherence issues, through the twice-weekly groups was an important part of the treatment in this study. The groups were based on the relationship between social support and better adherence, on but also included communication skills and ventilation of feelings. Stress management techniques, were included to improve "the patient's sense of relaxation, concentration, and awareness" (Ornish *et al.*, 1990) and covered stretching exercises, meditation and progressive relaxation.

Direct measures of adherence in this study demonstrated reduction in fat and dietary cholesterol intake among the treated group. The validity of these changes are supported by the significant reductions in total and LDL cholesterol (reduced by 24% and 37% respectively). Clinical results were also positive, with participants in the experimental treatment showing significant regression of their coronary artery lesions. Taken together, these results demonstrate the ability of free-living individuals to sustain severe restrictions on their dietary intake over the period of a year. The generalizability of this, however, must remain questionable as fewer than half those originally identified as being clinically eligible for the trial were subsequently recruited.

Another trial with a clinical population is the STARS (St Thomas' Atherosclerosis Regression Study) which also investigated the effects on clinical outcome of dietary change and lipid lowering medication among clinically ill patients (Watts *et al.*, 1992). The participants in STARS were 90 males, among which there was a larger percentage of smokers than among Ornish's participants, and had higher baseline levels of total cholesterol. The participants were randomly assigned to control, low-fat diet or low-fat diet and a lipid-lowering drug (cholestyramine). Fat intake was restricted to 27% of energy, with additional prescriptions of weight reducing diets for those with a BMI in excess of 25 kg/m2. There was no apparent direct measure of adherence, nor were direct attempts made to influence adherence, although general enquiries were made and encouragement given at follow-up visits with the clinician. Prospective participants were, however, given a trial of the lipid-lowering drug used in addition to diet in one condition of the trial, to check tolerance and responsiveness to it.

Changes in both lipid levels and coronary angiography analyses results suggest good adherence to the prescribed dietary changes. Total and LDL cholesterol levels were significantly reduced in the diet group (14% and 16% respectively) and there were also favourable angiographic changes. In addition, significantly fewer treated participants experienced cardiovascular events, such as myocardial infarction. This again demonstrates the ability of clinical populations to change their dietary behaviour. Both studies achieved good levels of behavioural dietary changes, although in the STARS study it was approximately half of the change achieved by Ornish's participants. In Ornish's study, it is supported by the correspondence between good adherence to the prescribed programme and cholesterol level changes. The more stringent treatment regime in the Ornish study may have been responsible for the very large reductions in cholesterol, but the additional components of the programme, such as exercise and stress management techniques, may either themselves be having a direct effect, or be improving adherence to the dietary changes prescribed. The ability of the participants in Ornish's study to adhere to a diet prescribing less than 10% of calories from fat supports the previous idea that clinical populations would show the best levels of adherence. Earlier, we suggested that the most likely causes for this would be incremental increases in perceived vulnerability, and hence motivation, and intensiveness of interventions. The two studies described in this section are both vastly different both in terms of the requirements of the diet and the intensity of the interventions, but clearly clinically ill participants are able to show good changes in clinical outcomes. What is clear, is that although often participants do not achieve the stated aims of a particular dietary changes, for example, reducing fat to less that 30%, 20% or 10% of fat, usually some study somewhere reports results to suggest that reducing fat to that absolute level can be achieved. An example of this is the reported inability of the participants in the Dietary Alternatives Study to adhere to the lowest level of fat reduction (18%), which seems to have been achieved by the participants in Ornish's trial. This may be the result of different intensity of interventions, although the Dietary Alternatives Study was certainly intensive, or perhaps it is related to participants wish to reset goals for themselves. Either way, it is not currently possible to elicit the answers to these issues from the available data.

FACTORS INFLUENCING ADHERENCE IN DIETARY TREATMENT

Taking together the data from all three populations, it becomes clear that at the very least adherence to diet at the group level is variable. Even when participants could be considered to be at high personal risk and highly motivated to change, the extent of changes achieved are often smaller than the goal level set. However, the differences observed in the outcomes of the trials suggests that there are some characteristics of both programmes and individuals which are more likely to be associated with improved outcomes. There are evidently aspects of both which are important in producing change and exploring these is a major goal if effective dietary behaviour change strategies are to be designed.

Few dietary intervention studies appear to involve explicit evaluations of the predictors of adherence, the Hypertension Prevention Trial and the Dietary Alternatives studies are notable exceptions to this. However, many studies make some attempt to compare those who do, with those who do not adhere to prescribed changes in a post-hoc fashion. An example of the latter is the ethnic differences observed in the 5 a Day campaign (with lower levels of change among Hispanic participants).

The health psychology literature suggests a number of factors which should have a significant effect upon adherence. These include individual characteristics, programme characteristics, setting, communication and environmental cues. However, in relation to diet, whilst the relationship between individual characteristics and adherence is sometimes reflected upon in intervention studies, they are rarely planned with the power or designs necessary to allow for the moderating effects of quite subtle variables. Even less likely is the design of a trial in which only adherence promoting variables vary between conditions, as usually the dietary intervention is also altered, for example a more stringent low-fat diet or added medication. Consequently, the main body of work in this area concerns the characteristics of participants. One frequently used method of classifying patients for the purposes of understanding their likely response to treatment is according to the "transtheoretical", or "stages of change" model (Prochaska and DiClemente, 1982; see Horne and Weinman, Chapter 2, for a description of the model). The model outlines five stages in relation health behaviour change: precontemplation – denial of the problem or responsibility for the problem; contemplation – awareness and concern about the problem but without an imminent plan of action; preparation (at times also referred to as decision) – an imminent plan for action is being drawn up with confidence that it will be successfully carried out; action – consistent and demonstrably successful behaviour change has been undertaken; and maintenance (at times also referred to as relapse) – long-term, successful behaviour change. This is not so relevant for studies of high risk and clinical populations, as usually the participants present themselves for screening or assessment. This may indicate that the majority of such participants are beyond the precontemplation stage. McCann and her colleagues (1996) used this model to predict the participation of hyperlipidaemic individuals in a dietary intervention to lower cholesterol in a workplace setting. In their sample of 772 people who were assessed and invited to take part in the treatment, those in preparation stage were significantly more likely to join, with 77.5% of them joining compared to 66.3% of contemplators, 61.4% of actors and 67.4% of maintainers.

The individual's appraisal of the costs and benefits of adopting a particular behaviour are important predictive elements of the likelihood of adopting a particular behaviour in the Health Belief Model (Becker, 1974; see Horne and Weinman, Chapter 2 for a description of the model). One of the few dietary interventions in which they were formally assessed was the Women's Health Trial. In a retrospective postal survey of 525 women who had been enrolled on the Women's Health Trial, Urban *et al.* (1992) examined the relationship of women's experience of the diet to maintenance at 5 to 20 months. The researchers constructed a 35 item questionnaire which represented the experience of the diet in six variables. Two factors which should promote adherence (general wellness and distaste for fat) and four which would deter (costliness, inconvenience, deprivation and dissatisfaction, and lack of family support) were assessed. Results showed perceived costliness to be the only experiential variable with a significant direct association upon long-term maintenance.

Characteristics associated with adherence to cholesterol lowering dietary interventions reported by Caggiula and Watson (1992) also demonstrated the importance of costs and benefits of treatment. A 35 item questionnaire measuring seven characteristics was used: (i) external environmental media; (ii) internal health locus of control; (iii) external locus of control; (iv) perceived costs and benefits; (v) perceived threat of disease; (vi) quality of care; and (vii) social support. Among the 264 participants in the MRFIT programme in Pittsburgh who were included in the analysis, costs and benefits were most predictive of adherence. An important finding in this study was the limited association between all the items measuring social support and adherence. However, there was a wide spread of predictive weights across the five items used to measure this construct.

Another concept which has been proposed as linked to the ability to initiate and maintain new behaviour is self-efficacy, which refers to the belief in one's own capability to meet challenges presented in specific situations (Bandura, 1977). The Dietary Alternatives Study included an investigation into the role of self-efficacy in adherence to diet among a sub-sample of 25 hyperlipidaemic men out of the original sample of 531 men (McCann *et al.*, 1996). Self-efficacy was assessed with a revised version of the Eating Self-Efficacy Scale (Glynn and Ruderman, 1986) which had two sub-scales: Negative Affect (NA) and Socially Acceptable Circumstances (SAC). As in the main study, dietary intake was measured by a four day food record.

Examination of the association between changes in Negative Affect scores, cholesterol levels and dietary saturated fat and cholesterol intake, showed a number of significant inter-correlations both at post-treatment and three month follow-up. However, a negative correlation was found between absolute pre-treatment NA self-efficacy scores and reduction in total cholesterol over the treatment period. SAC sub-scale scores were not associated with changes in dietary intake or cholesterol levels. The authors suggest that the findings reflect the importance of a realistic approach to achieving dietary changes, but the sample size was so small that is seems unlikely that the study had the power to detect a moderating effect of self-efficacy.

Social support, and its role in promoting behaviour, has been investigated in the context of a number of health issues, notably mental health problems such as depression (Brown, Harris and Copeland, 1977). It was also examined in relation to the adoption of low-fat diets (Bovbjerg *et al.*, 1995) in an investigation of the relationship between spousal support and adherence in the Dietary Alternatives Study. The intervention included elements designed to improve spousal support for dietary changes, and so it is uncertain as to whether the results presented reflect the baseline levels of support or the effect of change. Complete data were collected on 254 participants (50% of baseline participants) and analysed. A self-report 17 item questionnaire, the Evaluation of Spouse Support (ESS), was developed for use in the trial. Additional general support was measured using the Interpersonal Support Evaluation List, a 40 item self-report scale assessing perception of available support. Whilst scores on the ESS was not associated with attainment of dietary goals during the active treatment period of the trial, there were significant relationships between ESS scores and goal attainment in the follow-up period. This may reflect social desirability effects of questionnaire completion, especially as improvement in social support was an important goal of the intervention, which tailed off with time. However, these results point to the possible value of including increases in social support as a means of increase adherence to dietary interventions.

The variables mostly closely associated with compliance (as they call it) on the Hypertension Prevention Trial (Jeffrey *et al.*, 1990; Schmid *et al.*, 1991) were baseline urine sodium and potassium and baseline weight. The stated purpose of the study was "to learn more about what factors may help discriminate between participants who will meet dietary treatment goals from those who do not" (Schmid *et al.*, 1991). The authors noted the fact that physiological variables seemed to be more related to adherence than other more behavioural variables, such as use of salt substitutes (Schmid *et al.*, 1991). This, however, might be because their measures of adherence were physiological and not behavioural, for example sodium adherence was defined as having a urine sodium excretion of less than or equal to 70 mEq/24hr. In general, attendance at treatment sessions was positively associated with adherence (Schmid *et al.*, 1991). A useful addition to this study was the collection of data related to adherence problems as reported to clinic staff. Jeffery *et al.* (1990) reported that 82% of the participants reported adherence problems at least once, and in just over half of the sessions attended adherence problems were discussed. The three most common attributions reported for lack of adherence were high risk situations, "character defects" and the complexity of the diet. In general the attributions could be classified as external, stable and uncontrollable, but no stable associations were found between attributions and dietary outcomes (Jeffery *et al.*, 1990).

This brief review of variables associated with varying outcome in dietary interventions is of most importance as an indication of future directions to be pursued to improve adherence. We address some of these ideas in the next section.

PROMOTING SUCCESSFUL DIETARY CHANGE

In clinical terms, it is of great importance to improve adherence to dietary advice. However, it is not clear that effective methods of accomplishing this have been established. Increasingly it is being suggested that simple recommendations about the dietary changes are not adequate methods for achieving change, and the poor outcome of the community studies certainly suggests that simple advice is inadequate. The challenge is therefore to understand and promote ways of improving the uptake of healthy eating. One important approach is a shift in focus away from the content of the dietary advice, onto the recipients of the interventions (Health Education Authority, 1995). Accompanying this refocusing is the suggestion that interventions should concentrate on those most likely to benefit from a given course of treatment at a given moment in time. Traditionally HPs approach their patients as though they were all equally ready to implement the treatments prescribed for them. The implication of the proposed change of focus is that the characteristics of individual clients should guide the treatment packages offered to them. It is in this area that perhaps the greatest contribution of the transtheoretical model (Prochaska and DiClemente, 1982) can be made.

In the literature on obesity treatment, Brownell and Wadden (1992) reviewed three possible screening processes. Firstly, the classification of individuals on the basis of their level of obesity, usually measured by percentage overweight or BMI. This approach was criticised on the basis that it takes no account of the cost implications of various treatments or the individual needs of the patient. Secondly, the stepped care approach uses the least intensive, expensive and dangerous interventions initially, with progression to other treatments on the basis of earlier treatment failures. When adopted in isolation, this may mean that individuals receive treatments most unlikely to be successful for them, with the associated risks of undermining important contributors to successful outcome such as self-efficacy. The third process is that of matching individuals to programmes on the basis of both client and programme factors, such as initial weight, goal weight and cost of the programme.

Schwartz and Brownell (1995) conducted a survey of obesity experts in order to generate hypotheses about fruitful matches to investigate. They found support for the idea that different degrees of overweight required different approaches. There is certainly evidence of individual and programme characteristics being associated with differential outcomes which might also be pursued (Shah *et al.,* 1990; Urban *et al.,* 1992).

Although it is not clear exactly what the crucial individual variables might be, there is increasing attention being paid to the association between individual characteristics and behavioural dietary adherence. Cross-sectional studies examining the relationships between individual characteristics and dietary behaviour, such as the Working Well Study (Kristal *et al.,* 1995) can be used to inform prospective intervention studies. For example, their measures of predisposing factors, such as motivation, were associated with actual and planned dietary behaviour and it will be interesting to examine their relationship with actual changes in dietary behaviour, when these data are available. The increasing attention given to measuring predictive variables in prospective studies is encouraging, but it is important that research also extended to programmes variables, for example the suggestion that inclusion of exercise is treatment packages for obesity not only has an independent effect on energy expenditure, but actually seems to be associated with better adherence to energy restriction diets among overweight women (Racette *et al.*, 1995).

McCann *et al.* (1990) highlight the high cognitive demands of adopting low-fat, low-cholesterol diets and its implications for adherence. On the basis of their own work on the Dietary Alternatives Study, and a review of the relevant literature, they drew out three key elements for effective dietary intervention programmes. Firstly, they suggest that basic behavioural techniques, including self-monitoring and goal-setting, should be introduced early in the programmes. Secondly, they propose that significant others should be encouraged to be actively involved, and finally, they suggest that specific strategies for the enhancement of self-efficacy should be developed and tested in clinical settings.

Broadening the net of pertinent variables to consider one issue infrequently commented upon is the role of health care personnel and the treatment setting in relation to adherence to dietary prescriptions. In a paper addressing increasing the effectiveness of the National Cholesterol Education Program, Southard *et al.* (1992) identified this as an important area for consideration. They argue that, in particular, physicians' lack of confidence in the ability of their patients to make changes may undermine dietary interventions in primary care settings. Such acknowledgements are part of an increasing acceptance of the role of the health care professional in mediating adherence.

Based on the idea of the importance of behavioural control to successful behaviour change, there have been some innovative attempts to present interventions within the context of ordinary patterns of eating. An example of this is the incorporation of quick service foods into diets prescribed for hypercholesterolaemic men (Davidson *et al.*, 1996). Although in this case the outcome was not favourable, it is important to be realistic in suggesting changes which can be integrated into the individual client's life.

Many studies address the initial phase of a dietary intervention: acquiring knowledge of a diet and beginning to adopt appropriate strategies. However, it is argued by many that the greatest challenge is in maintaining such changes once they have been made (Robison *et al.*, 1995: Brownell and Cohen, 1995). Relapse prevention methods are increasingly being integrated into clinical programmes, such as Brownell's (1994) LEARN Program for Weight Control. The expense of providing longer-term interventions, or even follow-up of participants, is a drawback of trying to organise and fund such work. However, given the need for dietary behaviour change to be sustained for the benefits to be felt this area is in urgent need of attention.

CONCLUSIONS

Changing the diet has the potential to offer many health benefits in terms of preventing and even possibly reversing health problems, but the problems of adherence mean that we are still a long way from delivering these. There are diverse attempts both to explain and increase adherence to dietary interventions.

Community studies have had poor results, but intensive interventions with clinical samples are generally much more effective. Goals are most likely to be achieved by clinically ill populations, which may be due to a number of factors such as perception of personal vulnerability, motivation and intensity of intervention. Some positive associations between individual and programme characteristics and adherence have been observed, but there are likely to be many other factors at work in this area which we are not yet aware of or able to measure. The disregard for definition and measurement issues in many of the studies in the area, as well as the loosely defined interventions adopted, result in the loss of valuable opportunities for teasing out subtle moderating variables, such as self-efficacy. There is hope that some of the current lines of enquiry, such as using screening and matching between clients and interventions may help to refine the balance between costs of providing these programmes and the benefits seen by clients. Practitioners and researchers working in this field need to consider all the relevant variables which may influence successful adherence to behavioural dietary change (individual characteristics, programme characteristics, treatment setting and delivery and general environment) as well as tailoring interventions to both initiate and maintain changes in the long-term.

REFERENCES

Bandura, A. (1977). Self efficacy: Towards a unifying theory of behavioral change. *Psychological Review* **84**, 191–215.

Becker, M.H. (1974) The health belief model and sick role behaviour. *Health Education Monograph* **2**, 409–419.

Bovbjerg, V.E., McCann. B.S., Brief. D.J., Follette, W.C., Retzlaff, B.M., Dowdy, A.A., Walden, C.E. and R.H. Knopp. (1995) Spouse support and long-term adherence to lipid-lowering diets. *American Journal of Epidemiology* **141**, 451–460.

Brown, G.W., Harris, T. and Copeland, J.R., (1977) Depression and loss. *British Journal of Psychiatry* **130**, 1–18..

Brownell, K.D. (1994) *The LEARN program for weight control, 6th edition*. Dallas: American Health Publishing Company.

Brownell, K.D. and Cohen, L.R. (1995) Adherence to dietary regimens 2: components of effective interventions. *Behavioral Medicine* **20**, 155–164.

Brownell, K.D. and Wadden, T.A. (1992) Etiology and treatment of obesity: understanding a serious, prevalent and refractory disorder. *Journal of Consulting and Clinical Psychology* **60**, 505–517..

Caggiula, A.W. and Watson, J.E. (1992) Characteristics associated with compliance to cholesterol lowering eating patterns. *Patient Education and Counseling* **19**, 33–41.

Cannon, G. (1992) *Food and health: the experts agree*. London: The Consumers Association.

Davidson, M.H., Kong, J.C., Drennan, K.B., Story, K. and Anderson, H. (1996) Efficacy of the National Cholesterol Education Program Step I Diet. *Archives of Internal Medicine* **156**, 305–312.

Denke, M.A. (1995) Review of human studies evaluating individual dietary responsiveness in patients with hypercholesterolaemia *The American Journal of Clinical Nutrition* **62**, 471S–477S.

Department of Health (1991) *The health of the nation*. London: HMSO.

Dolecek, T.A., Milas, N.C., Van Horn, L.V., Farrand, M.E., Gorder, D.E., Duchene, A.G., Dyer, J.R., Stone, P.A.. and Randall, B.L. (1986) A long-term nutrition intervention experience: lipid responses and dietary adherence patterns in the multiple risk factor intervention trial. *Journal of The American Dietetic Association* **86**, 752–758.

dynamic approach and Norman and Connor (1996) suggest that future developments need to focus on identifying the social cognition factors that are relevant at each stage. Some attempts have been made towards this in the field of exercise research (e.g. Courneya, 1995; Godin, 1993). For example, Godin (1993) describes one study which examines the stages of change of adults randomly recruited from the general population and attempts to differentiate individuals according to the TPB variables. He found that PBC was higher among those contemplating than those starting to take exercise. He suggests that at this stage people are optimistic about exercise, perceiving a fairly high level of control. Godin suggests that, since they perceive few barriers and large benefits, it is not surprising if they become disillusioned when barriers start to emerge. He further suggests that interventions geared to increasing realism and lowering expectations and adopting goals which are not too demanding may be helpful at this stage. This seems particularly pertinent to exercise in medical settings where such unrealistic expectations seem common (see above). As people start to take action, interventions to maintain or boost perceived control may be more appropriate.

FUTURE DIRECTIONS FOR RESEARCH AND PRACTICE IN EXERCISE PRESCRIBING

A typical person referred for an exercise prescription in the UK may be a woman who is over 50, overweight, possibly with high blood pressure and /or depression and low self esteem. She is probably fairly inactive and has never seen herself as the sporty type. She associates sport with traumatic school experiences such as coming last in the skipping race and failing to be picked for the under-14 team. She has an image of gyms as being for slim and muscular young people clad in small and body revealing strips of lycra. It has seldom crossed her mind that exercise or gyms are relevant to her as she considers she is quite active enough in the course of household tasks. She has perhaps gone to her doctor suffering from symptoms such as tiredness or depression expecting relief in the usual form of medication. Suddenly her doctor suggests that instead of medication she will be prescribed exercise and that she is advised to go to work-out in a gym twice a week. Although she has never thought about it much before, her doctor sells the idea well and she becomes convinced that exercise could be the answer, it will help her lose weight, become fitter, get her out of the house and help her meet people. So despite some reservations, she goes along to the gym and finds she is quite unprepared for the reality. She is unsure of her way around and finds it difficult to remember the instructions about how to operate the unfamiliar equipment. She may feel embarrassed and out of place. She may find that exercise makes her hot and sweaty and it hurts. The pain is even worse the next day. Her initial confidence starts to wane. She may fear that exercise is not a suitable form of treatment and may even damage her health. She gets symptoms of breathlessness and aches and pains which are worse than those that took her to the doctor in the first place.

The theories and models discussed above take into account many elements present in the above description. They would suggest that the probability of her succeeding is low. She may not have a positive attitude to exercise and has low SE. She may not perceive any social pressure or support from family and friends (who may indeed perceive that her attending a gym is quite inappropriate). In terms of the Transtheoretical Model, she is suddenly pushed in a very short time from the precontemplation stage to the action stage. However, these general models and even models particularly designed for exercise do not encompass all elements that may be relevant. Ajzen (1991) himself suggests the possibility of adding additional predictors to the TPB, and other variables have been suggested in different contexts. For example, the role of self identity in healthy eating is discussed by Sparks and Shepherd (1992). The importance of not seeing yourself as "the sporty type", for example, is clearly likely to be relevant but so far does not seem to have received much research.

The rather obvious factor of lack of enjoyment or negative feelings associated with exercise has also not been adequately considered in research studies. In a study using a card-sort task, Eves (1995) found that while sport and exercise were associated with health they were also associated with items which were perceived negatively, such as "effort", and not with positive items such as "having fun". Wankel (1993) has also suggested that this factor deserves more attention and that ways in which enjoyment may be increased include providing opportunities for social interaction, developing flexible programmes to cater for individual interests and encouraging skill development and realistic goal achievement .

One limitation of much of the research that has looked at exercise in a medical context is that it has drawn too exclusively on approaches used in exercise psychology. These do not take into account the fact that different variables may come into play when exercise is recommended as a treatment rather than as a health promotion, although it is documented that the individual's representation of health may be very different from their representation of illness (see Radley, 1994). Maintaining health is more likely to be seen as the responsibility of the individual, treating illness as the responsibility of the doctor. Models looking at adherence with medical treatment do not yet seem to have been applied to exercise prescription e.g. Leventhal's Self Regulation model (Leventhal, Diefenbach and Leventhal, 1992). Leventhal and Cameron, (1987) suggests that "different people will construct different representations of the same illness threat and may see different action plans as appropriate for the containment of the threat." See Horne and Weinman, Chapter 2 for a full description of the model. There is clearly scope for integrating these approaches into studies of exercise adherence.

The theoretical challenge is to successfully develop and test models to guide action in exercise prescriptions and this chapter has attempted to outline some of the many possible approaches. Meanwhile existing models and research studies, albeit limited, do suggest some approaches that may increase adherence. Much of the work done points to the need for more gradual introduction to exercise incorporating preparatory work particularly where people have not previously even contemplated exercising. This would include overcoming barriers by helping with planning, setting realistic goals and establishing a realistic level of self-efficacy. This is in keeping with the 1994 Physical Activity Guidelines for adults in England which emphasises the value of moderate levels of exercise compatible with everyday routines e.g. walking or cycling to work. Earlier, more energetic recommendations are still seen as valid but accepted as unrealistic for many (Department of Health, 1995). Exercise prescriptions incorporating such gradual introductions to exercise are clearly one way in which people may be encouraged to overcome barriers and develop SE.

REFERENCES

Ajzen, I. (1985) From intentions to action: a theory of planned behavior. In J. Kuhl and J. Beckman (eds.) *Action control: from cognitions to behavior.* New York: Springer.

Ajzen, I. (1991) The theory of planned behavior. *Organisational Behavior and Human Decision Processes* **50**, 179–211.

ASCM (American College of Sports Medicine) (1986) *Guidelines for exercise testing and exercise prescription* (3rd edition). Philadelphia: Lea and Febiger.

Bagozzi, R.P. and Warshaw, P.R. (1990) Trying to consume. *Journal of Consumer Research* **17**, 127–140.

Bandura, A. (1977) Self efficacy: towards a unifying theory of behavioral change. *Psychological Review* **84**, 191–215.

Beardon, P., McGilchrist, M., McKendrick, A., McDevitt, D. and McDonald, T. (1993) Primary non-compliance with prescribed medication in primary care. *British Medical Journal* **307**, 846–848.

Biddle, S., Fox, K. and Edmunds, L. (1994) *Physical activity promotion in primary health care in England: final research report for the Health Education Authority.* London: Health Education Authority.

Blair, S.N., Kohl, H.W., Gordon, N.F. and Paffenbarger Jr, R.S. (1992) How much exercise is good for health? *Annual Review of Public Health* **13**, 99–126.

Blair, S.N., Kohl, H.W., Paffenbarger, R.S., Clark, D.G., Cooper, K.H. and Gibbons, L.W. (1989) Physical fitness and all cause mortality: a prospective study of healthy men and women. *Journal of the American Medical Association* **262**, 2395–2401.

Chapman, T. (1996) *Directory of GP-referred exercise schemes in England.* Chichester Institute of Higher Education.

Clarke, P. and Eves, F. (1997) Applying the transtheoretical model to the study of exercise on prescription. *Journal of Health Psychology* **2**, 195–207.

Conner, M. and Norman, P. (1996) *Predicting health behaviour.* Buckingham: Open University Press.

Connor, M. and Sparks, P. (1996) The theory of planned behavior and health behaviours. In M. Connor and P. Norman (eds.)

Predicting Health Behavior. Buckingham: Open University Press.

Courneya, K. (1995) Understanding readiness for regular physical activity in older individuals: an application of the theory of planned behavior. *Health Psychology* **14**, 80–87.

Department of Health (1992) *The health of the nation: a strategy for England.* London: HMSO.

Department of Health (1995) *More people, more active, more often: physical activity in England, a consultation document.* London: Department of Health.

Dishman, R.K. (1982) Compliance/adherence in health related exercise. *Health Psychology* **3**, 237–267.

Dzewaltowski, D.A., Noble, J.M. and Shaw, J.M. (1990) Physical activity participation: social cognitive theory versus the theories of reasoned action and planned behavior. *Journal of Sport and Exercise Psychology* **12**, 388–405.

Eves, F. (1995) Lay representations of exercise and health: the importance of feelings. In J. Rodriguez-Marin (ed.) *Health psychology and quality of life research.* Alicante: University of Alicante.

Ewart, C.K. (1992) The role of self-efficacy in recovery from heart attack. In R. Schwarzer (ed.) *Self efficacy: thought control of action* Washington, DC: Hemisphere.

Fishbein, M. and Ajzen, I. (1975) *Belief, attitude, intention and behavior.* New York: Wiley.

Godin, G. (1993) The theories of reasoned action and planned behavior:overview of findings, emerging research problems and usefulness for exercise promotion. *Journal of Applied Sport Psychology* **5**, 141–157.

Godin, G., Valois, P., Jobin, J. and Ross, A. (1991) Prediction of intention to exercise in individuals who have suffered from coronary heart disease. *Journal of Clinical Psychology* **47**, 762–772.

Godin, G., Vezina, L. and LeClerc, O. (1989) Factors influencing the intention of pregnant women to exercise after giving birth. *Public Health Reports* **104**, 188–195.

Gollwitzer, P.M. (1993) Goal achievement: the role of intentions. In W. Stroebe and M. Hewstone (eds.) *European Review of Social Psychology. Volume 4.* Chichester: John Wiley and Sons.

Hammond, J.M., Brodie, D.A., Bundred, P.E. and Cummins, A. (1995) *Exercise on prescription: an evaluation. A guide for similar schemes based upon the work of the Life Project and the University of Liverpool.* University of Liverpool.

HEA (1992) *Allied Dunbar National Fitness Survey.* London: Sports Council and Health Education Authority.

Janis, I.L. and Mann, L. (1977) *Decision making.* New York: Macmillan.

Jones, F. and Harris, P. (1995) Exercise prescription: the psychological predictors and benefits of compliance. Presented at The 9th Conference of the European Health Psychology Society, August, Bergen.

Jones, F. and Harris, P. (1995b) The use of repertory grid technique in exercise psychology. In C. Robson, B. Cripps, and H. Steinberg (eds.) *Quality and quantity: research methods in sport and exercise psychology. An occasional publication for the Sport and Exercise Psychology Section of the British Psychological Society.* Leicester: BPS.

Jones, F. and Harris, P. (1996) 'I want to be younger, slimmer, fitter..' A repertory grid study of expectations of participants in an exercise prescription scheme. Presented at the 10th Conference of the European Health Psychology Society. September, Dublin.

Kaplan, R.M., Atkins, C.J. and Reinsch, S. (1984) Specific efficacy expectations mediate exercise compliance in patients with COPD. *Health Psychology* **3**, 223–242.

Kendzierski, D. (1990) Decision making versus decision implementation: an action control approach to exercise adoption and adherence. *Journal of Applied Social Psychology* **20**, 27–45.

Leventhal, H. and Cameron, L. (1987) Behavioral theories and the problem of compliance. *Patient Education and Counselling* **10**, 117–138.

Leventhal, H., Diefenbach, M. and Leventhal, A.H. (1992) Illness cognition: using common sense to understand treatment adherence and to affect cognition interactions. Special issue: cognitive issues in health psychology. *Cognitive Therapy and Research* **16**, 143–163.

Lord, J. (1994) *Exercise on prescription: does it work.* Stockport: Stockport Health Commission..

Marcus, B.H., Banspach, S.W., Lefebvre, R.C., Rossi, J.S., Carleton, R.A. and Abrams, D.B. (1992a) Using the stages of change model to increase the adoption of physical activity among community participants. *American Journal of Health Promotion* **6**, 424–429.

Marcus, B.H., Selby, V.C., Niaura, R. S. and Rossi, J.S. (1992b) Self-efficacy and the Stages of Exercise Behavior Change. *Research Quarterly for Exercise and Sport* **63**, 60–66.

Mason, P. and Sills, M. (1994) *Helping people change Trainer's Manual: core and physical activity modules*. London: Health Education Authority.

McAuley, E. (1992) The role of efficacy cognitions in the prediction of exercise behavior in middle-aged adults. *Journal of Behavioral Medicine* **15**, 65–88.

Norman, P. and Connor, M. (1996) The role of social cognition models in predicting health behaviours: future directions. In M. Conner and P. Norman (eds.) *Predicting health behaviour*. Buckingham: Open University Press.

Norman, P. and Smith, L. (1995) The theory of planned behaviour and exercise: an investigation into the role of prior behaviour, behavioral intentions and attitude variability. *European Journal of Social Psychology* **25**, 403–501.

Patrick, K., Sallis, J.F., Long, B., Calfas, K.J., Wooten, W., Heath, G. and Pratt, M. (1994) A new tool for encouraging activity: project PACE. *The Physician and Sports Medicine* **22**, 45–55.

Prochaska, J.O. and DiClemente, C.C. (1983) Stages and process of self-change of smoking: toward an integrative model of change. *Journal of Consulting and Clinical Psychology* **51**, 390–395.

Prochaska, J.O. and Marcus, B.H. (1994) The transtheoretical model: applications to exercise. In R.K. Dishman (ed.) *Goals in exercise adherence* Champaign, IL: Human Kinetics.

Radley, A. (1994) *Making sense of illness: the social psychology of health and disease*. London: Sage.

Schwarzer, R. (1992) Self-efficacy in the adoption and maintenance of health behavior: theoretical approaches and a new model. In R. Schwarzer (ed.) *Self efficacy: thought control of action*. London: Hemisphere.

Schwarzer, R. and Fuchs, R. (1996) Self efficacy and health behaviours. In M. Conner and P. Norman (eds.) *Predicting health behaviour*. Buckingham: Open University Press.

Sonstroem, R.J. (1988) Psychological Models. In R. Dishman K, (ed.) *Exercise adherence: its impact on public health*. Champaign, IL.: Human Kinetics..

Sparks, P. and Shepherd, R. (1992) Self identity and the theory of planned behaviour: assessing the role of identification with 'green consumerism'. *Social Psychology Quarterly* **55**, 388–389.

Taylor, A.H. (1996) *Evaluating GP exercise prescription schemes: findings from a randomised control trial*. Brighton: Chelsea School Research Centre, University of Brighton.

Terry, D.J. and O'Leary, J.E. (1995) The theory of planned behaviour: The effects of perceived behavioral control and self-efficacy. *British Journal of Social Psychology* **34**, 199–220.

Wankel, L.M. (1993) The importance of enjoyment to adherence and psychological benefits from physical activity. *International Journal of Sport Psychology* **24**, 151–169.

Weinstein, N.D. (1988) The Precaution adoption process. *Health Psychology* **7**, 355–386.

Yordy, G.A. and Lent, R.W. (1993) Predicting aerobic exercise participation: social cognitive, reasoned action and planned behavior models. *Journal of Sport and Exercise Psychology* **15**, 363–374.

14

Adherence to Physiotherapy

E.M. Sluijs, J.J. Kerssens J. van der Zee and L.B. Myers

Physiotherapy (or physical therapy) is concerned with patients' mobility and its main objective is the rehabilitation of patients' movement dysfunctions. More than 90% of patients referred for physiotherapy in primary care suffer from diseases or disorders of the musculoskeletal system (Kerssens and Groenewegen, 1990). Symptoms, complaints, and injuries of the back, neck, shoulder and knee account for more than half of referrals. Around 30% of the disorders treated by physiotherapists appear to be chronic and there is a high recurrence rate (Knibbe, 1987). Part of this recurrence might be avoided if patients would adhere to their prescribed exercises. Indeed, research indicates that the overall effectiveness of physiotherapy may be enhanced by improving patients' adherence (Friedrich, Cermak and Maderbacher, 1996; Ice, 1985). As well as prescribing effective treatments for musculoskeletal dysfunctions, physiotherapists can make recommendations for regular exercise in order to promote overall fitness and, hence, reduce disease risks (Bouchard *et al.*, 1988; Hayne, 1988; Huhn and Volski, 1985; Lorish *et al.*, 1996; Lyne, 1986; Norton, 1986).

The main type of interventions undertaken by physiotherapists include massage, physical modalities (e.g. ultrasound, interferential therapy and shortwave therapy), exercise and advice to patients. Massage and physical modalities are usually applied to reduce pain, regulate muscle tone and reduce swelling (Dekker *et al.*, 1993). Patients play a passive role in these treatments. In contrast, there are a number of treatments which require patients to change their behaviour, hence patients play an active role. These treatments are exercise, instructions and following physiotherapist advice. They are applied to improve muscle strength, posture, range of motion and many other impairments and disabilities (Dekker *et al.*, 1993). Because the majority of physiotherapy treatments consist of combined interventions, patients' *active* co-operation and adherence is required.

This chapter provides a general overview of non-adherence to physiotherapy. Research on this topic is extremely limited, therefore the majority of the chapter describes an ongoing research program in the Netherlands which has been developed to improve patient education and adherence to physiotherapy.

NON-ADHERENCE IN PHYSIOTHERAPY

Exact rates of adherence to physiotherapy are unknown. However, most studies of multidisciplinary treatment programs which include physiotherapy indicate that as many as one third to two thirds of patients are not adherent to prescribed exercise, including low back programs, back schools (i.e. back care education), preventive fitness programs, exercises for rheumatoid arthritis and cardiac rehabilitation (Campen and Sluijs, 1989; Deyo, 1982; Dishman, 1982, 1988; Feinberg, 1988; Oldridge, 1988; Sikorsky, 1985; Spelman, 1984).

A study of patients in the USA who were solely having physiotherapy indicated a high level of adherence (Gahimer and Domholdt, 1996). Physiotherapists audiotaped entire treatments of 37 patients, resulting in 173 audiotaped sessions. Over 80% of patients reported having changed their behaviour as a result of instructions and education given by the physiotherapist. However, it is unclear whether these changes actually occurred or whether patients merely gave the desired response, because the authors "did not have any mechanism to measure behavioral changes beyond patient self report" (Gahimer and Domholdt, 1996).

In our second study (for a description of the studies, see below), adherence measurements have been restricted to an exercise regimen prescribed by physiotherapists (Sluijs, Kok and van der Zee, 1993a). Patients were asked questions such as: "did you manage to exercise regularly last week?" Of the 1178 patients who were instructed to perform home exercises, 35% reported that they fully adhered, 41% reported that they were partly adherent (exercising "now and then") and 22% reported that they were totally non-adherent. These figures may be an overestimation for two reasons. Firstly, the figures are based on patients' self-report (see Myers and Midence, Chapter 1, for a discussion of measurements of adherence). Secondly, the questionnaire was given to patients half way through their treatment when they were undertaking short-term supervised physiotherapy (Haynes, Wang and Da Mota Gomes, 1987; Oldridge, 1988). It is well recognised that adherence drops dramatically in the case of long-term physiotherapy (Green, 1987; Mazucca, 1982; Turk, Salovey and Litt, 1986). Long-term adherence to physiotherapy is usually defined as maintaining the change of behavior after treatment with a physiotherapist had ended (Sluijs and Knibbe, 1991).

Research indicates that physiotherapists are clearly aware of a drop in adherence to long-term unsupervised physiotherapy after treatment with the physiotherapist has stopped. A sample of 222 physiotherapists estimated that approximately 64% of their patients adhered with a home exercise regimen during the treatment period, but that only 23% of their patients continued to do so after treatment has stopped (Sluijs, 1991 a).

Although the problem of non-adherence has long been recognised in the physiotherapy literature (Croft, 1980; Mayo, 1978; Wagstaff, 1982) there is limited systematic research in the area. For example, measures of patient adherence are frequently absent in research about exercise programs (Belcon, Haynes and Tugwell, 1984; Evans *et al.*, 1987; Lindequist *et al.*, 1984; Mellin, Järvikoski and Verkasalo, 1984; Snook, 1987). This is a severe limitation, as the effects of such exercise programs largely depend upon patients adhering to the program (Feinstein, 1979). A recent overview of 16 randomised clinical trials concerning the efficacy of back schools (Koes *et al.*, 1994) showed that adherence was measured in only one study (Mellin *et al.*, 1990). Consequently, no firm conclusions can be made about the effectiveness of such programs and about the effectiveness of (physiotherapy) exercises (Koes *et al.*, 1991). Similarly, to the authors' knowledge, there have been no systematic attempts to find effective methods which enhance patients' adherence to physiotherapy. Indeed, it is only in recent years that modules about patient education have been added to the training curriculum and modules about non-adherence are still rare (Schultz, Wellard and Swerissen, 1988).

OUTLINES OF THE RESEARCH PROGRAM

The ultimate goal of the current research program is to include effective adherence enhancing skills in physiotherapy training and practice (Netherlands Institute for Primary Health Care, NIVEL, 1996). The research programme has consisted of three studies (see below). Currently, the effects of a number of adherence enhancing strategies in physiotherapy are being investigated (study three, results to be reported elsewhere). However, at the start of the research program in 1988, it was unknown what instructions and advice patients received from physiotherapists. Thus, it was also unknown to which regimen patients were supposed to adhere. Therefore, a number of fundamental questions had to be posed. In successive studies the following questions have been addressed.

- Which exercises, instructions and advice do physiotherapists prescribe?
- What problems do physiotherapists encounter when educating patients?
- Which factors are related to (and are possibly causes of) patients' non-adherence to physiotherapy?
- Which theories are useful to enhance understanding (and improving) long-term adherence to physiotherapy?
- Which strategies can be used to enhance adherence? And are these strategies applicable in physiotherapy?

OUTLINE OF PROGRAMME

Study one: Six physiotherapists audiotaped the entire course of treatment of 25 patients (mean number of sessions audiotaped per patient = 9). These recordings were used to: (i) develop a checklist of educational activities and (ii) analyse the way in which these educational activities were spread throughout the entire course of treatment. (Results are reported in Sluijs, 1991b; 1991c).

Study two: Data were collected from physiotherapists and patients. (i) Two hundred and twenty two physiotherapists completed a questionnaire about their views on patient education and adherence, (response rate 74%). (ii) Eighty four physiotherapists (response rate 28%) audiotaped treatment sessions of 1837 patients (mean number of sessions audiotaped per physiotherapist = 22). (iii) Patients were given a questionnaire by the physiotherapist upon completion of the audiotaped session (response rate 92%). The questionnaire included items concerning perception of patients illness and prognosis, their degree of adherence to the exercise regimen; problems they encountered when exercising and problems they encountered in following advice. Patients were told that the study concerned therapist-patient communication and that their physiotherapist would not see their answers. Results of this study have been reported elsewhere (Sluijs, 1993; Sluijs and Hermans, 1990; Sluijs *et al.*, 1993a; Sluijs and Kuijper, 1990; Sluijs, van der Zee, and Kok, 1993b).

Study three: The aim of the study is to assess the effects of adherence-enhancing strategies applied by physiotherapists on patients' adherence. Nineteen physiotherapists (response rate, 79%) completed training in adherence-enhancing strategies. Patients were chosen who were suffering from back pain. Adherence was assessed before physiotherapists received adherence-enhancing training. Adherence was measured with a new measuring instrument using a combination of adherence measures (to be described elsewhere). Currently adherence is being measured again after physiotherapists received training, to assess the effects of the training on adherence.

EXERCISES, INSTRUCTIONS AND ADVICE IN PHYSIOTHERAPY

The concept of "patient education" is often used to denote exercises, instructions and advice given by physiotherapists. The aim of patient education is to influence patients' knowledge and health behavior. In fact, physiotherapists are continuously trying to help patients change their behavior For example, by explaining to them the necessity to (i) improve (bad) posture or movement; (ii) perform home-exercises; (iii) take appropriate rest; (iv) make adaptations at work or at home; (v) reduce stress; (vi) keep fit and (vii) adopt a healthy lifestyle. Physiotherapists generally consider patient education as an essential part of treatment (Leathley, 1988). The amount of information, instructions and advice actually given by physiotherapists can be seen in Table 1. The figures are the result of 1837 audiotaped treatment sessions (Study two, reported in Sluijs, 1991a).

Table 1 The number of treatment sessions with education and mean number of educational remarks per session compared with Gahimer and Domholdt (1996)

	Percentage of treatment sessions with education	Mean number of educational remarks (Gahimer and Domholdt, 1996, study in parenthesis)
Teaching about illness	80	5.4 (4.7)
Exercise instructions	64	6.1 (4.0)
Advice (posture etc.)	69	4.8 (2.5)
Health (lifestyle) education	23	1.1 (0.4)
Psychosocial counselling	23	2.7 (0.2)
Total education	97	20.1 (11.8)

These results indicate that educational activity took place in almost all treatment sessions (97%). Similarly, in over three quarters of the sessions (80%), physiotherapists taught patients about their illness (diagnosis, causes, prognoses). In nearly two thirds of sessions both home exercises were prescribed (64%) and patients were given advice, for example about changing posture, taking rest or making adaptations (69%).

Gahimer and Domholdt (1996) replicated study one and concluded that their results were consistent with our findings. Results illustrated in Table 1 highlight that physiotherapists ask their patients to change their behaviour in many respects. Some physiotherapists seem to expect the impossible from patients. For example, one woman received a total of 23 pieces of advice in 15 sessions, as well as 98 exercise instructions and other information about her illness! (Sluijs, 1991 c). On the basis of these findings, it has been recommended previously that information and instructions should be spread over sessions to prevent overloading the patient (Sluijs, 1991 c). In addition, Meichenbaum and Turk, (1987) have concluded that adherence is more likely when attainable goals are set by mutual arrangement with the patient. Grueninger (1995) recommends to ask the patient: "what are you willing to do?" and "how are you going to try? "

PROBLEMS PHYSIOTHERAPISTS ENCOUNTER IN EDUCATING PATIENTS

Although patient education is part of their daily work, results from study two indicated that more than half of physiotherapists (52%) appeared to encounter problems when they tried to educate their patients (see Sluijs and Kuijper, 1990; Lyne and Phillipson, 1986). Table 2 shows the causes of the problems according to the physiotherapists (Sluijs and Kuijper, 1990).

Table 2 Number of problems encountered by physiotherapists and attributed to five categories of causes.

Source of Problem and Problem		Percentage problems
Patient:	Lack of interest	31
Physiotherapist:	lack of communication skills	31
Structural:	lack of leaflets, time or money	15
Type of illness		13
Other health professionals:	lack of multidisciplinary rapport	9
Other		1
Total problems		100

Thirty one percent of problems were attributed to the patient. Patients' lack of interest and knowledge was frequently mentioned: "patients don't feel responsible for their health;" "patients are reluctant to change;" patients are unmotivated" and "how do you teach pelvis tilting when patients don't even know they have a pelvis?" The physiotherapists attributed an equal number of problems to their own lack of communication skills. A physiotherapist remarked: "educating and motivating patients is very difficult and requires extra skills which –until now –have hardly been taught in the vocational training". Physiotherapists also indicated that patient information should be consistent between health professionals (HPs) and that patients should not be confronted with confusing or contradicting information. Previous research has indicated that contradictory information decreases the credibility of HPs together with patient adherence (DiMatteo and DiNicola, 1982; Nordin, 1995).

FACTORS RELATED TO PATIENTS' NON-ADHERENCE TO PHYSIOTHERAPY

Efforts to enhance adherence in physiotherapy should be based on knowledge about determinants of behavior and possible causes of non-adherence. Scheme 1 gives an overview of statistically significant factors related to patients' non-adherence with physiotherapy exercises (Sluijs *et al.*, 1993a): Subgroups of adherent and non-adherent patients were compared, using a stepwise discriminant analysis (these nine variables predicted 73% of non-adherent patients and 94% of adherent patients).

Scheme 1 Factors related to non-adherence with physical therapeutic exercises

Barriers	Barriers to perform exercises perceived and encountered by the patients.
Positive feedback	Lack of positive feedback from the physiotherapist.
Helplessness	Patients' feelings of helplessness.
Characteristics of the illness	–Pain: little or no pain encountered by the patient;
	–Disabilities: little or no disabilities encountered;
	–Seriousness: non-serious illnesses.
Type of diseases	–Multiple pathology;
	–Systemic diseases;
	–Chronic diseases.

First, patients' non-adherence was for the greater part explained by barriers that patients perceived and encountered when they tried to exercise regularly. Second, adherence appeared to be lower when positive feedback was lacking, in cases of slow or little progress, or when physiotherapists did not recognise or appreciate patients' efforts. Positive feedback is usually a motivating factor for adherence and viceversa (Lindström *et al.*, 1992). Furthermore, when some patients feel helpless in changing their behavior or influencing their health, their adherence declines. These findings are in line with general research findings about non-adherence and are predicted by theoretical models (e.g. the Health Belief Model, Janz and Becker, 1984; Self-Efficacy, Bandura, 1977 and Self-Regulatory Theory; Leventhal, Meyer and Nerenz, 1980). See Horne and Weinman, Chapter 2 for a description of these theoretical models. On the basis of these theories (and our research results) it is assumed that adherence will improve when barriers are overcome, when patients receive feedback and when patients' feelings of self-efficacy or self-esteem increases.

Unfortunately, patients' adherence also appears to be related to factors beyond physiotherapists control. For example, lower adherence levels are seen in patients with chronic conditions. However, adherence is higher in patients suffering considerable discomfort from their complaints. The possibility of overcoming discomfort or disabilities seems to be a strong motivating factor for adherence. Conversely, when recovery is impossible and patients suffer from chronic conditions, adherence appears to compete with many other priorities in their lives (Gerber and Nehemkis, 1986). Therefore, it appears that patients with chronic diseases are more likely to be non-adherent.

Can barriers perceived by patients be overcome? Table 3 shows barriers reported by patients to (i) performing exercises and (ii) following physiotherapist's advice (study two and Sluijs and Hermans, 1990).

Table 3 Type of barriers reported by patients who were instructed to exercise (n=1207) and by patients who were instructed to follow other advice (n=901)

Barriers to physiotherapy exercises (reported by 31% of patients)	%	Barriers to following advice (reported by 38% of patients)	%
Lack of time	32	Feasibility /practicality of advice	25
Pain and discomfort	25	Difficulty in changing lifestyle	16
Forgetting	17	Pain and discomfort	16
Lack of perseverance / motivation	13	Difficulty in giving up activities	9
Exercises are difficult to perform	3	Forgetting	6
Exercises not helping	3	Lack of perseverance / motivation	4
Other	7	Lack of time	4
		Other	19

For performing exercises, the most common barriers reported were lack of time and the fact that exercising may be painful, whereas, for following advice, feasibility of advice plus the difficulties of changing one's lifestyle were the most commonly reported barriers. Patients remarked that changing one's behavior is far from easy and changing one's routines is rather difficult. Below are some examples of patients' remarks: "As I am a nurse, lifting is unavoidable;" "teaching requires my utmost attention so I cannot attend to my posture;" "it is nearly impossible to change old habits;" "the swimming pool is closed when I am free" and, "to give up tennis would be a disaster for me".

Obviously, there is no single solution to these problems, as problems differ for each patient. Consequently, many authors recommend tailoring exercises and advice to patients' particular situations and routines as much as possible (Meichenbaum and Turk, 1987; Craig Fisher, 1990). For example, exercises may be integrated into patients' daily activities (walking, cycling, sports) to prevent adherence problems. In addition, Bartlett (1982) recommends discussion of potential barriers or problems which patients foresee and to seek resolutions by mutual co-operation with the patient.

In study two a comparison was made between audiotaped physiotherapy sessions and patient self-report. Our most striking study result was that patients seldom reported adherence problems. Although two thirds of physiotherapists routinely asked about patients' adherence, most patients did not either report non-adherence or the barriers they encountered: only in 5% of sessions were such problems discussed. For example, one patient wrote that "driving ten hours a day prevented him from exercising". However, during the audiotaped physiotherapy session, the physiotherapist asked "how about your exercises?" The patient answered: "no problem."

We concluded from these findings that it is not non-adherence *per se* which is the core of the problem but the fact that *non-adherence and connected adherence problems remains hidden and undiscussed*. Therefore, if the physiotherapist is not aware that there is a problem s/he cannot begin to address and possibly resolve any problems. It has been suggested that more exploring questions are needed together with a good therapist-patient relationship to discuss problems surrounding non-adherence (Bartlett *et al.*, 1990).

ADHERENCE TO SHORT-TERM AND LONG-TERM PHYSIOTHERAPY

Physiotherapists are not optimistic about long-term adherence to physiotherapy. Some estimated that 50% of their patients will maintain long-term exercising after treatment has stopped, whereas others expected none of their patients to be able to do so. The average expectation was found to be 23% (Sluijs *et al.*, 1993b). Comparably low figures are found in research on keeping to a diet, loosing weight, life style changes and health behavior (Cameron and Best, 1987; Dolan-Mullen, Green and Persinger, 1985; Haynes, Taylor and Sackett, 1979; Posavac, 1980). In other forms of long term medical care, adherence has been shown to sharply decline when the HP is no longer readily available to support the patient (Mullen, Green and Persinger, 1985).

According to Sluijs and Knibbe (1991) the decline of long-term adherence to physiotherapy may be understood on the basis of five differences between short-term and long-term adherence, which are set out in Scheme 2.

Scheme 2 Differences between adherence to short-term (supervised) and long-term (unsupervised) physiotherapy (Sluijs and Knibbe, 1991)

Supervision	Short-term physiotherapy is supervised; in long-term physiotherapy the supporting and stimulating role of the physiotherapist is absent.
Curative	Measures during short-term physiotherapy are curative in nature and aim at success in the shortest time possible; long term-physiotherapy usually concerns preventive measures;
Goal attainment	Goal attainment can easily be assessed both by the physiotherapist and the patient (recovery, disappearance of pain and symptoms); whereas the aim of long-term physiotherapy is that nothing will happen (no recurrence of the complaints);
Recovery	Expected recovery can be a strong motivation to adhere; but this factor is lacking in preventive measures (and also in chronic conditions);
Cues	Symptoms often function as cues or triggers that remind the patient to adhere; other triggers must be found to adhere in long-term adherence.

According to this scheme, adherence to long-term preventive measures must do without the support of the therapist and without the rewarding recovery and the triggering symptoms. In short, without the "reinforcements" and "cues" which are assumed to be driving forces in behavioral therapy. Theories of self-management or self-regulation may help us to understand and stimulate adherence to long-term therapy (Holroyd and Creer, 1986; Leventhal, Zimmerman and Gutmann, 1984; Mahowald *et al.*, 1988). These often define adherence to long-term therapy as self-management or self-care behaviours as patients must regulate their own health behavior.

To develop the expertise of adherence-enhancing skills, a manual was written with the help of expert physiotherapists (Sluijs, 1993). This manual describes eleven strategies to enhance adherence, based on patients' adherence problems, on the educational problems reported by physiotherapists and on theoretical insights. Subsequently, we investigated whether or not these strategies could be applied by physiotherapists. The results of training are described in the next section.

APPLICABILITY OF ADHERENCE ENHANCING SKILLS IN PHYSIOTHERAPY

Two groups of physiotherapists were trained in the application of adherence enhancing skills (study 3). The purpose of this study was to assess the effects of these strategies on patient adherence. This research is ongoing. The degree of patient adherence will be measured during the year before and after the therapists are trained. Adherence to short-term and long-term physiotherapy will be measured by questionnaires containing a number of self-care activities (DiMatteo *et al.*, 1993).

Nineteen physiotherapists were trained by two experienced trainers (psychotherapists). Training was based on the manual mentioned above and involved seven training sessions, each of four hours duration. At the end of the course, participants rated the degree in which they had learned to apply eleven adherence enhancing strategies (see Table 4).

Physiotherapists learned most about the utilization of positive feedback where patients efforts were rewarded for progress. In addition, many physiotherapists learned to establish good rapport with the patient and discuss non-adherence. However, the majority of physiotherapists considered that learning these skills, although most valuable, is complex. As a result, they reported to have learned 'little' about the practical application of most strategies. Whether or not what they learned is sufficient to improve patient adherence remains to be seen.

Table 4 Contingency table of number of physiotherapists (N=19) reporting to have learned either *none little or much* about adherence-enhancing strategies

	none	little	much
Establish good rapport with the patient	0	10	9
Acquire knowledge about patient's perceptions and selfcare	1	13	5
Inquire into and discuss patient's (non)adherence	1	10	8
Tailor regimen to patient's particular situation	2	10	7
Inquire into the cause of adherence problems and resolve them	1	12	6
Provide positive feedback for efforts and about progress	0	5	14
Teach patient to use cues, triggers or reminders	4	12	3
Teach patient to translate and generalise advice	5	7	7
Enhance patient's feelings of self-efficacy/ self-esteem	1	12	6
Follow a multidisciplinary approach to support adherence	4	9	6
Follow a planned and systematic approach (goal setting)	4	11	4

From the results of this initial training programme a number of suggestions were made for future training. The main conclusion was that, according to the trainers, the duration of the training was too short to cover all areas important to adherence. Apart from teaching training skills, other areas had to be discussed including the physiotherapists attitude towards adherence, their feelings about non-adherence and basic communication skill.

CONCLUSIONS

The effects of physiotherapy largely depend on patients' adherence to treatment. Adherence to physiotherapy means that patients have to change their behavior and lifestyle. Adherence-enhancing skills, discussed in this chapter, may presumably facilitate patients' adherence to short-term physiotherapy. Strategies we selected have been based on our research highlighting patients' adherence problems and from various theories of self-management or self-regulation (e.g. Holroyd and Creer, 1986; Leventhal *et al.*, 1984; Mahowald *et al.*, 1988).

However, more research is needed into long-term adherence and in this chapter we have discussed many problems associated with such adherence. It is extremely difficult for a physiotherapist to attempt to bring about long-term life-style changes which are required for long-term physiotherapy. Consequently, it is obvious that the physiotherapy profession needs to develop various effective adherence-enhancing strategies to improve adherence to long-term physiotherapy.

Unfortunately, the most effective strategy to enhance adherence until now has proven to be prolonged supervision and follow-up, in particular with chronic conditions. However, the usual aim of supervised physiotherapy is to finish treatment in the shortest time possible, which is at odds with endeavours to enhance adherence to long-term physiotherapy.

The adherence literature indicates that a gap exists between research and practice. Bartlett (1982) states that the clinical application of adherence-enhancing strategies in medical practice lags fifteen years behind research. That is one of the reasons why, in the current research program, serious efforts have been made to implement our results thus far into physiotherapy practice. Nevertheless, we expect that more research is needed to detect the most effective strategies for physiotherapy. Considering that our research program started in 1988, a period of ten years from research to implementation in practice seems unavoidable.

Acknowledgements

Thanks to the other members of the research team: J.J. Knibbe, I.M. J. Hermans and P.F.M. Verhaak.

REFERENCES

Bandura, A. (1977) Self-efficacy: toward a unifying theory of behavior change. *Psychological Review* **84**, 191–215.
Bartlett, E.E. (1982) Behavioral diagnosis: a practical approach to patient education. *Patient Counselling and Health Education* **4**, 29–35.

Bartlett, E.E., Higginbotham, J.C., Cohen-Cole, S. and Bird, J. (1990) How do primary care residents manage patient non-adherence? *Patient Education and Counselling* **16**, 53–60.

Belcon, M.C., Haynes, R.B. and Tugwell, P. (1984) A critical review of compliance studies in rheumatoid arthritis. *Arthritis and Rheumatism* **27**, 1227–1233.

Bouchard, C., Shephard, R.J., Stephens, T., Sutton, J.R. and Mc-Pherson, B.D. (eds.) (1988) *Exercise, fitness and health. a consensus of current knowledge.* Champaign: Human Kinetics Books.

Cameron, R., and Best, J.A. (1987) Promoting adherence to health behavior change interventions: recent findings from behavioral research. *Patient Education and Counselling* **10**, 139–154.

Campen, C. van. and Sluijs, E.M. (1989) *Patient compliance: a survey of reviews (1979–1989)* Utrecht: NIVEL.

Craig Fisher, A. (1990) Adherence to sports injury rehabilitation programmes. *Sports Medicine* **9**, 151–158.

Croft, J.J. (1980) Interviewing in physical therapy. *Physical Therapy* **60**, 1033–1036.

Dekker, J., Baar, M.E. van, Curfs, E.Chr. and Kerssens, J.J. (1993) Diagnosis and treatment in physical therapy: an investigation of their relationhip. *Physical Therapy* **73**, 568–577.

Deyo, R. A. (1982) Compliance with therapeutic regimens in arthritis: issues, current status, and a future agenda. *Seminars in Arthritis and Rheumatism* **12**, 233–244.

DiMatteo, M.R, and DiNicola, D.D. (1982) *Achieving patient compliance: the psychology of the medical practitioner's role.* New York: Pergamon Press.

Dimatteo, M.R., Sherbourne, C.D., Hays, R.D., Ordway, L., Kravitz, R.L., McGlynn, E.A., Kaplan, S. and Rogers, W.H. (1993) Physicians' characteristics influence patients' adherence to medical treatment: results from the Medical Outcome Study. *Health Psychology* **12**, 93–102.

Dishman, R.K. (1982) Compliance/adherence in health-related exercise. *Health Psychology* **1**, 237–267.

Dishman, R.K. (1988) *Exercise adherence: its impact on public health.* Champaign: Human Kinetics Books.

Dolan-Mullen, P.D., Green, L. W. and Persinger, G S. (1985) Clinical trials of patient education for chronic conditions: a comparative meta-analysis of intervention types. *Preventive Medicine* **14**, 753–781.

Evans, C., Gilbert, J.R., Taylor, W. and Hildebrand, A. (1987) A randomized controlled trial of flexion exercises, education, and bed rest for patients with acute low back pain. *Physiotherapy Canada* **39**, 96–101.

Feinberg, J. (1988) The effect of patient-practitioner interaction on compliance: a review of the literature and application in rheumatoid arthritis. *Patient Education and Counselling* **11**, 171–187.

Feinstein, A.R. (1979) "Compliance bias" and the interpretation of therapeutic trials. In R.B. Haynes, D.W. Taylor and D.L. Sackett (eds.) *Compliance in health care.* Baltimore: Johns Hopkins University Press.

Friedrich, M., Cermak, T. and Maderbacher, P. (1996) The effects of brochure use versus therapist teaching on patients performing therapeutic exercise and on changes in impairment status. *Physical Therapy* **76**, 1082–1088.

Gahimer, J.E. and Domholdt, E. (1996) Amount of patient education in physical therapy practice and perceived effects. *Physical Therapy* **76**, 1089–1096.

Gerber, K.E. and Nehemkis, A.M. (eds.) (1986) *Compliance: the dilemma of the chronically ill.* New York: Springer Publishing Company.

Green, C.A. (1987) What can patient health education coordinators learn from ten years of compliance research? *Patient Education and Counselling* **10**, 167–174.

Grueninger, U.J. (1995) Arterial hypertension: lessons from patient education. *Patient Education and Counselling* **26**, 37–55.

Hayne, C.R. (1988) The preventive role of physiotherapy in the National Health Service and industry. *Physiotherapy* **74**, 2–3.

Haynes, R.B., Taylor, D.W. and Sackett, D.L. (eds.) (1979) *Compliance in health care.* Baltimore: Johns Hopkins University Press.

Haynes, R.B., Wang, E. and Da Mota Gomes, M. (1987) A critical review of interventions to improve compliance with prescribed medications. *Patient Education and Counselling* **10**, 155–166.

Holroyd, K.A. and Creer, T.L. (eds.) (1986) *Self-management of chronic disease: handbook of clinical interventions and research.* Orlando: Academic Press.

Huhn, R.R. and Volski, R.V. (1985) Primary prevention programs for business industry: role of physical therapists. *Physical Therapy* **65**, 1840–1844.

Ice, R. (1985) Long-term compliance. *Physical Therapy* **65**, 1832–1839.

Janz, N.K. and Becker, M.H. (1984) The health belief model: a decade later. *Health Education Quarterly* **11**, 1–47.

Karoly, P. (1980) Operant Methods. In F.H. Kanfer, and A.P. Goldstein (eds.) *Helping people change: a textbook of methods; 2nd. edition.* New York: Pergamon Press.

Kerssens, J.J. and Groenewegen, P.P. (1990) Referrals to physiotherapy: the relation between the number of referrals, the indication for referral and the inclination to refer. *Social Science and Medicine* **30**, 797–804.

Knapp, D.N. (1988) Behavioral management techniques and exercise promotion. In R. K. Dishman (ed.) *Exercise adherence: its impact on public health.* Champaign: Human Kinetics Books.

Knibbe, J.J. (1987) Fysiotherapie en secundaire preventie van lage rugklachten: literatuurstudie naar mogelijkheden en beperkingen (Physical therapy and secondary prevention of low back pain) *Nederlands Tijdschrift voor Fysiotherapie* **97**, 175–183.

Koes, B. W., Bouter, L.M., Beckerman, H., Heijden, G.J.M.G. van der. and Knipschild, P.G. (1991) Physiotherapy exercises and back pain: a blind review. *British Medical Journal* **302**, 1572–1576.

Koes, B.W., Tulder, M. W. van, Windt, D.A. W. M. van der, and Bouter, L.M. (1994) The efficacy of back schools: a review of randomized clinical trials. *Journal of Clinical Epidemiology* **47**, 851–862 ..

Leathley, M. (1988) Physiotherapists and health education: report of a survey. *Physiotherapy* **74**, 218–220.

Leventhal, H., Meyer, D, and Nerenz, D (1980) The common sense representation of illness danger. In S. Rachman (ed.) *Contributions to medical psychology.* Oxford: Pergamon Press.

Leventhal, H., Zimmerman, R., and Gutmann, M. (1984) Compliance: a self-regulation perspective. In W. D. Gentry (ed.) *Handbook of behavioral medicine.* New York: The Guildford Press.

Lindequist, S., Lundberg, B., Wikmark, R., Bergstad, B., Lööf, G. and Ottermark, A.C. (1984) Information and regime at low back pain. *Scandinavian Journal of Rehabilitation Medicine* **16**, 113–116.

Lindström, I., Ohlund, C., Eek, C., Wallin, L., Peterson, L.E., Fordyce, W.E. and Nachemson, A.L. (1992) The effect of graded activity on patients with subacute low back pain: a randomized prospective study with an operant-conditioning behavioral approach. *Physical Therapy* **72**, 279/39–293/53.

Lorish, C., Francis, K., Jensen, G. and Sluijs, E.M. (1996) Enhancing the health status of patients by increasing adherence top therapeutic and voluntary exercise. In *Physical therapy course materials. a compendium of conference handouts.* Alexandria: American Physical Therapy Association.

Lyne, P.A. (1986) The professions allied to medicine: their potential contribution to health education. *Physiotherapy* **72**, 8–10.

Lyne, P.A. and Phillipson, C. (1986) The barriers to health education. *Physiotherapy* **72**, 10–12.

Mahowald, M.L., Steveken, M.E., Young, M. and Ytterberg, S.R. (1988) The Minnesota Arthritis-Training Program: emphasis on self-management, not compliance. *Patient Education and Counselling* **11**, 235–241.

Mayo, N.E. (1978) Patient compliance: practical implications for physical therapists: a review of the literature. *Physical Therapy* **58**, 1083–1090.

Mazucca, S.A. (1982) Does patient education in chronic disease have therapeutic value? *Journal of Chronic Diseases* **35**, 521–529.

Meichenbaum, D. and Turk, D.C. (1987) *Facilitating treatment adherence. a practitioners guidebook.* New York: Plenum Press.

Mellin, G., Härkäpää, K., Hurri, H. and Järvikoski, A. (1990) A controlled study on the outcome of inpatient and outpatient treatment of low back pain. Part IV. *Scandinavian Journal of Rehabilitation Medicine* **22**, 189–194.

Mellin, G., Järvikoski, A. and Verkasalo, M. (1984) Treatment of patients with chronic low back pain: comparison between rehabilitation centre and outpatient care. *Scandinavian Journal of Rehabilitation Medicine* **16**, 77–84.

Mullen, P.D., Green, L.W. and Persinger, G.S. (1985) Clinical trials of patient education for chronic conditions: a comparative meta-analysis of intervention types. *Preventive Medicine* **14**, 753–781.

NIVEL (1996) Research programme Utrecht: NIVEL.

Nordin, M. (1995) Back pain: lessons from patient education. *Patient Education and Counselling* **26**, 67–70.

Norton, S. (1986) Support for physiotherapists in health education. *Physiotherapy* **72**, 5–7.

Oldridge, N.B. (1988) Compliance with exercise in cardiac rehabilitation. In R.K. Dishman (ed.) *Exercise adherence: its impact on public health.*.Champaign: Human Kinetics Books.

Posavac, E.J. (1980) Evaluations of patient education programs: a meta-analysis. *Evaluation and the Health Professions* **3**, 47–62.

Schultz, C.L., Wellard, R. and Swerissen, H. (1988) Communication and interpersonal helping skills: an essential component in physiotherapy education? *The Australian Journal of Physiotherapy* **34**, 75–80.

Sikorsky, J.M. (1985) A rationalized approach to physiotherapy for low back pain. *Spine* **10**, 571–579.

Sluijs, E.M. (1991a) Patient education in physical therapy. Utrecht: NIVEL, Dissertation..

Sluijs, E.M. (1991b) A checklist to assess patient education in physical therapy practice: development and reliability. *Physical Therapy* **71**, 561/17–569/25.

Sluijs, E.M. (1991c) Patient education in physiotherapy: towards a planned approach. *Physiotherapy* **77**, 503–508.

Sluijs, E.M. (1993) Therapietrouw door voorlichting. Een handleiding voor patientenvoorlichting in de fysiotherapie. (A manual for patient education and adherence in physical therapy) Utrecht, LCGVO.

Sluijs, E.M. and Hermans, I.M.J. (1990) Problemen die patiënten ervaren bij het doen van huiswerkoefeningen en bij het opvolgen van adviezen: een inventarisatie (Problems that patients encounter in exercising and following advice) *Nederlands Tijdschrift voor Fysiotherapie* **100**, 175–179.

Sluijs, E.M. and Knibbe, J.J. (1991) Patient compliance with exercise: different theoretical approaches to short-term and long-term compliance. *Patient Education and Counselling* **17**, 191–204.

Sluijs, E.M., Kok, G.J. and Zee, J. van der. (1993a) Correlates of exercise compliance in physical therapy. *Physical Therapy* **73**, 771/41–782/52.

Sluijs, E.M. and Kuijper, E.B. (1990) Problemen die fysiotherapeuten ervaren bij het geven van voorlichting aan patienten: een inventarisatie (Problems physical therapists encounter in educating patients) *Nederlands Tijdschrift voor Fysiotherapie* **100**, 128–132.

Sluijs, E.M., Zee, J. van der. and Kok, G.J. (1993b) Differences between physical therapists in attention paid to educational activities. *Physiotherapy Theory and Practice* **9**, 103–117.

Snook, S.H. (1987) Approaches to the control of back pain in industry: job design, job placement and education/training. *Occupational Medicine: State of the Art Reviews* **3**, 45–61.

Spelman, M.R. (1984) Back pain: how health education affects patient compliance with treatment. *Occupational Health Nursing* **32**, 649–651.

Turk, D.C., Salovey, P., and Litt, M.D. (1986) Adherence: a cognitive-behavioral perspective. In K.E. Gerber, A.M. Nehemkis (eds.) *Compliance: the dilemma of the chronically ill.* New York: Springer Publishing Company.

Wagstaff, G.F. (1982). A small dose of commonsense – communication, persuasion and physioherapy. *Physiotherapy* **68**, 327–329.

Adherence in specific conditions

15

Adherence and Asthma

Christopher Hand

> *God and the Doctor we alike adore*
> *But only when in danger, not before;*
> *The danger o'er, both are requited,*
> *God is forgotten and the Doctor slighted.*

John Owen's (1560–1622) poem sits on my desk at home as a constant reminder that the doctor only plays a small part in patients' lives. Its relevance to this chapter is that it was given to me by a man who had asthma that was well controlled. His son Charles, however, had terrible asthma and home visits for acute asthma were frequent. These were often emergency visits in the night and accompanied by panic. Why was this? Looking at his medical record revealed the answer: numerous prescriptions for his reliever inhaler (a β_2-agonist) and very few for his preventer inhaler (in his case a corticosteroid or steroid inhaler). Yet, I had carefully explained to him the merits of prevention. That was 10 years ago.

This chapter looks at why patients with asthma do not always follow "medical" advice. Patients are not the only ones who fail to follow advice: health professionals (HPs) are no different. By looking at the problem from various peoples' viewpoints, I intend to draw together some of the more recent literature on adherence and asthma. In doing so, I hope to provide some possible solutions to the problem. The volume of literature on asthma has exploded in recent years and inevitably there has had to be some selection. I have tried to draw from as wide a range of evidence as possible to provide the reader with something that will be of relevance to them.

THE RATIONALE FOR TREATMENT

The emphasis in asthma care has shifted from symptom relief to the prevention of asthma, based on the knowledge that asthma is an inflammatory process (Barnes, 1989), and that over reliance on β_2-agonists may be harmful (Taylor *et al.*, 1992). The rationale for preventive treatment is that reversible airflow obstruction may be a precursor of progressive and irreversible decline in lung function (Carpenter *et al.*, 1989). Whilst the relieving effects of β_2-agonists are immediate and readily appreciated, the antiinflammatory effect of corticosteroids (steroids) are delayed and less easily perceived. Djukanovic *et al.* (1992) demonstrated that steroids produce some improvement in symptoms by two weeks, but this was not significant until four weeks, and histological signs of inflammation were still present at six weeks. The full benefit of inhaled steroids may not be apparent for as long as a year (Dompeling *et al.*, 1992), indicating that prolonged treatment and evaluation is required.

ADHERENCE

Adherence to What?

The effective management of asthma is a complex process and involves both patient and HP in a number of tasks which include:

- recognising asthma,
- monitoring asthma symptoms and severity,
- avoiding trigger factors,
- managing acute attacks,
- attending follow-up appointments,
- collecting further supplies of treatment,
- using inhalers correctly,
- taking optimal asthma medication.

Problems with adherence can occur at any of these points and may be partly responsible for the continuing morbidity and mortality from asthma.

Where is the Problem with Adherence?

Recognising asthma

Many patients appear not to perceive the symptoms of asthma (Barnes, 1992). The proportion has been be found to be as high as 60% (Kendrick *et al.*, 1993) and as low as 15% (Rubinfield and Pain, 1976). Patients also appear willing to tolerate symptoms (Quirk and Jones, 1990), particularly older people (Renwick and Connolly, 1996). Asthma that is not perceived may not be taken to the doctor in the first place or adequately dealt with even when it has been diagnosed, and failure to recognise serious symptoms is known to be a factor in deaths from asthma (Johnson *et al.*, 1984). Delays and errors in diagnosis and treatment, however, cannot always be blamed on patients; doctors are also responsible for not recognising asthma (Charlton *et al.*, 1991a; Kolnaar *et al.*, 1994) and for poor management (Gellert *et al.*, 1990; Wareham *et al.*, 1993). There is recent evidence that both under diagnosis and under treatment may be a particular problem in some ethnic groups (Duran-Tuleria *et al.*, 1996).

Monitoring asthma symptoms and severity

While it is possible to monitor asthma with symptom diaries and peak flow meters, many patients have difficulty in maintaining the motivation to keep up the recordings. Of the 60 participants in the Malo *et al.* (1993) study in which patients were asked to record either symptoms or peak flow rates in a simple diary, 40 finished the diary and peak flow periods, but only 20 managed to complete both periods over 18 months. Chowienczyk *et al.* (1994) found that about a quarter of peak flow diary entries were either invented or done retrospectively when they used a peak flow meter containing an electronic timing device that was unknown to the patient. Teenagers appear to be less reliable in their recording than adults (Wonham *et al.*, 1996). Reliability of peak flow recording can be improved using an electronic diary card with an alarm reminder (Kidd *et al.*, 1993). We should conclude that some patients will experience difficulties in keeping records reliably, which will reduce their chances of anticipating asthma episodes.

Diaries and peak flow records may, however, not be as useful as originally thought. The Grampian Asthma Study of Integrated Care (1994) concluded that the effectiveness of peak flow meters as self monitoring devices remains in doubt, except for patients with more severe asthma. If the relative importance of diaries and peak flow meters remains to be determined, is it reasonable to expect all patients to record these details all of the time? Some degree of flexibility would seem to be sensible and rigid adherence unnecessary (Jones *et al.*, 1995).

There may even be some dangers in relying on peak flow meters which are not as accurate as first thought (Miller *et al.*, 1992). Some of the commonly used meters do not perform in a linear manner. For example, the mini-Wright peak flow meter has a tendency to under-read at low and high values and to overread in the middle range, resulting in potential under treatment of patients following self-management advice. Underdiagnosis is also a possibility if meters are relied upon for diagnosis. Measuring the forced expiratory volume in one second (FEV_1) with a spirometer would seem advisable in uncertain cases.

Avoiding trigger factors

Avoiding potential allergens and other environmental precipitants, such as smoke, is suggested as part of asthma management (British Thoracic Society, 1993). Adherence to smoking advice is notoriously low, with success rates as low as 5% at one year being reported (Slama, 1990). Smoking cessation in asthma patients has received less attention than other preventive measures, but as many as two out of three patients would like to give up (Fitzmaurice and Bradley, 1994). A recent unpublished telephone survey of general practitioners (GPs) revealed that over 90% of them said that they gave advice about house dust mite avoidance, but the quality of advice was generally inadequate, judging by the small number of different strategies offered to the patients. Conventional instruction in house dust mite education is more effective in reducing mite allergen levels and patient symptoms if supplemented with computer instruction (Huss *et al.*, 1992).

Education alone will not ensure adherence as socio-economic factors influence the uptake of advice (Denson-Lino *et al.*, 1993).

Managing acute attacks

Patients may make serious errors in their management of acute attacks of asthma (Sibbald, 1989). The national asthma attack audit, organised by the GPs in Asthma Group (Neville *et al.*, 1993), reported that one in three patients had a particularly severe attack of asthma. This would imply that even the patients of GPs with an interest in asthma still delay in calling their doctor in an acute attack, although the assumption does not take into account that some of the attacks may have come on very suddenly. More worrying, however, was that doctors also mismanaged acute asthma. Their self-reported management was at variance with recommended guidelines, with underuse of nebulised bronchodilators and systemic steroids in all grades of clinical severity. This has major implications for future guidelines and GP education.

Attending follow-up appointments

Demographic variables associated with low and non-attendance rates for outpatient appointments include younger age, low educational attainment, lower socio-economic and ethnic minority status. In New Zealand, McClellan and Garrett (1989) reported low and non-attendance at their hospital asthma clinic to be higher amongst Maoris (44.7%) and Pacific Islanders (31.6%), with even higher rates in those referred from the accident and emergency department (66%). Poor education and low socio-economic class were considered more important than ethnicity per se. Whilst this may be a rather special situation, the general conclusions agree with other studies. Yoon *et al.* (1991) found that women, non-smokers and those whose attending physician was involved in their programme of asthma education, were more likely to attend the programme. Less than half of those invited (43%) completed the programme, and they represented 31% of those eligible. These figures are representative of other intervention studies. The authors' claim that many asthmatic patients recovering from a severe exacerbation of asthma will not participate in a hospital based education programme, puts a big responsibility upon those working in primary care. Even in general practice, some patients will not attend educational sessions (Hilton, 1986), making opportunistic education very important.

Coping with the workload caused by asthma, which is increasing in prevalence, is going to be an important factor in providing optimal care for patients in the community (Martys, 1992). Charlton *et al.* (1991b) have shown what effect a nurse-run asthma clinic can have on workload and patient morbidity in general practice. Those who attended showed significant improvements in their asthma, but over half did not attend the clinic or complete one year of follow up. This further emphasises the fact that patients who attend such clinics may be more motivated to improve their asthma, making interpretation of intervention studies difficult.

Collecting further supplies of treatment

Patients often run out of inhalers or continue to use them after they have delivered their licensed number of doses, and many of them do not have an inhaler in reserve (Williams *et al.*, 1993). Hand and Bradley (1996) demonstrated that reputed ease in obtaining inhalers was more highly correlated with beclomethasone (a preventer inhaler) use than with salbutamol (a reliever inhaler) use. They concluded that the inconvenience of collecting an inhaler presents less of a barrier to action where the benefits are obvious and immediate (symptom relief) compared to when they are less tangible and delayed (symptom prevention). In Australia, Gibson *et al.* (1993) found that over the counter purchase of salbutamol was associated with infrequent consultations with the doctor and undertreatment of asthma. Presumably, there were fewer opportunities to obtain the additional drugs that were necessary for optimum control of asthma when the doctor was bypassed. Attention to the consumer-friendliness of obtaining inhalers may be one simple way to increase the use of preventive treatment.

Using inhalers correctly

The factors that affect the dose of drug delivered from an inhaler are complex (Everard *et al.*, 1995). There is general agreement, however, that patients' inhaler technique often leaves much to be desired (Crompton, 1982), and can be improved with instruction (Horsley and Bailie, 1988). Unfortunately, improvements in technique decay over time unless regular reinforcement is given. Children and the elderly have more problems with using inhalers, but they can be overcome to a large extent by the use of spacer devices, such as a volumatic, which act as a reservoir between the inhaler and the patient, and new types of inhaler (Jackson and Lipworth, 1995). Adherence to treatment may be dependent upon acceptability of the inhaler to patients (Harvey and Williams, 1992). Efficient delivery systems, such as a turbohaler which is triggered when the patient breathes in, are usually more expensive. They may, however, not only improve control of asthma, but may allow dose reduction ("step-down" therapy) and possibly reduce overall prescribing costs (Jackson and Lipworth, 1995). Doctors are no better than patients in using inhalers correctly (Guidry *et al.*, 1992).

Taking optimal asthma medication

Methods for monitoring adherence to asthma medication. The methods used for assessing adherence have been summarised from both a North American (Rand and Wise, 1994) and European perspective (Cochrane, 1995). Usually, the patient's use of treatment is compared with a regime prescribed by the doctor. There is an underlying assumption here that the advised regime is not only appropriate for the individual patient, but that varying from the regime is unacceptable. While this assumption may be a requirement for clinical trials, it may not be necessary for everyday practice.

Prescription monitoring. Patient self-report has been shown to be unreliable when patients' own estimates of their treatment use are compared to those obtained by more objective means (Hyland *et al.*, 1993). When prescription monitoring is performed, approximately one in four patients have been found to overestimate preventer use and underestimate reliever use (Hand and Bradley, 1996). Whilst this is probably the most common method of assessment in both primary and secondary care, it can be unreliable since some patients "test-fire" their inhalers and many have spare inhalers, some of which are only partly used. On the other hand, some pharmaceutical companies overfill inhalers so that they contain more doses than stated. When pharmacy claims are compared with the data in medical records (Kelloway *et al.*, 1994), patients appear to be significantly more adherent to taking tablets than preventive inhalers. Unfortunately, current oral preparations for preventing asthma have more side-effects than inhaled medication, although new tablet treatments are being developed.

The disadvantage of these approaches is that they assume that the medical record contains the optimal regime and that patients who collect medications are going to use them. The advantage is that, with the advent of computerised prescribing and dispensing records, patients' intended use can be monitored very easily. If medication is not being ordered or collected, this can be discussed with the patient, providing they attend for medical advice. Regular audit of asthma prescriptions and medical records can be used to identify nonattenders (Barritt and Staples, 1991).

Patients ordering large numbers of β_2-agonist inhalers (Spitzer et al., 1992), or showing a pattern of increasing use of these inhalers (Suissa et al., 1994), are at risk of either death from asthma or a life-threatening attack of asthma. There is still controversy as to whether β_2-agonists can be harmful and whether high use causes death or just reflects more severe asthma. It is possible that there may be a difference between different levels of severity of asthma (van Schayck et al., 1995a). It would seem prudent to review patients ordering more than two β_2-agonist inhalers a month with the purpose of either starting or increasing preventive treatment or checking adherence to their regime.

Counting pills and weighing inhalers are more objective methods of assessing adherence, but they do not distinguish between true use and "dumping". In one clinical trial using a microprocessor monitoring device attached to the preventer inhaler, 14% of patients were observed to deliberately empty their inhalers by repeated actuation just before attending for follow up (Rand et al., 1992). A similar phenomenon is observed when microprocessor pill dispensers are used. Whether dumping is peculiar to trials or really occurs in practice is difficult to know, but what it does reflect is the strong desire that some patients have to please their doctor and the need to be seen in a good light. A more open doctor-patient relationship might be one solution to this problem, and doctors need to find ways of enabling patients to discuss the difficulties they have in adhering to treatment regimes. Even if this is achieved, there may still be difficulties as some patients have a very poor awareness of their own adherence (Price, 1995a).

Asking questions. Although clinical judgement has been shown to be a poor method of assessing adherence, with doctors generally overestimating the degree to which patients take their medication as advised, asking patients directly about adherence is associated with improved adherence (Hall *et al.*, 1988). Further research needs to be done to develop valid and reliable methods of assessing adherence (Rand and Wise, 1994), but a few simple questions could easily be asked either in the consultation or given to the patient as a short questionnaire before being seen by the doctor or nurse (Bailey *et al.*, 1990).

Monitoring drug levels. Monitoring drug levels provides an accurate objective method of determining whether or not the patient has taken their medication. Whilst this is straightforward for theophylline (a bronchodilator) it is more difficult for inhaled drugs (Horn *et al.*, 1989). Horn *et al.* (1990) were able to demonstrate in patients who responded to inhaled salbutamol (a reliever), that urine levels rose to a higher level than in those patients who failed to respond. Drug levels, however, only provide information about adherence in the period just before sampling and tell us nothing about the pattern of use over the preceding months.

Electronic monitoring. Electronic devices that record both the number of doses and the date and time at which they were taken have been available since the mid 1980s. They are the most objective method of assessing adherence to inhaled treatment and they are able to demonstrate different patterns of inhaler use. The findings of those studies that have used them have shown that adherence is even less than anticipated. In one of the first studies, Spector *et al.* (1986) used a Nebulizer Chronolog to assess the efficacy of a new inhaled anti-inflammatory preparation (a preventer) and found that only one in six participants used the treatment on at least 70% of the days. Underusage greatly exceeded overusage, and younger participants and male participants were less likely to use the inhaler appropriately. They also found that patients failed to write the truth in their diaries with overreporting of appropriate usage more than 50% of the times. Rand *et al.* (1992), however, showed that while 73% of patients reported using their bronchodilator inhaler (reliever) an average of two puffs three times a day, the chronolog data showed that only 15% of the participants actually used the inhaler this much. Comparing the two measures of adherence revealed that inhaler weighing overestimated the amount of treatment taken by more than 30%.

Bosley *et al.* (1994;1995) compared the adherence of an inhaled steroid (budesonide) with an inhaled β_2-agonist (terbutaline) and a combined preparation, using a Turbohaler Inhalation Computer (TIC). Unfortunately, nearly one in three data sets were lost because of TIC malfunction. The average adherence was 60–70%, and only 15% of patients had good adherence, taking the drugs as prescribed for more than 80% of the days. No significant difference was found between treatments and the authors concluded that adherence was patient dependent and not drug dependent. Patients' self-report and clinicians' impressions of adherence were not good predictors of actual adherence as measured by the computers. The important issue to arise from this study was the number of different patterns of adherence that were observed. Some patients took both drugs once a day, some were fully adherent with the treatment regime at irregular intervals, and others tended to be adherent just before and immediately after clinic visits.

The participants in this study, however, were encouraged to take both the preventer and reliever inhalers on a regular basis and to use another reliever (salbutamol) for rescue relief. It is not entirely surprising that if advised to take two treatments on a regular basis, the pattern of adherence will be the same, regardless of the different mechanisms of action of the two drugs. It is possible that there may be differences in patterns of adherence between relieving treatment and preventive treatment which relates to the different beliefs that patients hold about the two types of inhaler (Hand and Bradley, 1996). Current guidelines advise regular preventive treatment and symptom relief treatment on an as needed basis. This raises the issue of how adherence to treatment for the relief of symptoms should be judged. For two inhaler treatments there are 81 possible combinations of inhaler use and patient report, as there are nine potential combinations for each inhaler (see table 1). If only objective measurements of use are considered, there are still nine possible combinations of behaviours.

Table 1 Potential adherence patterns

Inhaler report	Inhaler use		
	Overuse	Use agrees	Underuse
Over report	1	2	3
Report agrees	4	5	6
Under report	7	8	9

In the studies described, the participants were aware that the device could measure the amount of drug taken but not that it could monitor the time that it was taken. When patients are made fully aware of the degree of monitoring, their adherence improves (Yeung *et al.*, 1994). How long this effect would last is not known.

What is optimal treatment and how should it be judged? What level of adherence with preventive treatment is necessary to maintain the patient in good health? Patients with less severe asthma may be able to get away with taking less medication than advised. A "step-down" approach to treatment is a relatively new concept (British Thoracic Society, 1993) and even periodic treatment regimens with inhaled steroids have been advocated by some authorities (van Schayck *et al.*, 1995b). As the effects of steroids are slow to wear off, however, the patient may think they have some leeway with their preventive treatment and are left with a false sense of security.

The dose of inhaled steroid needed to suppress symptoms may be less than the dose required to suppress inflammation. A direct comparison can be made here with other chronic diseases where symptoms only occur if the condition is either very severe (hypertension) or poorly controlled (diabetes). Current management of these latter conditions is aimed at getting the best possible control using objective measures of assessment (blood pressure and blood sugar) to prevent complications such as stroke or blindness. If we rely heavily on the reporting of symptoms for the control of asthma, we may satisfy our patients in the short term but may not help them in the long term if complications, such as chronic obstructive airways disease, develop. Tirimanna *et al.* (1996) suggest that measuring FEV_1 may be better for monitoring long-term changes in lung function than peak flow. Most GPs and nurses currently use peak flow meters rather than spirometers for monitoring asthma. Asthma specific quality of life measures may prove to be a useful addition (Juniper *et al.*, 1992).

Why is there a Problem?

Patient factors

Situations. There are perfectly understandable reasons why patients do not take their treatment. Dolce *et al.* (1991) found 14 reasons for 78 outpatients with chronic obstructive pulmonary disease (COPD) missing their medication in the previous month. Poor adherence was most strongly associated with situational factors rather than demographic variables. Four out of 10 patients felt good and either decided not to take their medication (21.8%) or forgot to take it (19.2%).

Patients' knowledge and beliefs. Concern about the effects of steroids is well documented. For example, two thirds of Barritt and Staples' (1991) patients expressed concern about the long term side-effects of treatment, general anxiety about being on steroids, dislike about needing to rely on drugs, and worry that if used too regularly the treatment might stop working, or become addictive. Osman *et al.* (1993) found that a dislike of asthma medication existed independently of whether the medication was for prophylaxis or relief, suggesting that steroid phobia is not the only explanation.

This view is supported by Hand and Bradley (1996) who discovered important differences in the beliefs that patients hold in relation to symptomatic and preventive use of inhaler treatment: perceived benefits of the inhalers, a positive attitude to using the inhalers and concern about side-effects had strong influences on the use of both reliever and preventer inhalers. Uncertainty about the inhalers, a negative attitude to using the inhalers, and the involvement of others in asthma management had less influence on inhaler use. Satisfaction with the doctor and the ease of obtaining an inhaler were more important issues for preventer use than for reliever use. These findings reflect what has frequently been reported in the adherence literature, that the doctor patient relationship and satisfaction with the quality of care provided have a crucial role in adherence to treatment.

The National Asthma Campaign (1990) reported that six in ten (59%) of patients wanted more information about asthma, and only one in five (22%) felt they had had a good discussion with their doctor or nurse when newly diagnosed. Acknowledging the patient's perspective of their illness and its treatment is an important step in negotiations with patients (Britten, 1994) and providing relevant information facilitates internal motivation to change (Williams *et al.*, 1991).

Psychological distress. One in four patients with asthma now say that their condition is so bad that it either totally controls their life or has a major effect on their well being (National Asthma Campaign, 1996). In the Bosley *et al.* study (1995), although adherence was not related to either the levels of anxiety or the number of interpersonal problems, 32% of participants felt ashamed, and 31% felt angry about asthma. Thirty two per cent of participants said something was stopping them from taking treatment and 23% reported specific concerns about the treatment (fear of side-effects, fear of becoming addicted). A regression model containing six variables predicted 74% of adherence (usually follows doctor's advice, avoidance of self-care, depression score, age and an interpersonal problems score). Drop-outs from their study were more likely to be younger and depressed. They concluded that psychological interventions may be helpful for some patients who are non-adherent.

Social aspects. Although there is little evidence that patient adherence is related to social class, adults in social classes 3 and 4 are approximately twice as likely to have severe asthma as those in classes 1 and 2 (Littlejohns and Macdonald, 1993). Although patients from lower social classes may receive inadequate treatment, environmental factors such as cigarette smoking and the standard of housing which influence the control of asthma (Connolly *et al.*, 1989) are also very important.

Social support systems are important in the self-management of chronic medical conditions. Patients with asthma report that lack of knowledge and unfavourable attitudes of family, friends and employers are a significant problem (Bailey *et al.*, 1990). Fireman *et al.* (1981) found that non-adherence was more likely to occur in the presence of family instability and disharmony and emphasised the need for enhancing family management skills. Given the social impact of asthma (Nocon and Booth, 1991) and the finding that adverse social circumstances are common in deaths from asthma (Wareham *et al.*, 1993), social interventions in asthma would seem to be a promising area for development. Simple support, such as the provision of a telephone for emergency use in acute asthma, might prevent unnecessary deaths. Involvement of family or close friends in the management of asthma would seem appropriate.

Health professional factors

The medical profession has been accused of failing to apply what it knows in the treatment of asthma (Keeley, 1993). Doctors have a tendency to overreliance on β_2-agonists, a reluctance to prescribe inhaled prophylactic therapy and suboptimal surveillance of lung function (Gellert *et al.*, 1990). There remain discrepancies between the views of doctors and patients as to what is an adequate explanation of asthma and between doctors' and patients' views about disease severity. Doctors need to understand the precise words and phrases that patients use if they are to improve communication and patient satisfaction (Modell *et al.*, 1983). There are, however, gaps in our knowledge about inhaled steroids and providing patients with accurate information is difficult (Geddes, 1992).

Nurses can provide effective education for patients with asthma (Maiman *et al.*, 1979) and feature in many of the intervention studies. Increasingly they are being relied upon to provide asthma services in both primary and secondary care, but deficiencies in nurse training have been highlighted (Barnes and Partridge, 1994). The role of pharmacists in monitoring inhaler technique and adherence to treatment has not yet reached its full potential.

Prescribing and management guidelines. A higher ratio of prophylaxis to bronchodilator prescribing is associated with lower admission rate to hospital (Griffiths *et al.*, 1996), and there is some evidence that there has been an increase in the prescribing of inhaled steroids (Warner, 1995). Appropriate prescribing has been shown to be related to the average age of GP principals in the practice, the presence of a GP trainer, the proportion of patients over 65, nursing hours available in the practice, and the presence of a practice manager (Sturdy *et al.*, 1995).

Providing feedback to doctors about their patients' asthma does not on its own lead to change in the outcome of clinical care (White *et al.*, 1995). Local guidelines coupled with practice based education can improve the care of patients with asthma (Feder *et al.*, 1995) and clinical audit of care based on guidelines has been shown to be effective in secondary care (Lim and Harrison, 1992). Diagnosis and treatment of childhood asthma in general practice can be favourably influenced by the use of an audit facilitator (Bryce *et al.*, 1995).

Treatment-related factors

Adherence to complex regimes is difficult for patients and taking doses at a high frequency is a particular issue for patients (Taggart, 1995). Every effort should be made to simplify the regime, both in the number of different drugs taken and also in the number of times a day that they have to be remembered. Adherence to inhaled therapy has been shown to be better with twice daily rather than four times daily regimes (Coutts *et al.*, 1992) and this is usually possible with inhaled steroids. There is some evidence to suggest that steroids may be as effective if taken once a day in mild to moderate stable asthma (Jones *et al.*, 1994). This may not be the case, with more severe asthma (Weiner *et al.*, 1995).

STRATEGIES FOR IMPROVING ADHERENCE

Early Educational Programmes

The educational programmes for childhood asthma that started in the USA in the 1970's and spread in the 1980's, set the scene for programmes that were developed in other parts of the world. Many of the first studies that were published were uncontrolled and relied upon self-reported measures of adherence. They did, however, have a sound basis in psychological theory. Bandura's concept of self-efficacy was one of the most influential (Tobin *et al.*, 1987), and the term self-management began to appear in the literature. The Health Belief Model (e.g. Becker, 1974) was also used to guide educational interventions which were evaluated in terms of hospital admissions, asthma exacerbations, adherence to treatment, days lost from school or work, as well as physiological measures of lung function (Radius *et al.*, 1978). Modest but cost-effective improvements were seen, and some studies reported lasting effects (Creer, 1987). In an early review of the field, Bartlett (1983) concluded that the most effective self-help approaches in childhood asthma included the principles of self-efficacy, information sharing, and patient involvement. While such programmes reported encouraging results, they were neither widely available nor widely used (Klingelhofer, 1987), and generalisation to normal clinical settings was hard, since the studies were usually from centres of excellence in hospitals with relatively low take-up rates and high numbers of drop-outs.

In British general practice, early attempts to produce improvements in asthma met with disappointing results. This was probably because they relied upon the assumption that transfer of information would produce behaviour change. This was an issue whether or not the education was provided individually (Hilton *et al.*, 1986) or in groups (White *et al.*, 1989). In a hospital setting, however, Beasley *et al.* (1989) were one of the first groups to demonstrate that a self-management plan guided by peak flow measurements could improve the control of asthma.

Although providing general information alone is not an effective way to change behaviour, patients clearly require some basic knowledge about asthma and its treatment. Giving them a choice of educational material would seem appropriate and allowing them to study it at home is an efficient use of time. Jenkinson *et al.* (1988) showed that patients learnt more from audiotapes but actually preferred the book that was provided. Partridge (1986), on the other hand, found that his patients preferred viewing videos to reading books or pamphlets.

Recent Studies in Self-Management Education

Providing information

There is so much to know about asthma and its treatment, that there is a danger of overloading the patient with information. However there is evidence that providing information can be effective provided that it is personalised and made specific. Written plans are recommended (British Thoracic Society, 1993; General Practitioners in Asthma Group, 1995) and advanced technology can be used to produce them. Osman *et al.* (1994) developed personalised computer booklets that encouraged patient questions and criticisms, and focused specifically on the management of symptoms. Their patients valued most highly what to do when breathless, and the decrease in hospital admissions, disturbed nights and reduction in days of restricted activity that were demonstrated, was achieved without any changes in the prescribing of bronchodilators or inhaled steroids. This suggests that the information given allowed patients to use their medication more effectively.

Providing individual education

An admission to hospital offers a critical opportunity to introduce asthma management skills. Taggart *et al.* (1991) provided inpatient education to a group of inner city children not reached by more traditional programmes. Discussions with a nurse in hospital with video tapes and written activity books were associated with an increased sense of personal control and an improved response to the early warning signs of asthma, with less emergency room use in the following 15 months. The trend towards shorter hospital admissions may, however, reduce these opportunities.

Social deprivation is a barrier to education, but Mayo *et al.* (1990) were able to demonstrate some important benefits for a particularly difficult group of adults with severe asthma in New York. They demonstrated a reduction in hospital admissions following a randomised crossover trial of patient education in which aggressive self-management strategies were compared to normal outpatient care. They were unable to determine which aspect of the programme was the most important for success, but thought that a face-to-face interaction with their medical care provider using an individualised approach was important. The increased use of inhaled steroids and the use of brief steroid courses almost certainly contributed to the success. The intervention was also cost-effective, halving the cost of care for those who attended.

Programmes that are successful in one context of care can be adapted for others. Charlton *et al.* (1994) used the programme that they had developed in primary care to use with children in a secondary care environment. Patients in the intervention group were more likely to report the correct response to an exacerbation of their asthma than the control group, resulting in fewer episodes of low peak flow, fewer school absences and fewer home visits from GPs. This was all achieved by a single 45 minute educational session with a nurse who demonstrated how peak flow measurements should guide the management of asthma. This compares very favourably with the single 3-hour educational session that was provided by Yoon *et al.* (1993).

Effective programmes do not have to be very complicated, and with some patient groups simplicity may be more appropriate. D'Souza *et al.* (1994) showed what can be done in a Maori community in which about half of the patients were not employed, were smokers and had no higher education. They used a simple credit card, which had symptom-based instructions on one side and peak flow-based instructions on the other. Not only did the regular use of inhaled steroids increase, but many patients also increased their inhaled steroids or started a course of steroid tablets on their own initiative.

Providing education with peer support

Education in groups can produce useful improvements in the way that patients manage their asthma, but the time input for both patients and professionals can be considerable. Mühlhauser *et al.* (1991) provided 20 hours of education by nurses in groups over 5 days for inpatients with moderate to severe asthma in a tertiary care hospital. Over 90% of patients completed the programme and adherence to maintenance drug therapy and management skills improved considerably. Despite self-initiated changes in drug regimes increasing dramatically, half the patients did not continue to monitor their peak flow.

Is education in groups more effective than one-to-one education in trying to produce change? Wilson *et al.* (1993) compared two forms of self-management education for adults with asthma in a controlled trial, although nearly half of those eligible did not take part. Small group education showed a trend towards greater improvements than individual education and cost less. Four 90–minute sessions in groups of six to eight people were provided, in which peer support and interaction allowed fears and concerns to be expressed. The authors concluded that careful analysis of patients actual problems should drive the objectives and content of educational programmes. One of the most important findings to come out of this study was that it took a year for the benefits to emerge, possibly due to prolonged effects of allergens and gradual response to steroids. The importance of prolonged follow up after educational interventions cannot be overstated.

There may be advantages in combining different forms of education. Windsor *et al.* (1990) used several approaches, combining a 30-minute one-to one session plus booklet, a 60-minute asthma support group session and two reinforcement telephone calls. They demonstrated a 44% improvement in adherence to medication and concluded that their programme was both effective and cost-effective, despite being very resource intensive.

Providing education with family involvement

Family involvement in educational programmes for children is common, but this is not the case for adults. Ignacio-Garcia and Gonzalez-Santos (1995) invited family members to the educational sessions of their intervention group at the hospital centre. They demonstrated that full adherence to a self-management plan guided by peak flow readings can actually lead to a total reduction in drug consumption. Allen *et al.* (1995) also encouraged a family member or friend to accompany each participant in their community programme. Although improvements occurred in knowledge and adherence, inadequacy of the medical treatment reduced potential benefits in morbidity. As with many programmes, it is difficult to identify exactly what aspect of the intervention was responsible for the improvements seen, as the different components are not controlled for in the studies. The theoretical grounds for including family support do, however, seem strong.

Guided self-management

The term guided self-management (Partridge, 1994) is a relatively new term in the asthma education literature and emphasises the partnership that should develop between patients and professionals. Lahdensuo *et al.* (1996), in a prospective and randomised trial, demonstrated that improvements in quality of life and reductions in incidents caused by asthma could be achieved by this approach. This study is important because the patients, who had mild to moderate asthma, were already well stabilised on inhaled steroids and nearly all of them completed the programme. Nurses and physiotherapists provided the education, which for the active intervention group was two-and-a-half hours, whereas controls only had one hour of contact. Although adherence was self-reported, the findings gives us a good insight into the level of adherence to self-management behaviours.

On the 141 occasions that the peak flow dropped below 85% of the optimal value, the inhaled steroid was doubled on 87 occasions (62% adherence), eighty five percent of patients starting within three days of the fall, and most (74%) starting on the first day. On the 13 occasions that the peak flow dropped below 70% of the optimal value, oral steroids were started on 10 occasions (77% adherence). Adherence was strongly related to severity of asthma symptoms. As the total amount of steroid inhaler used was much the same, and the spirometric values remained completely stable in both groups, what was it that made the difference? Although the authors listed possible reasons, they were unable to determine which was the most important.

There is also an issue concerning the amount of contact that patients have with HPs. In nearly all studies this has not been controlled for, giving the intervention group an unfair advantage in terms of time. Kotses *et al.* (1995) avoided this problem by using a control group that was on a six month waiting list before receiving the education. Their self-management programme improved morbidity by learning and performing self-management skills and actually reduced medication in a group whose asthma was under control. The programme was not only intensive but required a detailed asthma diary to be kept. A year after the training, patients reported increased use of self-management skills, but more objective improvements in cognitive measures were also seen. The feasibility of patients maintaining this level of participation for a year is reflected in the fact that one in three patients declined to take part in the study, and one in ten dropped out of the study before it had finished. Patient motivation appears to be a key factor in adherence.

Despite the common-sense appeal of self-management plans, there is some debate as to whether they are effective in reducing morbidity. Hoskins *et al.* (1996) found that, even in a randomised trial, GPs exhibited an "enthusiast bias" issuing plans to patients with uncontrolled asthma rather than to all patients who were eligible to receive them. Targeting intensive asthma care on those with the highest morbidity from asthma would seem a more appropriate use of resources (Jones *et al.*, 1992).

Making education more effective

The importance of communication in patient management and education has received a great deal of attention. Bailey *et al.* (1990) took the unusual step of observing consultations prior to their randomised control trial to improve self-management practices. They identified several barriers to effective communication prior to their education programme and, taking the findings into consideration, used a combination of educational interventions: individual counselling, a skills orientated work book, a support group, follow-up telephone calls, and clinic visits. This approach found favour with the patients as four times as many dropped out of the usual care group as dropped out of the intervention group. Self-report scales developed for measuring adherence to medication and inhaler use showed substantially better adherence in the self-management group.

FUTURE PROGRAMMES FOR IMPROVING ADHERENCE IN ASTHMA

Training in Self-Management or Education for Personal Development?

What has been provided for patients to date can be more accurately described as skills training rather than education. The emphasis has been on specific actions in specific situations rather than a deeper understanding of the meaning of illness. Patients are instructed how to use an inhaler properly and how to avoid asthma precipitants. They are advised to increase the dose of the inhaled steroids and reliever inhaler if their peak flow readings drop below a certain point (usually 70% of their best or optimal value) or at the start of a cold or if troublesome symptoms develop. If their peak flow drops too low (usually 50% of their best or optimal value) or if their β_2-agonist inhaler fails to give relief, they are strongly recommended to start oral steroids and contact their doctor. The action levels, the doses used, and the duration of increased dosage vary from programme to programme. The term guided self-management accurately describes this process, but the essence is still the expert telling the novice what to do, with little or no opportunity for the individual to discover things for themselves.

Self-help, self-control, self-efficacy, self-regulation and self-determination are closely related psychosocial concepts that have received much attention in the self-management health education literature. They are mirrored by the educational principles of adult, self-directed learning (Knowles 1980), which seem to have had rather less influence on patient education although they have been applied increasingly in professional education. Other important principles include differences in individual learning styles, active as opposed to passive participation, the value of problem-based learning, personal reflection, and the motivation to learn. This would suggest that giving patients the choice of educational materials, allowing active involvement in decision making, enabling patients to think about and discuss their problems, and finding ways of motivating patients to change are all promising areas for incorporating into asthma management programmes.

Bandura's social learning theory (1977), which has already been applied extensively in health education programmes, states that corrective learning occurs through:

1. an individual's successful accomplishments
2. their vicarious experiences
3. verbal persuasion
4. decreased emotional arousal.

The usual HP interventions occur at level 3 and sometimes level 4. Working in groups can reach level 2, but we need to find more effective ways of enabling level 1 as this has the most powerful effect. The common thread between theories of education and social psychology lies in the individual experience of the patient. This is the area that HPs need to explore before deciding any intervention with the patient. A variety of social cognition models can predict health behaviour (Conner and Norman, 1996) and developments in this area could help us to define those aspects of patient thinking and behaviour that can lead to success.

Should Motivation be Assessed before Providing Education?

Behavioural change needs to be negotiated and assessing whether patients are ready to change or not may be more effective than simply giving advice (Rollnick *et al.*, 1993). Humans have an intrinsic need to be self determining and will accept more responsibility for behaviour change when motivated internally rather than externally (Williams *et al.*, 1991). In the doctor-patient relationship, this internal motivation for change can be facilitated when doctors *allow choice,* provide *relevant information,* and acknowledge the *patient's perspective* (my italics). The language used by HPs to suggest change can affect peoples' internal motivation and subsequent behaviour change. The theory suggests that when they emphasise what people *should* do, people tend to be *less* internally motivated, and either rebel or comply (or say they do) to please. Indeed there is good evidence for provider-controlling behaviours being associated with lower internal motivation, less behaviour change and poorer health outcomes than autonomy-supportive measures (Williams *et al.*, 1991).

Better Education or Better Communication?

Partridge (1995) has summarised the key components needed for delivering optimal care to patients with asthma, and rightly emphasises the importance of good communication in education. Evidence from both the communication literature (Lipkin *et al.*, 1995) and the motivation literature suggests that the words and phrases used by HPs are crucial. Questions are an important component of the consultation (Tuckett *et al.*, 1985), but what questions should be asked, and how should they be asked? In return, how can we enable patients to ask questions? Acknowledging the likelihood of nonadherence would seem an important first step, showing patients that we realise they may not be able to do all the things asked of them. When we answer their questions, it may well be that the actual words we choose may be just as important as the choice of drug, and the amount of time spent as important as the dose of drug prescribed.

Variations in consultation style are well described and, given that some professionals are more effective than others at providing education, HPs should receive education that improves their communication skills. These generic skills can be used in areas other than asthma.

Secondary or Primary care?

It could be argued that scarce resources should be concentrated on intensive secondary care programmes helping those with the most severe disease. On the other hand, it might be more effective and efficient to make small changes to most, if not all, people with asthma on the grounds that a small shift in the health of a population is of more benefit than a large shift in a small number of high risk patients (Rose, 1992). However, there is evidence that adherence to inhaler therapy is greater in patients who have ever seen a chest physician (Dekker *et al.*, 1993), but the implications for hospital care if every one with asthma was referred would be enormous. Clearly what is needed is greater collaboration between primary and secondary care with the development of joint clinical guidelines, and audit and research programmes at the primary-secondary care interface.

What Kind of Health Professional?

There is also evidence that in hospital, chest specialists have better patient outcomes than their generalist counterparts (Bucknall *et al.*, 1988), which raises the issue as to whether there might be some advantage in GPs also specialising within their practices. This trend has been resisted in the past, but the formation of the GPs in Asthma Group in the UK has already had some influence on asthma care (General Practitioners in Asthma Group, 1995) and this is likely to increase as more HPs join.

Another question relates to who should be providing the education. Nurses have been partners in providing patient education from the very beginning (Maiman *et al.*, 1979), and nurse-run clinics have become the norm in British general practice since the advent of the 1990 contract. It is probably no longer possible to prove or disprove their clinical effectiveness (Jones and Mullee, 1995). They have, however, been shown to have an effect on morbidity, although it is not known which component of care has the greatest impact (Charlton *et al.*, 1991b). This has been demonstrated both in primary and secondary care. There is some evidence that patients prefer to get their information from their doctor (National Asthma Campaign, 1996), but success probably relies less on the type of HP than on the relationship they have with the patient and on the quality of their communication skills.

Individual Care with Continuity or Management by Teams with Consistency?

There is a move for more care to be provided by multidisciplinary teams than by individual HPs, with shared care already being standard in antenatal, psychiatric and diabetes care. This trend is likely to spread to asthma care as the organisation of health services evolves in response to changes in working patterns and difficulties in personnel recruitment and training. The main problem is going to be making sure that the message is consistent, and multidisciplinary education for HPs would seem to have something to offer here. The role of other HPs, such as pharmacists, health psychologists and physiotherapists, has yet to be fully exploited in the primary care management of asthma.

Group or Individual Approach?

Whilst the one-to-one doctor-patient relationship has been one of the great strengths of British general practice, the peer support that comes from working in groups can enable behavioural change and is cost-effective. There is an extensive literature demonstrating that there are advantages in using a peer modelling approach rather than one that relies upon mastery. Not all patients would want to join a group, but those who do should at least be given the opportunity. This requires a degree of organisational flexibility which should be possible in primary care, and might bring benefits in time saved in consultations. What is not known, however, is how often such groups should meet and for how long. Attendance is likely to decrease as the number of meetings increases.

Structured or Unstructured Education?

While some studies have shown that structured patient education can be effective (Charlton *et al.*, 1991b), is it flexible enough for the individual? It is tempting to give patients more information than they actually want or need (Bailey *et al.*, 1990). Patients probably need to know less about the pathophysiology of their disease and more about integrating the new demands into their own daily routines (Mazzuca, 1982). There is a need to find out what elements of the structure are the most useful (Partridge, 1995) and combine these with an approach that allows variation to accommodate individual problems. There needs to be a compromise between the educational aims of the doctor and the patient.

Whatever education is offered, there are going to be some patients who are reluctant to accept it and will not attend special asthma clinics. Every patient contact should be used as an potential opportunity for education (Hilton, 1986), although assessing motivation to learn (change) might be the most appropriate first step.

How Much Time Should be Invested and With Whom?

Clinicians are faced with a dilemma about the most effective way to allocate resources. Should more time be spent at the very beginning when asthma is first diagnosed when, perhaps, patients may be more amenable to change as their personal experience is not great, or should the time be spent equally on all people with asthma? Although investment at an early stage of the illness may well pay dividends, the amount of time that is effective and the optimal time for follow-up is not known. Long-term effectiveness may get sacrificed for gains in short-term efficiency.

New Pharmacological Treatments or Old?

New drugs for asthma that have recently been developed include long-acting β_2-agonists (salmeterol and eformoterol) and inhaled steroids that are believed to have less systemic effects (fluticasone). Inevitably newer treatments are initially more expensive, but studies are needed to test their cost-effectiveness, which may be dependant upon patient acceptability and adherence. The early signs are promising with the costs of treatment increasing but the overall costs of care decreasing (Price, 1995b). Treatments in tablet form, such as the newly developed leukotriene inhibitors, may simplify management and improve adherence. New inhaler devices, using environmentally friendly propellants, may also make taking treatment easier.

FUTURE RESEARCH

Most of the studies of educating patients in self-management skills have relied on subjective methods of assessing adherence. The improvements in demonstrated outcome have been assumed to be due to either increased adherence in taking medication or some other change in behaviour. Given the findings from studies that have used electronic monitoring, it is clear that future studies looking at medication adherence and the use of peak flow meters need to utilise more sophisticated methods of assessment. Whether it will be possible to conduct such studies with current devices, which do not appear to totally reliable, remains to be seen. It is likely, however, that the technology for monitoring will improve.

Long term studies of adherence are uncommon and, given the fact that asthma is a chronic condition that lasts for years, it is important to know how adherence changes over time. Given the problems of recruitment and attendance, let alone cost, such studies may not be feasible. If they are possible anywhere it is in primary care especially in those countries, such as Great Britain, that have an individual list of patients. In this context, adherence will almost certainly have to be measured subjectively, using computerised repeat prescribing and dispensing data to corroborate the patient's story. What we need to find out is how best to improve communication so that we can assess patients' adherence to medication and self-management behaviours. Questioning appears a crucial issue to investigate as the responses, whether obtained indirectly by questionnaire or directly in the consultation, can be used for assessing motivation and providing education.

The other area that needs to be clarified is the core components of treatment packages needed to improve self-management practices. We need to dissect out the most effective and efficient components of the "black box" of asthma care. There are probably some very simple things that can be said that will improve patient adherence and can be applied widely. Enquiring about the effects of asthma on daily living rather than about symptoms (Quirk and Jones, 1990), asking the patient if they are satisfied with their treatment, offering more information if it is wanted, checking inhaler technique and improving the system for obtaining supplies of treatment, may be all that is needed for the vast majority of patients. More intensive self-management programmes could be reserved for more resistant cases.

There is a move to start treating asthma with inhaled steroids at a much earlier stage in the disease on the grounds that this might prevent the development of asthma. If early treatment proves to be effective, strategies for ensuring that the evidence is put into action by HPs will need to be developed. Alternative ways of providing education for improving HPs' management of asthma is an area that needs to be studied to find out which are most effective. Developments in information technology will undoubtedly have an influence on this process and their full potential remains to be seen. No doubt patients will be able to access the same evidence as professionals.

CONCLUDING REMARKS

We have known for some time that a patient/illness centred and behaviour based approach is more effective than a doctor/disease centred and knowledge based approach in improving adherence, physiological progress and long-term health outcomes (Mazzuca, 1982). The shift in emphasis has been gradual and very much reflects the even slower changes in the education of HPs. Until most HPs experience the benefits of adult educational principles themselves, they are unlikely to be persuaded that they should be applied to patients. The challenge for us all is to see that education empowers the individual (Rogers, 1969), whether this is a patient or a professional.

POSTSCRIPT

How's Charles? I thought you might ask. I saw him the other week, having not seen him for ages. He's fine: no asthma and a massive peak flow of 650 (better than average). "Why do you think is your asthma so much better?" I asked. "Well", he replied "My life is so much more settled now. I've got a job and I'm going to get married." Sure enough, on the computer screen were regular prescriptions for his preventer inhaler. "Not a lot to do with doctors" I thought!

ACKNOWLEDGEMENT

I should like to thank Professor Shirley Pearce for reading earlier drafts of this chapter and for her helpful comments.

REFERENCES

Allen, R.M., Jones, M.P. and Oldenberg, B. (1995) Randomised trial of an asthma-self management programme for adults. *Thorax* **50**, 731–738.

Bailey, W.C., Richards, J.M., Brooks, C.M. and Soong, S. (1990) A randomized trial to improve self-management practices of adults with asthma. *Archives of Internal Medicine* **150**, 1664–1668.

Bandura, A. (1977) Self-efficacy: toward a unifying theory of behavioral change. *Psychological Review* **84**, 191–215.

Barnes, G. and Partridge, M.R. (1994) Community asthma clinics. *Quality in Health Care* **3**, 133–136.

Barnes, P.J. (1989) A new approach to the treatment of asthma. *New England Journal of Medicine* **321**, 1517–1527.

Barnes, P.J. (1992) Poorly perceived asthma. *Thorax* **47**, 408–409.

Barritt, P.W. and Staples, E.B. (1991) Measuring success in asthma care: a repeat audit. *British Journal of General Practice* **41**, 232–236.

Bartlett, E.E. (1983) Educational self-help approaches in childhood asthma. *Journal of Allergy and Clinical Immunology* **72**, 545–554.

Beasley, R., Cushley, M. and Holgate, S.T. (1989) A self management plan in the treatment of adult asthma. *Thorax* **44**, 200–204.

Becker, M.H. (1974) The Health Belief Model and sick role behavior. *Health Education Monographs* **2**, 409–419.

Bosley, C.M., Fosbury, J.A. and Cochrane, G.M. (1995) The psychological factors associated with poor compliance with treatment in asthma. *European Respiratory Journal* **8**, 899–904.

Bosley, C.M., Parry, D.T. and Cochrane, G.M. (1994) Patient compliance with inhaled medication. Does combining beta-agonists with corticosteroids improve compliance? *European Respiratory Journal* **7**, 504–509.

British Thoracic Society. (1993) Guidelines on the management of asthma. *Thorax* **48**, S1–S24.

Britten, N. (1994) Patients' ideas about medicines: a qualitative study in a general practice population. *British Journal of General Practice* **44**, 465–468.

Bryce, F.P., Neville, R.G., Crombie, I.K., Clark, R.A. and McKenzie, P. (1995) Controlled trial of an audit facilitator in diagnosis and treatment of childhood asthma in general practice. *British Medical Journal* **310**, 838–842.

Bucknall, C.E., Robertson, C., Moran, F. and Stevenson, R.D. (1988) Differences in hospital asthma management. *Lancet* **i**, 748–750.

Carpenter, L., Beral, V., Strachan, D., Ebi-Kryston, K.L. and Inskip, H. (1989) Respiratory symptoms as predictors of 27 year mortality in a representative sample of British adults. *British Medical Journal* **299**, 357–361.

Charlton, I., Jones, K. and Bain, J. (1991a) Delay in diagnosis of childhood asthma and its influence on respiratory consultation rates. *Archives of Disease in Childhood* **66**, 633–635.

Charlton, I., Charlton, G., Broomfield, J. and Mullee, M.A. (1991b) Audit of the effect of a nurse run asthma clinic on workload and patient morbidity in a general practice. *British Journal of General Practice* **41**, 227–231.

Charlton, I., Antoniou, A.G., Atkinson, J., Campbell, M.J., Chapman, E., Mackintosh, T. and Schapira, D. (1994) Asthma at the interface: bridging the gap between general practice and a district general hospital. *Archives of Disease in Childhood* **70**, 313–318.

Chowienczyk, P.J., Parkin, D.H., Lawson, C.P. and Cochrane, G.M. (1994) Do asthmatic patients correctly record home spirometry measurements? *British Medical Journal* **309**, 1618.

Cochrane, G.M. (1995) Compliance in asthma: a European perspective. *European Respiratory Review* **26**, 116–119.

Conner, M. and Norman, P. (eds.) (1996) *Predicting health behaviour*. Buckingham: Open University Press.

Connolly, C.K., Chan, N.S. and Prescott, R.J. (1989) The influence of social factors on the control of asthma. *Postgraduate Medical Journal* **65**, 282–285.

Coutts, J.A., Gibson, N.A. and Paton, J.Y. (1992) Measuring compliance with inhaled medication in asthma. *Archives of Disease in Childhood* **67**, 332–333.

Creer, T.L. (1987) Living with asthma: replications and extensions. *Health Education Quarterly* **14**, 319–331.

Crompton, G.K. (1982) Problems patients have using pressurised aerosol inhalers. *European Journal of Respiratory Diseases* (Supplement 119) **63**, 101–104.

Dekker, F.W., Dielman, F.E., Kaptein, A.A. and Milder, J.D. (1993) Compliance with pulmonary medication in general practice. *European Respiratory Journal* **6**, 886–890.

Denson-Lino, J.M., Willies-Jacobo, L.J., Rosas, A., O'Connor, R.D. and Wilson, N.W. (1993) Effect of economic status on the use of house dust mite avoidance measures in asthmatic children. *Annals of Allergy* **71**, 130–132.

Djukanovic, R., Wilson, J.W., Britten, K.M., Wilson, S.J., Walls, A.F., Roche, W.R., Howarth, P.H. and Holgate, S.T. (1992) Effect of an inhaled corticosteroid on airway inflammation and symptoms in asthma. *American Reviews of Respiratory Diseases* **145**, 669–674.

Dolce, J.J., Crisp, C., Manzella, B., Richards, J.M., Hardin, M. and Bailey, W.C. (1991) Medication adherence patterns in chronic obstructive pulmonary disease. *Chest* **99**, 837–841.

Dompeling, E., van Schayck, C.P., Molema, J., Folgering, H., van Grunsven, P.M. and van Weel, C. (1992) Inhaled beclomethasone improves the course of asthma and COPD. *European Respiratory Journal* **5**, 945–952.

D'Souza, W., Crane, J., Burgess, C., Te Karu, H., Fox, C., Harper, M., Robson, B., Howden-Chapman, P., Crossland, L., Woodman, K., Pearce, N., Pomare, E. and Beasley, R. (1994) Community-based asthma care: trial of a "credit card" asthma self-management plan. *European Respiratory Journal* **7**, 1260–1265.

Duran-Tuleria, E., Rona, R.J., Chinn, S. and Burney, P. (1996) Influence of ethnic group on asthma treatment in children in 1990–1: national cross sectional study. *British Medical Journal* **313**, 148–152.

Everard, M.L., Devadason, S.G., Summers, Q.A. and Le Souëf, P.N. (1995) Factors affecting total and "respirable" dose delivered by a salbutamol metered dose inhaler. *Thorax* **50**, 746–749.

Feder, G., Griffiths, C., Highton, C., Eldridge, S., Spence, M. and Southgate, L. (1995) Do clinical guidelines introduced with practice based education improve care of asthmatic and diabetic patients? A randomised controlled trial in general practices in east London. *British Medical Journal* **311**, 1473–1478.

Fireman, P., Friday, G.A., Gira, C., Vierthaler, W.A. and Michaels, L. (1981) Teaching self-management skills to asthmatic children and their parents in an ambulatory care setting. *Pediatrics* **68**, 341–348.

Fitzmaurice, D.A. and Bradley, C.P. (1994) Helping asthma patients to stop smoking. *British Journal of General Practice* **44,** 533.

Geddes, D.M. (1992) Inhaled corticosteroids: risks and benefits. *Thorax* **47**, 404–407.

Gellert, A.R., Gellert, S.L. and Iliffe, S.R. (1990) Prevalence and management of asthma in a London inner city general practice. *British Journal of General Practice* **40**, 197–201.

General Practitioners in Asthma Group. (1995) *Asthma: improving compliance, reducing the burden.* London: Shire Hall Publishing.

Gibson, P., Henry, D., Francis, L., Cruickshank, D., Dupen, F., Higginbotham, N., Henry, R. and Sutherland, D. (1993) Association between availability of non-prescription β₂-agonist inhalers and undertreatment of asthma. *British Medical Journal* **306**, 1514–1518.

Grampian Asthma Study of Integrated Care (GRASSIC). (1994) Effectiveness of routine self monitoring of peak flow in patients with asthma. *British Medical Journal* **308**, 564–567.

Griffiths, C., Naish, J., Sturdy, P. and Pereira, F. (1996) Prescribing and hospital admissions for asthma in east London. *British Medical Journal* **312**, 481–482.

Guidry, G.G., Brown, W.D., Stogner, S.W. and George, R.B. (1992) Incorrect use of metered dose inhalers by medical personnel. *Chest* **101**, 31–33.

Hall, J.A., Roter, D.L. and Katz, N.R. (1988) Meta-analysis of correlates of provider behavior in medical encounters. *Medical Care* **26**, 657–675.

Hand, C.H. and Bradley, C. (1996) Health beliefs of adults with asthma: toward an understanding of the difference between symptomatic and preventive use of inhaler treatment. *Journal of Asthma* **33**, 331–338.

Harvey, J. and Williams, J.G. (1992) Randomised cross-over comparison of five inhaler systems for bronchodilator therapy. *British Journal of Clinical Practice* **46**, 249–251.

Hilton, S. (1986) Patient education in asthma. *Family Practice* **3**, 44–48.

Hilton, S., Sibbald, B. Anderson, H.R. and Freeling, P. (1986) Controlled evaluation of patient education on asthma morbidity in general practice. *Lancet* **i**, 26–29.

Horn, C.R., Essex, E., Hill, P. and Cochrane, G.M. (1989) Does urinary salbutamol reflect compliance with aerosol regimen in patients with asthma? *Respiratory Medicine* **83**, 15–18.

Horn, C.R., Clark, T.J.H. and Cochrane, G.M. (1990) Compliance with inhaled therapy and morbidity from asthma. *Respiratory Medicine* **84**, 67–70.

Horsley, M.G. and Bailie, G.R. (1988) Risk factors for inadequate use of pressurised aerosol inhalers. *Journal of Clinical Pharmacy and Therapeutics* **13**, 139–143.

Hoskins, G., Neville, R.G., Smith, B. and Clark, R.A. (1996) Do self-management plans reduce morbidity in patients with asthma? *British Journal of General Practice* **46**, 169–171.

Huss, K., Squire, E.N. Jr., Carpenter, G.B., Smith, L.J., Huss, R.W., Salata, K., Salerno, M., Agostinelli, D. and Hershey, J. (1992) Effective education of adults with asthma who are allergic to dust mites. *Journal of Allergy and Clinical Immunology* **89**, 836–43.

Hyland, M.E., Kenyon, C.A.P., Allen, R. and Howarth, P. (1993) Diary keeping in asthma: comparison of written and electronic methods. *British Medical Journal* **306**, 487–489.

Ignacio-Garcia, J.M. and Gonzalez-Santos, P. (1995) Asthma self-management education program by home monitoring of peak expiratory flow. *American Journal of Respiratory and Critical Care Medicine* **151**, 353–359.

Jackson, C. and Lipworth, B. (1995) Optimizing inhaled drug delivery in patients with asthma. *British Journal of General Practice* **45**, 683–687.

Jenkinson, D., Davison, J., Jones, S. and Hawtin P. (1988) Comparison of effects of a self management booklet and audiocassette for patients with asthma. *British Medical Journal* **297**, 267–270.

Johnson, A.J., Nunn, A.J., Somner, A.R., Stableforth, D.E. and Stewart, C.J. (1984) Circumstances of death from asthma. *British Medical Journal* **288**, 1870–1872.

Jones, A.H., Langdon, C.G., Lee, P.S., Lingham, S.A., Nankani, J.P., Follows, R.M.A., Tollemar, U. and Richardson, P.D.I. (1994) Pulmicort Turbohaler once daily as initial prophylactic therapy for asthma. *Respiratory Medicine* **88**, 293–299.

Jones, K.P., Charlton, I.H., Middleton, M., Preece, W.J. and Hill, A.P. (1992) Targeting asthma care in general practice using a morbidity index. *British Medical Journal* **304**, 1353–1356.

Jones, K.P. and Mullee, M.A. (1995) Proactive, nurse-run asthma care in general practice reduces asthma morbidity: scientific fact or medical assumption? *British Journal of General Practice* **45**, 497–499.

Jones, K.P., Mullee, M.A., Middleton, M., Chapman, E., Holgate, S.T. and the British Thoracic Society Research Committee. (1995) Peak flow based asthma self-management: a randomised controlled trial in general practice. *Thorax* **50**, 851–857.

Juniper, E.F., Guyatt, G.H., Epstein, R.S., Ferrie, P.J., Jaeschke, R. and Hiller, T.K. (1992) Evaluation of impairment of health related quality of life in asthma: development of a questionnaire for use in clinical trials. *Thorax* **47**, 76–83.

Keeley, D. (1993) How to achieve better outcome in treatment of asthma in general practice. *British Medical Journal* **307**, 1261–1263.

Kelloway, J.S., Wyatt, R.A. and Adlis, S.A. (1994) Comparison of patients' compliance with prescribed oral and inhaled asthma medications. *Archives of Internal Medicine* **154**, 1349–1352.

Kendrick, A.H., Higgs, C.M.B., Whitfield, M.J. and Laszlo, G. (1993) Accuracy of perception of severity of asthma: patients treated in general practice. *British Medical Journal* **307**, 422–424.

Kidd, R.J.G., Kolbe, J. and Cochrane, G.M. (1993) Reliability of New Zealand adult asthmatics in recording peak expiratory flow rates. *European Respiratory Journal* **6**, 275S.

Klingelhofer, E.L. (1987) Compliance with medical regimens, self-management programs, and self-care in childhood asthma. *Clinical Review of Allergy* **5**, 231–247.

Knowles, M.S. (1980) *The modern practice of education: from pedagogy to androgogy.* Chicago: Follett.

Kolnaar, B.G.M., Beissel, E., van den Bosch, W.J.H.M., Folgering, H., van den Hoogen, H.J.M. and van Weel, C. (1994) Asthma in adolescents and young adults: screening outcome versus diagnosis in general practice. *Family Practice* **11**, 133–140.

Kotses, H., Bernstein, I.L., Bernstein, D.I., Reynolds, R.V.C., Korbee, L., Wigal, J.K., Ganson, E., Stout, C. and Creer, T.L. (1995) A self-management program for adult asthma. Part 1: development and evaluation. *Journal of Allergy and Clinical Immunology* **95**, 529–540.

Lahdensuo, A., Haahtela, T., Herrala, J., Kava, T., Kiviranta, K., Kuusisto, P., Perämäki, E., Poussa, T., Saarelainen, S. and Svahn, T. (1996) Randomised comparison of guided self management and traditional treatment of asthma over one year. *British Medical Journal* **312**, 748–752.

Lim, K.L. and Harrison, B.D.W. (1992) A criterion based audit of in-patient asthma care. *Journal of the Royal College of Physicians of London* **26**, 71–75.

Lipkin, M., Putman, S. and Lazare, A. (eds.). (1995) *The medical interview.* New York: Springer.

Littlejohns, P. and Macdonald, L.D. (1993) The relationship between severe asthma and social class. *Respiratory Medicine* **87**, 139–143.

Maiman, L.A., Green, L.W., Gibson, G. and MacKenzie, E.J. (1979) Education for self-treatment by adult asthmatics. *Journal of the American Medical Association* **241**, 1919–1922.

Malo, J-L., L'Archeveque, J., Trudeau, C., d'Aquino, C. and Cartier, A. (1993) Should we monitor peak expiratory flow rates or record symptoms with a simple diary in the management of asthma? *Journal of Allergy and Clinical Immunology* **91**, 702–709.

Martys, C.R. (1992) Asthma care in Darley Dale: general practitioner audit. *British Medical Journal* **304**, 758–760.

Mayo, P.H., Richman, J. and Harris, H.W. (1990) Results of a program to reduce admissions for adult asthma. *Annals of Internal Medicine* **112**, 864–871.

Mazzuca, S.A. (1982) Does patient education in chronic disease have therapeutic value? *Journal of Chronic Diseases* **35**, 521–529.

McClellan, V.E. and Garrett, J.E. (1989) Attendance failure at Middlemore Hospital asthma clinic. *New Zealand Medical Journal* **102**, 211–213.

Miller, M.R., Dickinson, S.A. and Hitchins, D.J. (1992) The accuracy of portable peak flow meters. *Thorax* **47**, 904–909.

Modell, M., Harding, J.M., Horder, E.J. and Williams, P. (1983) Improving the care of asthmatic patients in general practice. *British Medical Journal* **286**, 2027–2030.

Mühlhauser, I., Richter, B., Kraut, D., Weske, G., Worth, H. and Berger, M. (1991) Evaluation of a structured treatment and teaching programme on asthma. *Journal of Internal Medicine* **230**, 157–164.

National Asthma Campaign/MORI poll. (1990) *Attitudes to Asthma.* London: National Asthma Campaign.

National Asthma Campaign. (1996) *Attitudes to Asthma.* London: National Asthma Campaign.

Neville, R.G., Clark, R.C., Hoskins, G. and Smith, B. for General Practitioners in Asthma Group. (1993) National asthma attack audit 1991–2. *British Medical Journal* **306**, 559–562.

Nocon, A. and Booth, T. (1991) The social impact of asthma. *Family Practice* **8**, 37–41.

Osman, L.M., Russell, I.T., Friend, J.A.R., Legge, J.S. and Douglas, J.G. (1993) Predicting patient attitudes to asthma medication. *Thorax* **48**, 827–830.

Osman, L.M., Abdalla, M.I., Beattie, J.A.G., Ross, S.J., Russell, I.T., Friend, J.A., Legge, J.S. and Douglas, J.G. on behalf of the

Grampian Asthma Study of Integrated Care (GRASSIC). (1994) Reducing hospital admission through computer supported education for asthma patients. *British Medical Journal* **308**, 568–571.

Partridge, M.R. (1986) Asthma education: more reading or more viewing? *Journal of the Royal Society of Medicine* **79**, 326–328.

Partridge, M.R. (1994) Asthma: guided self management. *British Medical Journal* **308**, 547–548.

Partridge, M.R. (1995) Delivering optimal care to the person with asthma: what are the key components and what do we mean by patient education? *European Respiratory Journal* **8**, 298–305.

Price, D.B. (1995a) Perceived asthma compliance related to symptom control and patient attitudes. *Thorax* **50 (Suppl 2)**, 53.

Price, D.B. (1995b) Patterns of prescribing of inhaled steroids over a seven year period in a general practice and its implications. *Thorax* **50**, 443.

Quirk, F.H. and Jones, P.W. (1990) Patients' perception of distress due to symptoms and effects of asthma on daily living and an investigation of possible influential factors. *Clinical Science* **79**, 17–21.

Radius, S.M., Becker, M.H., Rosenstock, I.M., Drachman, R.H., Schuberth, K.C. and Teets, K.C. (1978) Factors influencing mothers' compliance with a medication regimen for asthmatic children. *The Journal of Asthma Research* **15**, 133–149.

Rand, C.S., Wise, R.A., Nides, M., Simmons, M.S., Bleecker, E.R., Kusek, J.W., Li, V.C. and Tashkin, D.P. (1992) Metered-dose inhaler adherence in a clinical trial. *American Reviews of Respiratory Disease* **146**, 1559–1564.

Rand, C.S. and Wise, R.A. (1994) Measuring adherence to asthma medication regimens. *American Journal of Respiratory and Critical Care Medicine* **149**, S69–76.

Renwick, D.S. and Connolly, M.J. (1996) Prevalence and treatment of chronic airways obstruction in adults over the age of 45. *Thorax* **51**, 164–168.

Rogers, C. (1969) *Freedom to learn for the 80s.* Columbus, Ohio: Merrill.

Rollnick, S., Kinnersley, P. and Stott, N. (1993) Methods of helping patients with behaviour change. *British Medical Journal* **307**, 188–190.

Rose, G. (1992) *The strategy of preventive medicine.* New York: Oxford University Press..

Rubinfield, A.R. and Pain, M.C.F. (1976) Perception of asthma. *Lancet* **i**, 882–884.

Sibbald, B. (1989) Patient self care in acute asthma. *Thorax* **44**, 97–101.

Slama, K., Redman, S., Perkins, J., Reid, A.L.A. and Sanson-Fisher, R.W. (1990) The effectiveness of two smoking cessation programmes for use in general practice: a randomised clinical trial. *British Medical Journal* **300**, 1707–1709.

Spector, S.L., Kinsman, R., Mawhinney, H., Siegel, S.C., Rachelefsky, G.S., Katz, R.M. and Rohr, A.S. (1986) Compliance of patients with asthma with an experimental aerolised medication: implications for controlled trials. *Journal of Allergy and Clinical Immunology* **77**, 65–70.

Spitzer, W.O., Suissa, S., Ernst, P., Horwitz, R.I., Habbick, B., Cockcroft, D., Boivin, J-F., McNutt, M., Buist, S. and Rebuck, A.S. (1992) The use of β_2-agonists and the risk of death and near death from asthma. *The New England Journal of Medicine* **326**, 501–506.

Sturdy, P., Naish, J., Pereira, F., Griffiths, C., Dolan, S., Toon, P. and Chambers, M. (1995) Characteristics of general practices that prescribe appropriately for asthma. *British Medical Journal* **311**, 547–548.

Suissa, S., Blais, L. and Ernst, P. (1994) Patterns of increasing β-agonist use and the risk of fatal or near-fatal asthma. *British Journal of General Practice* **7**, 1602–1609.

Taggart, V.S. (1995) Implementation of the guidelines: a patient's perspective. *European Respiratory Review* **5**, 112–115.

Taggart, V.S., Zuckerman, A.E., Sly, R.M., Steinmueller, C., Newman, G., O'Brien, R.W., Schneider, S. and Bellanti, J.A. (1991) You can control asthma: evaluation of an asthma education program for hospitalised inner-city children. *Patient Education and Counseling* **17**, 35–47.

Taylor, D.R., Sears, M.R., Herbison, G.P., Flannery, E.M., Print, C.G., Lake, D.C., Yates, D.M., Lucas, M.K. and Li, Q. (1992) Regular inhaled β_2-agonist in asthma: effects on exacerbations and lung function. *Thorax* **48**, 134–138.

Tirimanna, P.R.S., den Otter, J.J., van Schayck, C.P., van Herwaarden, C.L.A., Folgering, H. and van Weel, C. (1996) Evaluation of the suitability of weekly peak flow expiratory flow rate measurements in monitoring annual decline in lung function among patients with asthma and chronic bronchitis. *British Journal of General Practice* **46**, 15–18.

Tobin, D.L., Wigal, J.K., Winder, J.A., Holroyd, K.A. and Creer, T.L. (1987) The "Asthma self-efficacy scale". *Annals of Allergy* **59**, 273–277.

Tuckett, D., Boulton, M., Olson, C. and Williams, A. (1985) *Meetings between experts: an approach to sharing ideas in medical consultations.* London: Tavistock.

van Schayck, C.P., Dompeling, E., van Herwaarden, C.L.A., Folgering, H., Akkermans, R.P., van den Broek, P.J.J.A. and van Weel, C. (1995a) Continuous and on demand use of bronchodilators in patients with non-steroid dependent asthma and chronic bronchitis: four-year follow-up randomized controlled study. *British Journal of General Practice* **45**, 239–244.

van Schayck, C.P., van den Broek, P.J.J.A., den Otter, J.J., van Herwaarden, C.L.A., Molema, J. and van Weel, C. (1995b) Periodic treatment regimes with inhaled steroids in asthma or chronic obstructive pulmonary disease: is it possible? *Journal of the American Medical Association* **274**, 161–164.

Wareham, N., Harrison, B.D.W., Jenkins, P.F., Nicholls, J. and Stableforth, D.E. A district confidential enquiry into deaths due to asthma. (1993) *Thorax* **48**, 1117–1120.

Warner, J.O. (1995) Review of prescribed treatment for children with asthma in 1990. *British Medical Journal* **311**, 663–666.

Weiner, P., Weiner, M. and Azgad, Y. (1995) Long term clinical comparison of single versus twice daily administration of inhaled budesonide in moderate asthma. *Thorax* **50**, 1270–1273.

White, P., Atherton, A., Hewett, G. and Howells, K. (1995) Using information from asthma patients: a trial of information feedback in primary care. *British Medical Journal* **311**, 1065–1069.

White, P., Pharoah, C.A., Anderson, H.R. and Freeling, P. (1989) Randomized controlled trial of small group education on the outcome of chronic asthma in general practice. *Journal of the Royal College of General Practice* **39**, 182–186.

Williams, G.C., Quill, T.E., Deci, E.L. and Ryan, R.M. (1991) "The facts concerning the recent carnival of smoking in Connecticut" and elsewhere. *Annals of Internal Medicine* **115**, 59–63.

Williams, D.J., Williams, A.C. and Kruchek, D.G. (1993) Problems in assessing contents of metered dose inhalers. *British Medical Journal* **307**, 771–772.

Wilson, S.R., German, D.F., Lulla, S., Chardon, L., Starr-Schneidkraut, N. and Arsham, G.M. (1993) A controlled trial of two forms of self-management education for adults with asthma. *American Journal of Medicine* **94**, 564–576.

Windsor, R.A., Bailey, W.C., Richards, J.M., Manzella, B., Soong, S-J. and Brooks, M. (1990) Evaluation of the efficacy and cost-effectiveness of health education methods to increase medication adherence among adults with asthma. *American Journal of Public Health* **80**, 1519–1521.

Wonham, K., Jenkins, J., Pillinger, J. and Jones, K. (1996) Compliance with completing peak flow charts. *Asthma in General Practice* **4**, 7–8.

Yeung, M., O'Connor, S.A., Parry, D.T. and Cochrane, G.M. (1994) Compliance with prescribed drug therapy in asthma. *Respiratory Medicine* **88**, 31–35.

Yoon, R., McKenzie, D.K., Miles, D.A. and Bauman, A. (1991) Characteristics of attenders and non-attenders at an asthma education programme. *Thorax* **46**, 886–890.

Yoon, R., McKenzie, D.K., Bauman, A. and Miles, D.A. (1993) Controlled trial evaluation of an asthma education programme for adults. *Thorax* **48**, 1110–1116.

16

Adherence and Diabetes

Laura Warren and Paula Hixenbaugh

THE NATURE OF THE DISEASE

Diabetes mellitus is one of the most psychologically and behaviourally demanding of the chronic medical diseases (Cox and Gonder-Frederick, 1992). It affects an estimated 3% of the adult British population, with a prevalence rate of 1,380,000 (British Diabetic Association, BDA 1996). However, prevalence increases with age. In the over 65 age group, 6% of the population are affected. The figures are comparable in all western societies (Shillitoe and Miles, 1989). In the USA an estimated 14 million people are affected (Molitch, 1991). More deaths are caused by diabetes than by lung cancer, breast cancer, motor accidents or infant mortality (Kelleher, 1988a).

Diabetes is caused by partial or complete failure of the pancreas to produce the hormone, insulin. As a result, the body is unable to convert glucose into energy and therefore, in order to sustain life and avoid serious medical complications such as blindness and kidney failure, the individual must undertake a complex and demanding treatment regimen aimed at self-regulating blood glucose (BG) levels. The treatment of diabetes and its complications takes up more than 8% of the total health care expenditure in the UK (Marks, 1996).

Those individuals that continue to produce some insulin are referred to as having non-insulin dependent diabetes (NIDDM).

They make up between 75 and 90% of the total diabetic population (BDA, 1996). The onset of NIDDM is typically diagnosed in middle age, with the prevalence increasing with age. It is characterised by a gradual, often asymptomatic onset, as a result of which approximately 20% of individuals show signs of medical complications at diagnosis (Shillitoe, 1991). There is a strong genetic component. Obesity and insufficient exercise are understood to contribute to onset and whilst it has been estimated that 90% of NIDDM's could be treated with diet and exercise only (Newburgh and Conn, 1979), the significant majority of patients have to take either hyperglycaemic oral agents (50%) or insulin injections (20%) to lower their BG levels. Whilst the former imposes restrictions on *how much* food can be eaten, the latter reduces autonomy over *when* food can be eaten.

Insulin dependent diabetes (IDDM), in contrast to NIDDM, typically develops before the age of 30 years, with a peak incidence during adolescence. In the last decade there has been a large increase in the incidence rate among the under five's (Gale, personal communication). Characterised by a failure to produce insulin, rather than insulin resistance, onset is sudden and symptoms (due to severe hyperglycaemia) are acute. Genetic, auto-immune and infection factors are thought to be involved in the development of IDDM (Cox, Gonder-Frederick and Saunders, 1991). Subsequent survival depends on daily insulin injections.

Diabetes is unique both in the degree to which the patients must assume responsibility for their treatment (Milton, 1989) and the degree to which it imposes a pattern on the lives of those affected, which governs their use of time and limits spontaneity in social life. The prescribed regimen is aimed at keeping the BG level as near normal as possible. It requires the individual not only to take tablets or insulin at regular intervals each day and take regular exercise, but also to adhere to a special diet, regulating food timing or intake to take account of levels of energy expended. Regular tests of blood or urine glucose must be undertaken to determine the "success" of their diabetes management. In instances where test readings are outside the recommended limits the person must firstly make a decision (rightly or wrongly) as to what caused the fluctuation (e.g. eating too much food, the timing of medication) and secondly, make an appropriate adjustment (e.g. increasing medication intake). Being able to make the appropriate adjustments means having to constantly monitor daily events (May, 1991).

Sustained hyperglycaemia, in the long-term, is associated with microvascular complications such as retinopathy (which can lead to blindness), estimated to affect 30% of people with diabetes; neuropathy (impaired nerve function), estimated to affect as many as 60% of people with diabetes and nephropathy (which can lead to kidney failure) which was found in one large British sample to have affected 6.8% of people with diabetes (BDA, 1988). Additionally, macrovascular complications (e.g. strokes and coronary heart disease) occur at a younger age and are more prevalent and extreme, compared to the non-diabetic population. Due to the long-term complications associated with diabetes, it is estimated that life expectancy, following diagnosis, is reduced by an average of 30% (Cox *et al.*, 1991).

Besides possible long-term complications, people with diabetes face the daily risk of hypoglycaemia (hypo), whereby blood glucose levels fall below the limit which the body can tolerate, causing cognitive, behavioural, mood and other disturbances. Whilst rare with NIDDM (as a side-effect of a particular group of oral agents, sulphonylureas), the risk with insulin therapy is significantly greater. As BG levels decrease, the symptoms become more severe and if not treated, seizures or a coma can occur. Severe hypoglycaemia is particularly common when BG levels are in tight control (Diabetes Control and Complications Trial, DCCT, 1993). Even so, the recent findings of the DCCT clearly highlight that tight metabolic control significantly prevents or delays the risk of long-term complications.

Due to the unique extent to which diabetes impinges on all areas of a person's life, psychological well-being is important for its successful management. Thus, psychosocial variables and their effects on regimen adherence and BG control have been the subject of a voluminous amount of research in recent decades. Early psychological diabetes research conducted during the 1970's searched in vain for the typical diabetic personality (Dunn and Turtle, 1981). From the early 1980's, a shift in attention occurred towards trying to determine the ultimate psychosocial predictor of adherence and/or control. Despite this change in direction, to date, research has been unable to propose an adequate explanation for non-adherence.

The aim of this chapter is to propose reasons why the psychosocial aspects of diabetes deserve to remain high on the list of the research and clinical agenda and to raise awareness of some important gaps in the literature. In the past decade or so we have not come far enough in addressing many conceptual issues that might advance our broader understanding of non-adherence to the diabetes regimen.

In many countries our societies are multi-cultural, yet little research exists which addresses the particular needs and experiences of different ethnic minorities. For example, in the UK there are large Asian and Afro-Caribbean diabetic populations. They have specific cultural problems and communication difficulties which need addressing. Similarly, relatively little is known about adults living with diabetes. A large amount of research has been conducted with children and adolescents, (for a review of diabetes in children and adolescents, see Bryon, Chapter 7). Yet, most people are diagnosed as adults *and* of course most children with diabetes will go on to be adults with diabetes. Recent research (Warren and Hixenbaugh, 1995) suggests that, regardless of the age of diagnosis, a very real and somewhat different set of problems affect people in adulthood. An in-depth review of the research literature by the authors in preparation for this chapter revealed that when adults have been studied most research has sampled only Caucasian, well-educated people. Because the needs and experiences of adults are in some respects different to those of children and because it is with regard to the adult population that we most need to move our understanding forward, this chapter will focus on diabetes in adulthood.

ADHERENCE AND ITS BARRIERS

Rates of non-adherence to the diabetes regimen are widely acknowledged to be high. This is not surprising given that it has all of the hallmarks of a treatment regimen which make non-adherence predictable. It is lifelong, complex and pervasive. However, research has demonstrated that adherence to one component is unrelated to another for both IDDM's and NIDDM's (Orme and Binik, 1989). Medication is in many cases the most frequently adhered to component, particularly in the case of insulin as it is vital for survival, even though the relationship between prescription and adherence is not considered to be linear (Kelleher, 1988a; Turk and Meichenbaum, 1991). In contrast, between 40% and 80% of people with diabetes under report their blood sugar levels on at least half of their recordings (Mazze *et al.*, 1984; Wilson and Endres, 1986). Comparably, non-adherence to the dietary components is understood to apply to as much as 75% of the diabetic population (Surwit, Scovern and Feinglos, 1982; Christensen *et al.*, 1983).

While the above statistics appear to suggest that determining the rate of patient non-adherence is straightforward, the area is fraught with difficulties: both conceptual and methodological. Conceptually, in spite of the fact that it has been known for some time that glycaemic control is not a reliable measure of adherence due to the interference of other variables such as time of day, severity of illness and appropriateness of the regimen (Peyrot and McMurry, 1985), it is still often the outcome measure of choice in adherence studies. While a handful of studies have managed to demonstrate a small (although significant) relationship between adherence and control (Harris and Linn, 1985; Brownlee-Duffeck *et al.*, 1987), most studies have shown that it is not possible to equate the two (Schafer, McCaul and Glasgow, 1986; Glasgow, McCaul and Schafer, 1987). Those that have shown a relationship have mostly used global measures of adherence. Additionally, it is not possible to ascertain the direction of causality. It could be that rather than adherence having led to better control, better control of blood glucose levels reinforced good adherence. Equally good adherence might not have led to good control (Cox *et al.*, 1986).

A further conceptual difficulty in measuring adherence lies in the fact that patients are not always given a specific regimen to follow. Advice, particularly with regard to diet and exercise, often can be vague and conflicting. In such situations, where an absolute standard does not exist, it is of limited value to talk of non-adherence (Glasgow, 1991).

When measuring rates of non-adherence many studies have used unverified self-reports. New technology has shown that self-report data can be unreliable, over reporting adherence (Christensen *et al.*, 1983; Wilson and Endres, 1986). However, when given the chance to report anonymously, non-adherence figures are much higher (Delameter *et al.*, 1988). Delamater and colleagues suggested that such discrepancies can be largely accounted for by how threatened patients feel about reporting non-adherence. This assertion is backed up by the findings of a recent UK survey whereby 43% of patients (i.e. 205, from a sample of 324 adults with either IDDM or NIDDM) reported that they were regularly untruthful to their health professionals (HPs) regarding their adherence: with a further 20% stating that they were dishonest on occasion. Patients most frequently cited their reasons as being the fear that the HPs would think that they did not take their diabetes seriously and the belief that the HPs would be angry with them (Warren and Hixenbaugh, 1995; 1996b). When conducting research, steps can be taken to make self-report data more reliable, such as having patients report anonymously, however, in the clinical situation health care providers need to be aware of their contribution to unreliable data by being less judgmental (Kurtz, 1990).

As well as impeding our understanding of non-adherence, Kurtz (1990) made the important point that for as long as patients are being untruthful to their HPs, any recommendations that are made on the basis of that information are unlikely to result in effective self-care. What this indicates is that the patient's viewpoint is of importance. To emphasise the point, there is a widely held belief, that patients make-up their self-monitored blood glucose (SMBG) results in order to present a more positive clinical profile. Studies which checked the accuracy of patient BG diaries with memory meters found that patients modifications were inclined towards omitting unacceptable readings and increasing favourable readings (Mazze *et al.*, 1984; Wilson and Endres, 1984). However, more recent evidence suggests that presenting a more positive profile is not the patients intention and that the information available from patients self-report data can be useful. A study of patients with IDDM (Gonder-Frederick *et al.*, 1988) found that not only were BG levels computed from patient diaries *not* significantly lower than those recorded by memory meters, but also that it was the *patients' belief* in the fact that they were using SMBG as often as they should (as opposed to actual frequency of monitoring) that was significantly related to metabolic control. In contrast, diary accuracy had *no* influence on either adherence or metabolic control. Such findings suggest, as the authors emphasised, that attention to the individual's viewpoint could greatly improve our ability to define, recognise and improve SMBG and other regimen components. Of course, this is unlikely to prove of value if the treatment components are considered in isolation to each other. Several studies have demonstrated that merely increasing the frequency of blood glucose monitoring is of negligible benefit if the results obtained are not used to modify other regimen behaviours (Mazze *et al.*, 1985; Marrero *et al.*, 1989).

The diabetes literature in terms of barriers to adherence is difficult to interpret. Three important issues are rarely considered. Firstly, the assumption is made that the prescribed regimen is always appropriate, however, evidence exists that disputes this assumption. Warren and Hixenbaugh (1996b) and Hiss (1986) in large community surveys in the UK and USA, respectively, found that between two thirds and three quarters of those sampled were of the opinion that their prescribed regimen was unsuitable for them. Thus, they rejected it in favour of a self-prescribed regimen that took account of the realities of life. Secondly, despite the fact that adherence to different regimen components is unrelated, most researchers still assume that some underlying assumption, such as a health belief, invariably determines responses to all treatment demands (Orme and Binik, 1989). Finally, researchers, when analysing their data, tended to "aggregate dissimilar patient groups" thereby increasing the possibility of erroneous results (Davis *et al.*, 1987). Studies in which detailed analysis has been undertaken (or which have used fairly homogenous samples), have revealed a number of potentially important relationships. These relationships suggest that different psychosocial variables may predict adherence according to type of diabetes and type of treatment (Davis *et al.*, 1987; Warren and Hixenbaugh, 1996a) and stage of the lifespan (Coates and Boore, 1995; Warren and Hixenbaugh, 1996a). For example, Warren and Hixenbaugh found while the most frequent predictors for patients with NIDDM were diabetes-related health beliefs, these did not predict non-adherence at all for patients with IDDM. Rather, in the case of patients with IDDM, perceived inappropriate psychological support from HPs and significant others was found to be the most reliable predictor of non-adherence. Further research is required to confirm the importance of these factors and to identify other potentially important patient differences.

The fact that studies to date have rarely been able to account for more than 25% of the variance in outcome, even when trying to account for heterogeneity (Bloom Cerkoney and Hart, 1980) suggests that sub-grouping needs further refining. Three possible factors are worthy of future investigation.

Firstly, given the role of genetics in diabetes onset, a significant proportion of the diabetic population will have experienced familial diabetes (quite possibly problematic) by the time of diagnosis. This variable has recently been found to statistically predict 1) failing to take medication and 2) consuming an inappropriate amount of food (Warren and Hixenbaugh, 1995; 1996b). More research is needed to confirm the role of family history and adherence. New patients in this group might well be in need of additional support at diagnosis.

Secondly, a further potential sub-group that should be considered separately are those patients who have had to change treatment: whether it be *beginning* tablets or insulin *or changing* tablet group or type of insulin. The latter is particularly important when patients have been prescribed sulphonylureas or human insulin which increase fears and/or frequency of hypoglycaemic attacks as these have been shown to be both prevalent (Warren and Hixenbaugh, 1995) and predictive of altering medication dose (Irvine, Cox and Gonder-Frederick, 1992). Researchers and HPs often make the assumption that patients on insulin adhere more to their regimen (particularly their medication) as they perceive the disease as more serious. However, Cohen *et al.* (1960) reviewed 73 cases of ketoacidosis and found that the most frequent precipitating factor was non-administration of insulin. Interestingly, over half the patients attributed the omission to psychological stress. What is not known is what caused the psychological stress. A great deal of additional time is afforded routinely to patients new to insulin. However, Warren and Hixenbaugh (1996b) found that while a significant proportion of study participants (94/324) patients had had to change to insulin, only 23% of those were of the opinion that the change had made their diabetes more difficult to manage. Importantly, it was this *belief,* rather than taking insulin per se (i.e. type of treatment), that significantly predicted non-administration of insulin. Furthermore, the belief that treatment change had made diabetes more difficult to manage was also held by the additional 14% of participants who had changed from diet to diet and tablets. For both of these potential patient groups, the belief was significantly predictive of non-adherence to many aspects of the diabetes regimen: although it is important to note that the patterns of non-adherence were not directly comparable. Further research is needed to confirm a possible link between the stress associated with regimen change and non-adherence. We also need to determine whether there is a point in time, in terms of duration of the disease, when people become resistant to the demands required from a change in treatment.

Thirdly, lifespan factors such as age and duration of diabetes need far more attention if we are to move towards a comprehensive understanding of adherence. While no conclusive evidence is available, one possible reason for researchers in the field not having been able to identify valid clinical predictors of adherence is lack of consideration of the dynamic nature of self-care. For example, in the case of the regimen component of SMBG, it was found that adults who were diagnosed as children or adolescents were significantly more likely to be non-adherent by *falsifying* readings, whereas for those diagnosed as adults non-adherence occurred in relation to *omitting* BG (or urine glucose) readings (Warren and Hixenbaugh, 1996b). Furthermore, it cannot be assumed, as is often the case, that barriers to adherence remain constant. Warren and Hixenbaugh (1996b) found that, for those in the age-group between 18 and 50 years, self-reported non-adherence was most likely in the company of *work colleagues* (33%), in contrast, people over 50 years of age most frequently reported that non-adherence occurred in the company of *friends* (28% -compared to 12% for work colleagues). Equally, men, in comparison to women, reported more non-adherence in the company of work colleagues as opposed to friends.

THE ROLE OF HEALTH BELIEFS

The Health Belief Model (HBM, e.g. Becker and Maiman, 1975), makes the assumption that perceived vulnerability to the disease, perceived seriousness of the disease, and degree of interest in health matters, when considered together, will determine an individual's level of adherence. These variables will also be affected by cues to action (which can be internal –such as thoughts; or external –such as prompts) and further will be modified by experience. According to the HBM it is the individual's *subjective* view of the components that is important. For a full description of the model, see Horne and Weinman, Chapter 2.

Despite a relatively sizeable database of diabetes related research, support for the model remains equivocal. While some studies have found that either individual components or combinations were positively related to adherence (Alogna, 1980; Bloom Cerkoney and Hart, 1980), other studies have failed to find support for the model (Harris and Linn, 1985). However, as yet, the relationship between health beliefs and adherence has not been demonstrated sufficiently to provide useful clinical predictors (Schlenk and Hart, 1984). May

(1991) and deWeerdt *et al.* (1989) have suggested that the model lacks the ability to demonstrate cause and effect. Indeed, May has gone as far as to suggest that levels of regimen adherence in fact *determine* health beliefs. If this is the case, then as behaviour varies across the regimen we cannot expect the model to be of any significant value. Shillitoe and Miles (1989) moved this conceptual argument one step further, asserting that due to the *changing relationship* between beliefs, behaviour and outcomes, information gleaned from the model is unlikely to be stable and, therefore, of predictive value, over time. Furthermore, Hochbaum (1983) has made the critical point that beliefs, *other* than health beliefs, are equally important.

Two factors could potentially improve the clinical predictiveness of the HBM. The first is to use validated diabetes specific scales (Lewis and Bradley, 1994). The use of these has met with some success when used in studies designed to try to understand differences in choice of treatment and to assess treatment efficacy. However, Lewis and Bradley noted that the relationship between health beliefs and adherence was found to be weakened by both lack of patient knowledge and the existence of competing priorities. Also, NIDDM specific measures of disease severity were found to be related to control in the *opposite* direction to that which the model would predict.

The second factor that could potentially strengthen the validity of the HBM is one that appears not to have been given consideration to date. It is possible that either 1) health beliefs change *predictably* over time and/or the duration of the disease, or that 2) health beliefs regarding diabetes remain static but that their relationship with behaviour alters systematically over time. For example, for the significant proportion of the population who go on to develop long-term complications (Leese, 1992; Marks, 1996), the onset of such complications, could be a time when the belief in personal vulnerability develops. Alternatively, whilst a pre-held belief in personal vulnerability could have increased adherence to certain aspects of the regimen *prior* to the appearance of complications, upon the onset of complications, the belief, although maybe still held, might well no longer act as a stimulus for adherence, given the fact that complications arose *despite* efforts to reduce that personal vulnerability (Warren and Hixenbaugh, 1996a). The fact that different studies have reported conflicting findings could be an artefact of the stage of the lifespan of the sample employed. For instance, in the study carried out by Alogna (1980) many of her participants were fairly newly diagnosed with 84% of them having been diagnosed for less than 12 years. Other research has divided the sample into age groups (Brownlee-Duffeck *et al.*, 1987). Under such conditions, data analysis revealed that for adolescents the only individual health belief variable to predict adherence was the perceived cost of adhering. However, for adults perceived benefits predicted adherence. When combining the sample, however, perceived susceptibility was significantly correlated with adherence, but in the *wrong direction*, such that increased perceived susceptibility was associated with decreased adherence. Thus, as well as the scales needing to be more specific, the populations with diabetes to which they apply need to be given greater consideration in order to confirm or refute the model's validity. This point could also apply to the *degree* to which these beliefs are held. Kurtz, (1990) has suggested that the relationship between the HBM components of perceived susceptibility and severity are curvilinearly related to adherence, such that too strong a belief (accompanied by excessive anxiety) or too weak a belief (accompanied by too little anxiety) would inhibit adherence. In the absence of such considerations the HBM is unlikely to develop into a reliable clinical predictor.

KNOWLEDGE: ITS ACQUISITION AND FUNCTION

Affording the patient knowledge about diabetes and its treatment is almost exclusively the only intervention aimed at enhancing adherence delivered as a routine part of diabetes care. The reasons for this are threefold. Firstly, those delivering health care rightly assume that a patient will be unable to follow the complex regimen in the absence of such an understanding. Secondly, the nature of medical training (coupled with time constraints within the clinic) means that HPs may not have the skills or resources to offer alternative forms of intervention which might further enhance patient adherence (Nichols, 1984; Shillitoe, 1991). Thirdly, research has revealed that patients frequently incorrectly perform a range of diabetes self-care activities (Strube, Yost and Haire-Joshu, 1993).

When the outcomes of additional education interventions have been evaluated, the benefits have been found to be limited to improving adherence to the medical aspects of the regimen i.e., adjusting insulin and SMBG (Rubin, Peyrot and Saudek, 1991). In a study designed to enhance psychosocial functioning, with a sample of older men with NIDDM, the beneficial effects were maximised when spouses were involved in the education program (Gilden *et al.*, 1989). However, the younger adults (aged 28–64 years) reported a *decrease* in quality of life.

Studies using a randomised design (Korhonen *et al.*, 1983; Rettig *et al.*, 1986; Wilson and Pratt, 1987) all showed that, while education programs increased knowledge about diabetes management, this increase did not lead to improved long-term glycaemic control or to reduced hospitalisations. Education programs, designed for those with established diabetes, need to take account of patients' control. A study conducted by Strube, Yost and Haire-Joshu (1993) found that when patients in poor control were given educational intervention, negative psychological reactions occurred. This most probably transpired due to the enhanced knowledge increasing self-blame and stress. Naturally, this could lead to further disruption in metabolic control. A meta-analysis of education studies (Brown, 1992) determined that *individualised* education, which accounted for each patient's needs, was preferential to group education. Importantly, length of education was not important: suggesting that quality was the key to improved adherence. This is significant from the point of view that most people have been found not to be willing or motivated enough to take extended periods of time out to partake in lengthy programs (Rubin *et al.*, 1991).

One final point that should be taken into consideration is the level of knowledge of the HPs and it's effect on patient adherence. Evidence exists to suggest that greater knowledge on the part of the physician is not predictive of success in managing their patients. Rather, certain beliefs, whether justified or not, are able to differentiate those patients who are well managed from those who are not (Weinberger, Cohen and Mazzuca, 1984). Weinberger and his colleagues suggested that the relationship between the development of such beliefs and successful patient management is dynamic, such that HPs with certain beliefs manage diabetes more successfully, which in turn reinforces those critical beliefs. Thus, just as some patients' attitudes need changing through education, the role of HPs' attitudes needs to be given consideration.

FAMILY/SOCIAL SUPPORT

Whilst many studies have examined how diabetes affects the family and indeed, how the family affects diabetes, virtually all investigations have focused on children with diabetes and their relationship with their mothers only. Most investigations have employed metabolic control as their dependent variable, rather than regimen adherence. Therefore, the complexities of family interactions and their relationship with adherence in adult populations with diabetes are not understood well enough to enable translation of the research findings into effective interventions, either to enhance adherence to the regimen, the psychosocial status of patients with diabetes, or to prevent psychosocial problems. However, both the existing research and clinical data pertaining to adults and children reinforce the fact that the impact of diabetes on the family cannot be overemphasised, due to it necessitating unwelcome changes in family routines and lifestyle. Although most studies have found chronic illness to have a negative effect on the family (Springer, 1985; Schafer *et al.*, 1986), others have found either positive, or no significant effects (Peyrot, McMurry and Hedges, 1988). Equally, all studies reveal substantial variability in the effects of chronic illness, illustrating that there is no single, intransigent response.

Most *general* social support research underscores the centrality of the marital relationship as a major source of support (Brown, 1978). However, it is important to recognise that many marital relationships are, at the same time, an active source of stress: the effect of which can be to reduce adherence to the regimen (Warren and Hixenbaugh 1995; Warren and Hixenbaugh, 1996b). This issue has been demonstrated to be particularly pertinent when one partner has diabetes. Lewis *et al.* (1989) carried out a study into the effect of family functioning, with chronic illness in the mother. They found that the presence of diabetes, in contrast to breast cancer, negatively affected marital adjustment. The authors determined that this was due to male partners with diabetes, in contrast to the partners of women with breast cancer, being unable to attribute behavioural and affective changes following diagnosis in terms of their illness. This finding also serves to underscore the possible problems arising from HPs underplaying the degree to which diabetes can affect daily functioning, in terms of the frequent occurrence of symptoms such as tiredness and mood changes. Indeed, 1 in 3 of the population of adults with IDDM or NIDDM surveyed by Warren and Hixenbaugh (1996b) believed that, as a result of feeling tired due to their diabetes, they made less effort towards the marital relationship.

In an effort to explain the mixed findings derived from family functioning studies, rather than simply examining *levels* of support, Bailey and Kahn (1993) in an interesting study of adults wth IDDM, examined how individuals with diabetes evaluate and respond to spousal help. They found that two factors were fundamental in shaping responses to spousal help: perceived need and perceived spousal motivation. They suggested that these perceptions might be responsive to change, with improved communication between partners. This could be achieved through intervention, with the aim of enhancing the quality of spousal interaction and thus, self-management behaviours. Several studies support this contention. Inclusion of significant others in health-care programs has been shown to significantly improve regimen adherence (Brownell *et al.*, 1978; Shenkel *et al.*, 1985–86). To maximise the effects, negotiation between the dyad (i.e., the ability of both partners to compromise) and appropriate interpersonal skills need to be addressed (Peyrot *et al.*, 1988). In order to avoid long-term problems, these issues need to be addressed at the point of diagnosis, as the way in which this initial crisis is handled has been found to influence future coping responses (Jensen, 1985).

If family communication is absent, support is unlikely to be in line with that is wanted by the patient. When this is the case, offers of support (in the form of reminders to take medication, eat less etc.) have been found to be taken as criticism and, therefore, resented. Research has determined that this "unwanted" support is related *directly* to non-adherence to the regimen (Warren and Hixenbaugh, 1995) and *indirectly* through it's relationship with depression, stress and anxiety (Manne and Zautra, 1989; Littlefield *et al.*, 1990; Bailey and Kahn, 1993; Warren and Hixenbaugh, 1995).

In summary, in the area of familial support, diabetes specific support, rather than global family functioning is deemed to be the best predictor of adherence. This is true with regard to medication taking, diet, glucose testing and exercise (Glasgow and Toobert, 1988).

While it is apparent that the social environment is important to the control of diabetes, the role of those outside of the family in this process is unclear. When assessing the role of friends, Kaplan and

Hartwell (1987), using global measures of support, found that for men with NIDDM, in contrast to women, good support was associated with poor control. When using diabetes specific measures, *perceived good support* for both men and women was found to be significantly related to *non-adherence* (Warren and Hixenbaugh, 1996b). The social support function of work colleagues is unknown, as is the impact of diabetes on the career.

While many critical questions remain unanswered in the area of social support, the research to date clearly indicates that it is the individual's *perceptions* of relationships and their nature and function, termed a "functional perspective" (Cohen and Lyme, 1985), rather than more "objective" measures such as network size, which are likely to give researchers and clinicians alike the best guidance in determining reasons for non-adherence to the regimen. Further research needs to be undertaken to investigate whether friends and work colleagues (and for that matter school and college associates) have a significant role to play in diabetes management. If they do, future interventions will have to give much more attention to the role of the community in terms of the barriers it creates to adherence.

THE ROLE OF THE HEALTH PROFESSIONAL

The notion of the patient as an active decision maker in terms of his or her own care is at the heart of recent changes in the health service in Britain. If HPs are to contribute effectively, with the patient's role having been redefined, they need to recognise that they will have to consider the *patient's viewpoint.*

Patients with diabetes have expressed a need for a more individual approach to treatment that takes account of their changing needs throughout the course of the disease (Hares *et al.*, 1992; Warren and Hixenbaugh, 1995). However, Hallett, (1994) has stated that "many HPs are still not listening closely enough to what people say their needs are". One way to meet patient needs could be to tailor advice to fit into patients existing beliefs and expectations and take into account the constraints imposed on individuals by their everyday lives (Donovan, 1995). This will be difficult to achieve for as long as medical training fails to shift its emphasis from the traditional biomedical approach to one that is biopsychosocial in it's orientation. As recently as 1991, Whitehouse in a large scale survey of UK medical schools, found that the routine training of communication skills designed to teach medical students to take account of the patient's viewpoint was still patchy, with some schools not even addressing such issues. Negative staff attitudes were cited as a major barrier. The situation was seen to be comparable in the USA.

The notion of patient participation implies that they are given the right to decline to follow advice or alter it without recrimination (Coates and Boore, 1995). Given that the prescription is often too general, many patients find themselves *having* to alter their prescribed regimen. Furthermore, it is still the case, far too often, that patients are faced with a potentially unsympathetic, angry or dismissive physician (Groen and Pelser, 1982; Warren and Hixenbaugh, 1995). In such cases patients will often withhold or make up information regarding self-care (DiMatteo and DiNicola, 1982). This is a well established barrier to adherence (Kurtz, 1990; Warren and Hixenbaugh, 1996b). One question that is frequently asked is why, under such circumstances, do people continue to attend clinic? The answer is that it probably makes them feel less vulnerable, i.e., they use it as a personal risk-reducing strategy. The recent survey by Warren and Hixenbaugh (1996b) found that the only significant predictor of avoiding clinic visits (from a broad range of demographic and psychosocial variables) was a perceived lack of psychological support from the health-care team. For suggestedly similar reasons, Jacobson et al., (1991) found that infrequent clinic attendees were those in poor control. Of course, this should not be taken to mean that those who attend clinic regularly are necessarily satisfied with their treatment. Equally, patient satisfaction should not be the only outcome measure of the adequacy of the doctor/patient relationship. This is because there are those that will be satisfied with less than optimal care and also because it has not been established whether, or in combination with which other factors, patient satisfaction leads to better adherence (Kaplan, Greenfield and Ware, 1989).

Three factors serve as potential barriers towards a shift in the role of the health professional. Firstly, the findings of the DCCT Research Group, whilst welcomed for their contribution to the understanding of ways by which to improve the long-term quality of life, have raised concerns that HPs will face an even greater pressure to focus the care of diabetes on metabolic control, *at the expense* of psychological well-being (Bradley, 1994) and quality of life in the short and medium term (Guppy, 1994). Secondly, being given the skills necessary to change their approach to treatment will only be of benefit provided health team members have the support they need to employ them. Thirdly, teaching HPs communication skills will not guarantee a change in their attitudes and beliefs, which were found by Gamsu and Bradley (1987) to contain a self-serving bias: such that the treatment *they* recommended was seen as responsible for positive outcomes, in contrast to negative outcomes, which instead were seen as the fault of the patient. Research needs to ascertain if, and how, these barriers to change might be overcome. One way of getting HPs to see regimen adherence from the patient's perspective might be to have them, during their training, mimic living as a person with diabetes. Two very enlightening studies, getting hospital staff to do just that (Welborn and Duncan, 1980; Warren-Boulton, Auslander and Gettinger, 1982) showed that regimen adherence was very low, diabetes problems were frequent and that participants were surprised at how much time the regimen took up. Welborn and Duncan reported that one participant abandoned the trial on day 3 —due to domestic tensions! An alternative strategy examined by Gillespie and Bradley (1988), ascertained that when, between them, doctor and patient discussed patient problems with the aim of reaching agreement about the nature and causes of problems being experienced, it was the doctors attributions that were changed to be more in line with the patients'. A trend towards better control was also noted. It is possible that over longer periods of time, during which a greater understanding could be built, the level of improvement could reach significance. This is worthy of future investigation.

One suggested reason for the discrepancy in doctor/patient attitudes and beliefs is that they have very different goals to treatment. In one study which examined these beliefs, the goal of treatment of the parents of children with diabetes was found to be related to beliefs about the short-term complication of hypos. In contrast, doctors goals were related to concern over long-term complications (Marteau *et al.*, 1987). This difference in beliefs was suggested by the authors to be due to differences between the groups in terms of exposure. This study serves to illustrate the point that doctor and patient should discuss the goals of treatment. If doctors wish patients' self-care to be more oriented towards achieving long-term goals, they will need to be candid with patients with regard to issues such as the risk of complications. Of course, this will be difficult unless they have the time and skills to give patients the support to come to terms with these issues. There were many instances in the survey by Warren and Hixenbaugh (1995) of patients citing complications of diabetes, such as heart problems and circulation problems as illnesses independent of diabetes. In addition, only 41% of those surveyed were of the opinion that they had been given an adequate explanation of complications.

In the last few decades we have become much more knowledgeable regarding effective ways of imparting knowledge and aiding patient recall, such as using concrete specific advice and checking patients understanding (see Sanson Fisher *et al.*, 1989). However, these skills are unlikely to make a clinically relevant impact on adherence unless these broader issues are addressed.

BEHAVIOURAL INTERVENTION

Some psychologists, rather than viewing non-adherence as being the result of some underlying attitude or belief, prefer to conceive of it as a behaviour problem (Gross, 1987). Based upon this assumption, they argue that clinicians should identify specific responses in need of alteration which will allow them to make use of well established behaviour modification techniques to increase adherence. This means that the HP should consider the consequences of a particular behaviour in terms of whether the patient associates that behaviour with reward or punishment. For instance, eating snacks prevents a hypo, therefore, because the behaviour (eating a snack) *relieves* the discomfort associated with a hypo, the outcome serves as a reward and so increases the frequency of occurrence (i.e. it reinforces the behaviour). In contrast, testing blood (or urine) glucose, as well as taking time to do, means having to draw attention to yourself regularly. Thus, the outcome is regarded as unpleasant (aversive) and so is likely to decrease the frequency of occurrence. However, even those components which are not aversive, such as taking medication in the form of tablets (patients with NIDDM), have a considerable rate of non-adherence (Wing *et al.*, 1985). Equally, for patients with NIDDM, SMBG does not have to be frequent (9 times per week) to be effective, yet, Wing *et al.*, (1984) found that adherence reduced over the course of a 37 week program to 60% of the sample. Thus, almost all components of the regimen can be seen as aversive and in the few cases where sub-components may not be perceived as aversive, adherence is still low. Unfortunately, one added barrier to self-care is that *good control* of diabetes in the short-term can bring unfavourable consequences in the form of hypo's. It is the role of the doctor to convince the patient that the discomfort or inconvenience in the short-term will bring rewards (by avoiding complications) in the long-term (Gross, 1987). In order to achieve this, reinforcements, such as praise for appropriate behaviour, must be immediate.

Many behavioural techniques have been tested, such as giving patients feedback and contracting, to try and improve adherence in both patients with IDDM and patients with NIDDM. Most have been in the area of dietary adherence and weight loss. However, there is not enough research to date to determine which are effective for all diabetic populations. This is because many of the studies have investigated only adults with IDDM or children. Furthermore, the majority have only used small numbers of participants, thus reducing their applicability. Also, importantly, many have shown no benefit of behavioural intervention over standard care. A further limitation of research in this area is that most of the investigations employed several methods concurrently, so it is impossible to determine which components worked for who. Equally, because participants were rarely followed up we know little about rates of relapse. When follow-ups were included, the results were not encouraging (Wing *et al.*, 1985). The best evidence for the effectiveness of behavioural interventions has been in the area of teaching social skills to children with the purpose of enabling them to resist peer pressure (Kaplan, Chadwick and Schimmel, 1985): although the exact nature of the intervention was not reported. This is an area that is worthy of investigation with adults: particularly as social pressure has been found to be a significant barrier to adherence for adults, regardless of gender or type of diabetes (Warren and Hixenbaugh, 1996a).

Another possible line of future enquiry would be to determine the benefit of spousal support in behavioural intervention. A well controlled study, investigating weight loss in people without diabetes, conducted by Brownell *et al.* (1978), found that obese men and women lost more weight and sustained the significant losses at 6 month follow-up when their spouses attended the (cognitive behavioural) program meetings with them. This was compared both to a group whose spouses were willing to attend but were not required to *and* to a group whose partners refused to attend. The aim of the program was to train both partners in behavioural techniques designed to reduce caloric intake and change dietary habits, for example, mutual monitoring of each others eating habits. It was stressed that joint effort was important. The *couple*, rather than the participant, was reinforced by the group leader for habit change, in order to enhance the spirit of *mutuality*. Evidence from within the field of diabetes suggests that it is encouraging the spirit of mutuality which was the key to the success of the intervention. A study by Wing *et al.* (1987) in which individuals with diabetes and their overweight spouses were involved in a similar program that did *not* foster the spirit of mutuality found that the *spouses* lost *more* weight than their partner with diabetes, possibly due to a competitive factor. Even though in the Brownell *et al.* study the partner was not needy of the treatment, the fact that he or she was able, through understanding, to support the partner, suggests that in diabetes education programs spousal support could be a beneficial addition.

To date, no single intervention has been shown to be useful on its own (Turk and Meichenbaum, 1991). The problem is that if multiple intervention techniques are needed to improve adherence to the multifaceted components of the regimen, the intervention could become unmanageable. For example, Wing *et al.* (1985) evaluated a behaviour modification program, employing numerous behavioural techniques, such as self-monitoring of caloric intake and exercise, goal setting, stimulus control and contingency contracts, with the aim of changing eating and exercise habits. This method was compared to a group receiving nutrition education and a standard care control group. While those people in the behaviour modification group had lost significantly more weight than the other two groups by the end of the study, it would be difficult to determine which of the techniques (or combination) used were responsible for the improvements. Furthermore, the gains were not sustained at 16 month follow-up. It would be problematic to ascertain whether the failure to sustain the initial gains was due either to there being too few behavioural strategies employed (or perhaps the wrong combination), or whether, in fact, there were *too many* techniques for patients (or at least for some patients) to manage on a long-term basis. Thus, when multiple strategies are evaluated simultaneously it is difficult to assess which of them, and in what combinations, are effective (Southam and Dunbar, 1986). However, because adherence to any one component of the diabetes regimen, in order to be successful, requires adherence to each of the other components simultaneously, multiple techniques are no doubt required. One possible way forward could be to devise modular programs whereby patients could select the parts of the intervention program that were acceptable to them (Bradley, 1994). This could not only potentially help to ascertain which particular modules were most effective, but would also greatly improve the cost-effectiveness of such treatments.

THE PATIENT'S PERSPECTIVE

The fact that the perceived social impact of diabetes has been shown to be significantly related to the risk of mortality (Davis, Hess and Hiss, 1988) and that patients beliefs and emotions affect their regimen adherence (Hampson, Glasgow and Toobert, 1990), serves as further evidence for the need to conduct additional research which takes account of the patient's perspective to determine whether it is amenable to change.

Qualitative research suggests that an individual's self-care routine, rather than being grounded in the theoretical principles of diabetes management imparted by HPs, is managed by learning to recognise patterns of their own physical, lifestyle and psychological responses to the disease, according to individual experience: in response to which the patient determines a self-care routine which works for them (Price, 1993). While Price reported that the HP's advice was deemed by patients to be important during the *initial* stages of the disease: this was gradually superseded by what she termed "body listening", which is a process of internal, subjective monitoring by the individual as to how they feel physically and in terms of their diabetes. Perhaps this finding was due largely to the fact that most patients still view their health care in terms of the inflexible and unrealistic medical model (Wikblad, 1991). Further research is needed to ascertain if this model can be applied to populations other than Caucasian people with IDDM.

The notion of people altering their regimen has been addressed by other researchers. Kelleher, (1988b) investigating adherence from the patient's perspective, found that patients who had altered their prescribed regimen in an effort to have their diabetes fit in with their life, rather than have their life fit in with their diabetes, were labelled by medics as "difficult patients". Again, they rejected the prescribed regimen because they felt that their own knowledge was more appropriate than the doctors generalised scientific knowledge. Interestingly, they were the only ones deemed to be coping both physically and psychologically with their regimen.

SUMMARY

Diabetes is a complex disease in terms of its management, which requires substantial motivation and effort on the part of the individual affected. Due to the fact that diabetes impinges on all areas of a person's life the potential barriers to adherence are numerous. Attempts to overcome these barriers require not only adequate patient education, but also understanding and psychosocial support from the HPs who are involved with patient management. Theoretical models from within field of health psychology have provided both researchers and clinicians with frameworks with which to understand, explain and predict non-adherence and furthermore, with tools with which to develop strategies to increase the commonly accepted poor rates of adherence. However, until very recently, neither researchers nor health care providers adequately considered the patient's perspective, which means that many potentially important factors that might aid our understanding have yet to be fully explored. The recent shift in emphasis within health care of the role of the patient, from one in which the patient is viewed as a passive recipient of advice, towards one in which the patient is encouraged to be an active participant in the care of their health, will no doubt result in a change of focus within diabetes research. Indeed, there is already evidence of such a change. There is also now much more stress on qualitative inquiry. These shifts should prove to be advantageous, not least because studies adopting such an approach can be more readily understood by HPs without psychological training. Equally, the patients themselves should more readily adhere to a regimen in which their preferences and difficulties have been considered and in which they have had input. In the absence of making the perspective of the patients (and indeed their families) the focus of clinical care and research, improving levels of adherence to the degree deemed necessary by the DCCT (1993) could prove an insurmountable challenge.

Acknowledgements

This work was partly supported by a research grant awarded to Laura Warren and Dr. Paula Hixenbaugh from Glaxo Wellcome UK Ltd.

REFERENCES

Alogna, M. (1980) Perception of severity of disease and health locus of control in compliant and non-compliant diabetic patients. *Diabetes Care* **3**, 533–534.

Bailey, B.J. and Kahn, A. (1993) Apportioning illness management authority: how diabetic individuals respond to help. *Qualitative Health Research* **3**, 55–73.

Becker, M.H. and Maiman, L.A. (1975) Sociobehavioural determinants of compliance. In D.L. Sackett and R.B. Haynes (eds.) *Compliance with therapeutic regimens.* Baltimore: John Hopkins University Press.

Bloom Cerkoney, K.A. and Hart, L.K. (1980) The relationship between the health belief model and compliance of persons with diabetes mellitus. *Diabetes Care* **3**, 594–598.

Bradley, C. (1994) Contributions of psychology to diabetes management. *British Journal of Clinical Psychology* **33**, 11–21.

British Diabetic Association, (1988) *Diabetes in the United Kingdom: a Report.*

British Diabetic Association, (1996) *Diabetes in the United Kingdom: a Report.*

Brown, B.B. (1978) Social and psychological correlates of help-seeking behaviour among adults. *American Journal of Community Psychology* **6**, 4, 425–439.

Brown, S. (1992) Meta-analysis of diabetes patient education research: variations in intervention effects across studies. *Researching in Nursing and Health* **15**, 409–419.

Brownell, K.D., Heckerman, C.L., Westlake, R.J., Hayes, S.C. and Monti, P.M. (1978) The effect of couples training and partner co-operativeness in the behavioural treatment of obesity. *Behaviour Research and Therapy* **16**, 323–333.

Brownlee-Duffeck, M., Peterson, L., Simonds, J., Goldstein, D., Kilo, C., and Hoette, S. (1987) The role of health beliefs and regimen adherence and metabolic control of adolescents and adults with diabetes mellitus. *Journal of Consulting and Clinical Psychology* **55**, 139–144.

Christensen, N.K., Terry, R.D., Wyatt, S., Pichert, J.W. and Lorenz, R.W. (1983). Quantitative assessment of dietary adherence in patients with insulin dependent diabetes mellitus. *Diabetes Care* **6**, 245–250..

Coates, V.E. and Boore, J.R. (1995) Self-management of chronic illness: implications for nursing. *International Journal of Nursing Studies* **32**, 628–640.

Cohen, S. and Lyme, S.L. (1985) Issues in the study and application of social support. In S. Cohen and S.L. Lyme (eds.) *Social support and health*. New York: Academic Press.

Cohen, A.S., Vance, V.K., Runyan, J.W. and Horwitz, D. (1960) Diabetic acidosis: an evaluation of the cause, course and therapy of 73 cases. *Annals of Internal Medicine* **52**, 55–86.

Cox, D.J. and Gonder-Frederick, L. (1992) Major developments in behavioural diabetes research. *Journal of Consulting and Clinical Psychology* **60**, 28–638.

Cox, D.J., Gonder-Frederick, L., Pohl, S. and Pennebaker, J.W. (1986) Diabetes. In K. Holroyd and T. Creer (eds.) *Self management of chronic disease: handbook of clinical interventions and research*. New York: Academic Press.

Cox, D.J., Gonder-Frederick, L. and Saunders, J.T. (1991) Diabetes: clinical issues and management. In J.J. Sweet, R.H. Rozensky and S.M. Tovain (eds.) *Handbook of clinical psychology in medical settings*. New York: Plenum.

Davis, W.K., Hess, G.E. and Hiss, R.G. (1988) Psychosocial correlates of survival in diabetes. *Diabetes Care* **11**, 538–545.

Davis, W.K., Hess, G.E., Van Harrison, R. and Hiss, R. G. (1987) Psychosocial adjustment to and control of diabetes mellitus: differences by type and treatment. *Health Psychology* **6**, 1–14.

Delameter, A.M., Kurtz, S.M., White, N.H. and Santiago, J.V. (1988) Effects of social demand on reports of self-monitored blood glucose in adolescents with type 1 diabetes mellitus. *Journal of Applied Social Psychology* **18**, 491–502.

DCCT Research Group, (1993) The effect of intensive treatment of diabetes on the development and progression of long-term complications in insulin-dependent diabetes mellitus. *New England Journal of Medicine* **329**, 977–986.

deWeerdt, I., Visser, A. and van der Veen, E. (1989) Attitude behaviour and theories in diabetes education programmes. *Patient Education and Counselling* **14**, 3–19.

DiMatteo, MR. and DiNicola, D.D. (1982) *Achieving patient compliance: The psychology of the medical practitioners role*. New York. Pergamon Press.

Donovan, J.L. (1995) Patient decision making: The missing ingredient in compliance research. *International Journal of Technology Assessment in Health Care* **11**, 443–455.

Dunn, S.M. and Turtle, J.R. (1981) The myth of the diabetic personality. *Diabetes Care* **4**, 640–647.

Gamsu, D.S. and Bradley, C. (1987) Clinical staff's attributions about diabetes: scale development and staff vs. patient comparisons. *Current Psychological Research and Reviews* **6**, 69–78.

Gilden, J.L., Hendryx, M., Casia, C. and Singh, S.P. (1989) The effectiveness of diabetes education programs for older patients and their spouses. *Journal of the American Geriatric Society* **37**, 1023–1030.

Gillespie, C.R. and Bradley, C. (1988) Causal attributions of doctor and patients in a diabetes clinic. *British Journal of Clinical Psychology* **27**, 67–76.

Glasgow, R.E. (1991) Compliance to diabetes regimens. In J.A. Cramer and B. Spiker (eds.) *Patient compliance in clinical trials*. New York: Raven Press.

Glasgow, R.E., McCaul, K.D. and Schafer, L.C. (1987) Self-care behaviours and glycaemic control in type 1 diabetes. *Journal of Chronic Diseases* **40**, 399–412.

Glasgow, R.E. and Toobert, D.J. (1988) Social environment and regimen adherence among type II diabetic patients. *Diabetes Care* **11**, 377–386.

Gonder-Frederick, L.A., Julian, M.A., Cox, D.J., Clarke, W.L. and Carter, W.R. (1988) Self-measurement of blood glucose: accuracy of self-reported data and adherence to recommended regimen. *Diabetes Care* **11**, 579–585.

Groen, J.J. and Pelser, H.E. (1982) Psychosocial aspects in the therapy of diabetes. *Paediatric and Adolescent Endocrinology* **10**, 168–177.

Gross, A.M. (1987) A behavioural approach to the compliance problems of young diabetics. *The Journal of Compliance in Health Care* **2**, 7–21.

Guppy, T. (1994) The DCCT results: My own view. *Balance* **140**, III.

Hallett, L. (1994) Are doctors communicating? *Balance* **140**, 12–15.

Hampson, S.E., Glasgow, R.E. and Toobert, D.J. (1990) Personal models of diabetes and their relations to self-care activities. *Health Psychology* **9**, 632–646.

Hares, T., Spencer, J., Gallaher, M., Bradshaw, C. and Webb, I. (1992) Diabetes care: who are the experts? *Quality in Health Care* **1**, 219–224.

Harris, R. and Linn, M.W. (1985) Health beliefs, compliance and control of diabetes mellitus. *Southern Medical Journal* **78**, 162–166.

Hiss, R.G. (1986) *Diabetes in communities.* Ann Arbor, MI: University of Michigan.

Hixenbaugh, P. and Warren, L. (1994) Psychological well-being and adherence in diabetic patients. Presented at the XXVI International Congress of Psychology. August, Montreal, Canada.

Hixenbaugh, P. and Warren, L. (1996) Counselling Psychology in the Treatment of Diabetes Mellitus: Establishing the Need. Presented at the British Psychological Society Counselling Division 3rd Annual Conference. April, York, UK.

Hochbaum, G.M. (1983) The Health Belief Model revisited. Presented at the AHPA meeting; November, Dallas, USA.

Irvine, A.A., Cox, D. and Gonder-Frederick, L. (1992) Fear of hypoglycaemia: relationship to physical and psychological symptoms in patients with insulin-dependent diabetes mellitus. *Health Psychology* **11**, 135–138.

Jacobson, A.M., Adler, A.G., Derby, L., Anderson, B.J. and Wolsdorf, J.I. (1991) Clinic attendance and glycaemic control. *Diabetes Care* **14**, 7, 599–601.

Jensen, S.B. (1985) Emotional aspects in diabetes mellitus: a study of somatopsychological reactions in 51 couples in which one partner has insulin-treated diabetes. *Journal of Psychosomatic Research* **29**, 353–359.

Kaplan, R.M., Chadwick, M.W. and Schimmel, L.E. (1985) Social learning intervention to promote metabolic control in type I diabetes mellitus: pilot experiment results. *Diabetes Care* **8**, 152–155.

Kaplan, S.H., Greenfield, S. and Ware, J.E. (1989) Assessing the effects of physician-patient interactions on the outcomes of chronic disease. *Medical Care* **27**, S110–S127.

Kaplan, R.M. and Hartwell, S.L. (1987) Differential effects of social support and social network on physiological and social outcomes in men and women with Type II diabetes mellitus. *Health Psychology* **16**, 387–398.

Kelleher, D. (1988a) *Diabetes.* London: Routledge.

Kelleher, D. (1988b) Coming to terms with diabetes: coping strategies and non-compliance. In R. Anderson and M. Bury (eds.) *Living with chronic illness: the experience of patients and their families.* London: Unwin Hyman.

Korhonen, T., Huttenen, J.K., Aro, A., Hentinen, M., Ihalainen, O., Majander, H., Siitoren, O., Uusitupa, M. and Pyorala, K (1983) A controlled trial of the effects of patient education in the treatment of insulin dependent diabetes. *Diabetes Care* **6**, 256–261.

Kurtz, S.M. (1990) Adherence to diabetes regimens: empirical status and clinical applications. *Diabetes Educator* **16**, 50–56.

Leese, B. (1992) The cost of diabetes and its complications. *Social Science and Medicine* **35**, 1303–1310.

Lewis, K.S. and Bradley, C. (1994) Measures of diabetes specific health beliefs. In C. Bradley (ed.) *Handbook of psychology and diabetes.* Harwood Academic Publishers.

Lewis, M.L., Woods, N.F., Hough, E.E. and Bensley, L.S. (1989). The family's functioning with chronic illness in the mother: the spouses perspective. *Social Science and Medicine,* **29** 1261–1269.

Littlefield, C.H., Rodin, G.M., Murray, M.A. and Craven, J.L. (1990) Influence of functional impairment and social support on depressive symptoms in persons with diabetes. *Health Psychology* **9**, 737–749.

Manne, S.L. and Zautra, A.J. (1989) Spouse criticism and support: their association with coping and psychological adjustment among women with rheumatoid arthritis. *Journal of Personality and Social Psychology* **56**, 608–617.

Marks, L. (1996) *Counting the cost: The real impact of non-insulin dependent diabetes.* A report by the King's Fund Policy Institute. London: British Diabetic Association.

Marrero, D.G., Kronz, K.K., Golden, M.P., Wright, J.C., Orr, D.P. and Fineberg, N.S. (1989) Clinical evaluation of computer-assisted self-monitoring of blood glucose system. *Diabetes Care* **12**, 345–350.

Marteau, T.M., Johnston, M., Baum. and Bloch, S. (1987) Goals of treatment in diabetes: a comparison of doctors and parents of children of diabetes. *Journal of Behavioural Medicine* **10**, 33–48.

May, B. (1991) Diabetes. In M. Pitts and K. Phillips (eds.) *The psychology of health: an introduction.* London: Routledge.

Mazze, R.S., Pasmantier, R., Murphy, J.A. and Shamoon, H. (1985) Self-monitoring of capillary blood glucose: changing the performance of individuals with diabetes. *Diabetes Care* **8**, 207–213.

Mazze, R.S., Shamoon, H., Pasmantier, R., Lucido, D., Murphy, J., Hartman, K., Kuykendall, V. and Lopatin, W. (1984) Reliability of blood glucose monitoring by patients with diabetes mellitus. *American Journal of Medicine* **77**, 211–217.

Milton, J. (1989) Brief psychotherapy with poorly controlled diabetics. *British Journal of Psychotherapy* **4**, 532–543.

Molitch, M. (1991) Changing those grim statistics. *Clinical Diabetes* **9**, 50–51.

Newburgh, L.H. and Conn, J.W. (1979) A new interpretation of hyperglycaemia in obese middle-aged persons. *Journal of the American Medical Association* **112**, 7–11.

Nichols, K.A. (1984) The nurse and the psychologist. *Nursing Times* **80**, 22–24.

Nichols, K.A. (1993) *Psychological Care in Physical Illness.* London: Chapman and Hall.

Orme, C.M. and Binik, Y.M. (1989) Consistency of adherence across regimen demands. *Health Psychology* **8**, 27–43.

Peyrot, M. and McMurry, J. (1985) Psychosocial factors in diabetes control: adjustment of insulin-treated adults. *Psychosomatic Medicine* **47**, 542–557.

Peyrot, M., McMurry, J.F. and Hedges, R. (1988) Marital adjustment to adult diabetes: interpersonal congruence and spouse satisfaction. *Journal of Marriage and the Family* **50**, 363–376.

Price, M.J. (1993) An experiential model of learning diabetes self-management. *Qualitative Health Research* **3**, 29–54.

Rettig, B.A., Shrauger, D.G., Recker, R.P., Gallaher, T.F. and Wiltse, H. (1986) A randomised study of the effects of a home diabetes education programme. *Diabetes Care* **9**, 173–178.

Rubin, R.R., Peyrot, M. and Saudek, C.D. (1991) Differential effect of diabetes education on self-regulation and life-style behaviours. *Diabetes Care* **14**, 335–338.

Sanson-Fisher, R.W., Campbell, E.M., Redman, S. and Hennrikus, D.J. (1989) Patient-provider interactions and patient outcomes. *Diabetes Educator* **15**, 134–138.

Schafer, L.C., McCaul, K.D. and Glasgow, R.E. (1986) Supportive and non-supportive family behaviours: Relationship to adherence and metabolic control in persons with type 1 diabetes. *Diabetes Care*, **9**, 179–185.

Schlenk, E.A. and Hart, L.K. (1984) Relationship between health locus of control, health value and social support and compliance with diabetes mellitus. *Diabetes Care* **7**, 566–574.

Shenkel, R.J., Rogers, J.P., Perfetto, G. and Levin, R.A. (1985–86) Importance of significant others in predicting co-operation with diabetic regimen. *International Journal of Psychiatry in Medicine* **15**, 149–155.

Shillitoe, R.W. (1991) Counselling in health care: diabetes mellitus. In H. Davis and L. Fallowfield (eds.) *Counselling and communication in health care*. London: Wiley.

Shillitoe, R.W. and Miles, D.W. (1989) Diabetes mellitus. In A. Broome (ed.) *Health psychology: processes and applications*. New York: Chapman Hall.

Southam, M.A. and Dunbar, J. (1986) Facilitating patient compliance with medical interventions. In K.Holroyd and T. Creer (eds.) *Self-management of chronic disease: handbook of clinical interventions and research*. New York: Academic Press..

Springer, J.R. (1985) The family with a chronically ill adult. *Family Therapy Collection*, **13**, 83–104.

Strube, M.J., Yost, J.H. and Haire-Joshu, D. (1993) Diabetes knowledge as a moderator of reactions to illness by patients with insulin-dependent diabetes. *Journal of Applied Social Psychology* **23**, 944–958.

Surwit, R., Scovern, A. and Feinglos, M. (1982) The role of behaviour in diabetes care. *Diabetes Care* **5**, 337–342.

Turk, D.C. and Meichenbaum, D. (1991) Adherence to self-care regimens: the patient's perspective. In J.J. Sweet, R.H. Rozensky and S.M. Tovain (eds.) *Handbook of clinical psychology in medical settings*. New York: Plenum.

Warren, L. and Hixenbaugh, P. (1995) Psychosocial needs and experiences of adults with diabetes: their relationship to regimen adherence from the patients perspective. *Proceedings of the British Psychological Society* **4**, 39.

Warren, L. and Hixenbaugh, P. (1996a) The role of health beliefs and locus of control on regimen adherence from a life-span perspective. *Proceedings of the British Psychological Society* **5**, 17.

Warren, L. and Hixenbaugh, P. (1996b) Adherence to the diabetes regimen: the role of the health-care team. *Unpublished manuscript.*

Warren-Boulton, E., Auslander, W.F. and Gettinger, J.M. (1982) Understanding diabetes routines: a professional training exercise. *Diabetes Care* **5**, 537–541.

Weinberger, M., Cohen, S.J. and Mazzuca, S.A. (1984) The role of physicians' knowledge and attitudes in effective diabetes management. *Social Science and Medicine* **19**, 965–969.

Welborn, T.A. and Duncan, N. (1980) Diabetic staff simulation of insulin-dependent diabetic life. *Diabetes Care* **3**, 679–681.

Whitehouse, C.R. (1991) Teaching of skills in United Kingdom medical schools. *Medical Education* **25**, 311–318.

Wikblad, K.F. (1991) Patients perspectives of diabetes care and education. *Journal of Advanced Nursing* **16**, 837–844.

Wilson, D.P. and Endres, R.K. (1984) Compliance with home glucose monitoring (HGM) in Type I diabetes mellitus. *Clinical Research* **32**, 883A.

Wilson, D.P. and Endres, R.K. (1986) Compliance with blood glucose monitoring in children with Type 1 diabetes mellitus. *Journal of Paediatrics* **108**, 1022–1024.

Wilson, W. and Pratt, C. (1987) The impact of education and peer support upon weight and glycaemic control of elderly persons with non-insulin dependent diabetes mellitus. *American Journal of Public Health* **77**, 634–635.

Wing, R.R, Epstein, L.H., Nowalk, M.P., Koeske, R. and Hagg, S. (1985). The relationship between behaviour change, weight loss and physiological improvements in patients with type II diabetes. *Journal of Consulting and Clinical Psychology*, **53**, 111–122.

Wing, R.R, Epstein, L.H., Nowalk, M.P., Scott, N., Koeske, R. and Hagg, S. (1984). Does self-monitoring of blood glucose improve dietary compliance for obese patients with Type II diabetes? *American Journal of Medicine,* **81,** 830–836.

Wing, R.R., Marcus, M.D., Epstein, L.H. and Salata, R. (1987). Type II diabetic subjects lose more weight than their overweight non-diabetic spouses. *Diabetes Care* **10,** 563–566.

17

Adherence in Children with Renal Disease

Anthony L. Schwartz

RENAL DISEASE

Problems of kidney function can be caused by anatomical abnormalities, acquired glomerular diseases or hereditary disorders. Acute renal failure develops when renal function has diminished to a point when body fluid homeostasis can no longer be maintained. The child may recover from this, depending on the cause which precipitated the renal failure, or it may become a chronic disorder. Chronic renal failure in children under five years of age is commonly the result of anatomical abnormalities, whereas after five years of age, acquired glomerular diseases or hereditary disorders predominate (Bergstein, 1992). Regardless of the cause of kidney damage, once a critical level of renal functional deterioration is reached, progression to end-stage renal failure is inevitable. However, the child may not feel unwell until kidney function is almost non-existent, and at this point dialysis may be required to remove excess fluid and waste from the blood. This may be in the form of continuous ambulatory peritoneal dialysis (CAPD), continuous cyclic peritoneal dialysis (CCPD) or haemodialysis. Ultimately, the goal for these young people is to undergo renal transplantation. Nevertheless, the requirement to adhere with ongoing treatment continues even after successful transplantation (see Myers and Midence, Chapter 1).

Haemodialysis usually takes place in hospital, whereas CAPD and CCPD are carried out at home. In general, children need regular haemodialysis sessions three times per week in order to survive. These haemodialysis sessions last about four hours. Along with dialysis, the child usually has dietary restrictions to maintain the potassium and phosphorous levels within limits, in addition there are limitations on the amount of fluid which can be taken. This is to prevent placing strain on the heart when there is too much fluid which cannot be removed during dialysis. In addition, there are several medications which are expected to be taken on a daily basis. Following kidney transplantation, a strict regime of immunosuppressive therapy needs to be maintained, which has a variety of unpleasant side-effects, some of which affect physical appearance.

The incidence of renal failure in children is considered to be between four and sixteen per year per million child population (Donckerwolcke, Chantler and Broyer, 1983). Young people with renal failure require ongoing medical treatments to maintain a relatively normal state of health. As is common with other children with a chronic or life-threatening illness, this affects the whole family and impacts on their development. Issues of coping and adaptation to the condition and adherence to the medical and nursing regimes are central. This chapter will discuss research in this field of applied psychology, and emphasise the child in the context of the family and system of health care, as this relates to treatment adhere.

POTENTIAL PSYCHOLOGICAL AND SOCIAL INFLUENCES IN ADHERENCE

Medical advances in the treatment of chronic illness have, over recent years, led to an increasing number of people surviving to adulthood. In the field of renal disease, dialysis and transplantation have improved outcome substantially. These advances have, however, not always been associated with psychological well-being and research has investigated psychosocial adjustment of these survivors of paediatric dialysis and transplant (Reynolds *et al.*, 1993).

Psychological well-being is of importance for child and family, whether or not the child has a chronic condition. As Brownbridge and Fielding (1994) note, for young people with renal disease, psychosocial factors take on an even greater importance because of their likely impact on the child's adherence to medical treatment regimes and, therefore, on the child's physical health.

The individual with renal disease is, according to Basch, Brown and Cantor (1981), affected at three levels; physical being, psychological being, and socio-behavioural. The bio-psycho-social nature is intertwined, and can be seen as part of a wider environment of the family and community. With the conceptualisation of the socio-ecological and systems models (Bronfenbrenner, 1979) the understanding of context and treatment-in-context raises further challenges to holistic care. The effects of a child's chronic illness work in a mutually interactive manner in the family. Rothenberg (1982) considers chronic illness to upset the "psychosocial metabolism" of the entire family. Two major areas of influence cited by the author are the affective issues for the child and family, and the socio-economic and physical environmental issues for the whole family. Kidney disease brings with it changed circumstances for the individual and the family, with an ongoing process of problem-solving, adaptation and adjustment. Research is needed to investigate treatment in the context of the child, family and treatment environment.

Renal disease has associated areas of concern, some of these are discussed below. These are: growth and body image; self-esteem and depression; parental stress and coping and general psychosocial adjustment. Whereas these features may not affect adherence directly, they add further issues which makes the burden of living with this illness more complex.

Growth And Body Image

The effects of renal disease on growth and physical appearance have been identified as a major concern for children on dialysis by Henning *et al.*, (1988) The authors also found educational under-functioning and considerable disruption to normal social and school activity. The difficulties in adhering to treatments which restrict their diet and fluid intake, or taking medications which affect their appearance are complicated by the desire to be similar to their peers. Issues of body-image arise particularly as a result of procedures and treatments that leave scars, a fistula, acne, lack of muscle and fat tissue, cushingoid features or delayed sexual development (Basch, Brown and Cantor, 1981). Whereas these may be a cause for concern at any age, they are acutely so for adolescents. Gorynski and Knight (1992) comment that many adolescent patients perceive their bodies as defective or even repulsive.

Self-Esteem And Depression

Problems associated with low self-esteem and depression have been found in children with renal disease (Bennett, 1994), although Brown-bridge and Fielding (1991) found a trend for children who had home haemodialysis or CAPD to have fewer depressive symptoms than children receiving haemodialysis in hospital. Attempts to enhance a sense of self-esteem and to foster peer relationships through establishing support groups of young people in similar circumstances have been reported in the literature (Gorynski and Knight, 1992). The use of activity or outward-bound experiences have also been suggested as a way of raising the self-esteem of young people with kidney disease (Schwartz, Tegg and Hewerdine, 1996).

Parental Stress And Coping

Issues of parental stress and coping are of great influence not only on the course of the medical treatment, but also for psychological development of the child (Hulstijn-Dirkmaat and Damhuis, 1994). These authors found that parents of dialysis patients greatly differed in the amount they experienced their child's treatment as a burden. Parents of children who were of school-going age experienced more stress than parents of younger children. Parents of children who had undergone a failed transplant were found to be particularly at risk. It was also observed that duration of treatment did not influence the amount of stress experienced. The authors proposed that the process of adaptation, the practical routine of dialysis treatment, and the personal control and involvement offer a structure and clarity to daily life. However, Reynolds *et al.* (1988), found that family life was particularly disrupted in families where a child was undergoing hospital haemodialysis, with practical issues such as the restrictions imposed by the child's condition or treatment substantially affecting their day-to-day life. Parents also reported that marriages had been affected.

General Psychosocial Adjustment

In renal disease in children, it is important to acknowledge the impact of a chronic illness on the stages of the family's life-cycle. Both family and individual development needs to be considered, as these will be affected as the child and family accommodate to the condition. Certain nodal points (e.g. adolescence) are likely to offer specific challenges. Brownbridge and Fielding (1994) report that adolescents tended to show poorer adherence than younger children and Shulman and Rubinroit (1987) consider adolescents with renal disease as being tied to a medical routine which interferes with common age-related activities. Adherence to treatment may become a battleground between parents and the adolescent (Frey, 1984).

Patterson (1988) proposed a model for viewing family adjustment and adaptation to stress which might be applied to understanding families with children who have kidney disease. The Family Adjustment and Adaptation Response Model (FAAR) examines the impact of chronic conditions on the family. It looks at what resources, coping behaviours, and meanings in the family facilitate successful adaptation. Using this framework, medical prescriptions may be seen as demands which place the family under stress to ensure improved kidney functioning. Patterson points out that there has been a disproportionate emphasis of research on how chronic conditions create dysfunction in families. She highlights the family system and the efforts to maintain balanced functioning through using its capabilities to meet the demands placed on it. In applying this to renal disease, one would need to examine the family's functioning over time as it goes through cycles of adjustment (with comparative stability), crisis, and adaptation.

PROBLEMS OF ADHERENCE

Inextricably interwoven with the above considerations, adherence to medical regimes has been identified as a major problem in the treatment of children with end stage renal failure (Fine, Salusky and Ettenger, 1987). A number of factors influence the individual as well as the family and treatment environment; these are postulated to have an effect on treatment adherence.

They include issues of developmental stage both in the child (Erikson, 1980) and in the family's life cycle, as well as the inter-relationships and dynamics within the wider context of home and hospital.

There are many areas of treatment which may present difficulties for children on dialysis. These include: (1) dietary constraints; (2) restrictions of fluid intake; (3) taking various medications. Issues concerning dialysis may include: (4) limitations it imposes in terms of family and social activities; (5) the time-consuming nature of treatments; (6) travel to and from hospital for haemodialysis; (7) periods away from school; (8) creating and accessing the fistula to set-up dialysis; (9) the side-effects of dialysis and (10) uncertain prognosis. These are situations which both individually and together stretch the individual's resources for adhering to the treatment regime. Therefore, taking these features into consideration, we might conclude that non-adherence with onerous treatment regimes is understandable and not preventable.

Interventions designed to modify difficulties associated with adherence problems need to be refined, although useful suggestions arise in contemporary therapeutic literature (Kuttner, 1989; Mauksch and Roesler, 1990; Rissman and Rissman, 1987). Therapeutic inter-ventions include educative approaches, support and supervision, and behavioural interventions such as anxiety management. The use of applied psychophysiology and biofeedback to reduce stress has also been described (Gagnon, Hudnall and Andrasik, 1992; Stroebel and Stroebel, 1984). Individual coping strategies and match-ing interventions with personal coping style have also been studied (Smith, Ackerson and Blotcky, 1989). Research on children's hospital experiences and medical procedures have shown these to be stress-ful for young people, although studies are equivocal about the negative impact of hospitalisation and ongoing treatments. Stressful situations may, in fact, afford the young person an opportunity to cope successfully with difficult situations (Hall and Stacey, 1979; Lansdown and Sokel, 1993; Prins, 1994; Ross and Ross, 1988). These studies have looked at children's views and understanding regarding medical treatment.

As mentioned earlier, creating and accessing the fistula to set up dialysis frequently causes significant distress and anxiety. Various psychological interventions are available to ameliorate this difficulty. With increased use of computers, applications such as those of Ultramind Ltd (London) which link galvanic skin response to imagery on the screen can be used. Recently, Morris and Lawson (1997) evaluated this application with children on haemodialysis to assist with adherence around fistula access. Indications are that the Inner Tuner™ programme allows for easy engagement of the child and the generalising of skills learnt from interactive software, thereby fostering procedural coping and adherence with treatment.

Brownbridge and Fielding (1994) investigated psychosocial adjustment and adherence to dialysis treatment regimes. They found low treatment adherence was associated with poor adjustment to diagnosis and dialysis by children and parents. In addition, they found anxiety and depression to be correlated with poor adjustment, as was the duration of dialysis. Family features such as low family socio-economic status and family structure were also correlated with poor adherence.

The findings of Brownbridge and Fielding (1994) highlight the importance of the provision of psychosocial support to children on dialysis and their families, as a part of a package of general health care. They suggest that psychosocial intervention may be useful in improving adherence with treatment regimes. In applying the model proposed by Patterson (1988), it would be necessary for the treatment team to consider the needs of the child and family at different stages in the process. They would, as is customary practice currently, consider together with the child and family which of a range of facilities might be helpful. Input would be likely to come from different professionals, focusing on biological, psychological or social issues. Issues of working in teams have been the focus of studies in organisational psychology, although there have been few papers concerning practical working in the field of renal work. Collier and Watson (1994) outline the functions of a multi-disciplinary paediatric renal team. McLoughlin and Hawkins (1994) describe the collaboration between a nursing sister and social worker, and Winkley (1990) describes the role of a psychiatrist as consultant to a renal team. Kaplan De-Nour and Czaczkes (1974) report how team issues influence patients' adherence in a small scale sample which shows that where there is a clear and realistic team opinion, patients adhere to treatment better.

Altschuler *et al.* (1991) point out that the impact of treatment needs to be seen in its context. They cite an example of adolescents with renal disease and discuss adherence within a nephrology unit for adolescents which is affected by a complex network of systems, including relationships between family members, and between family and medical staff. They concluded that the views which different members of the family have about the illness, its effects, and ways of executing the treatment regimes, the treatment context and the views of the professionals are relevant to treatment.

Nevertheless, the focus has primarily been on the individual with the acknowledgement of the wider system and its participants. Rissman and Rissman (1987) comment that it appears that the context in which non-adherence occurs is rarely considered, and that interventions are based on the assumption that non-adherence is due to a deficit in the patient. These authors highlight that attempts at enhancing adherence fail to take account of the myriad of factors that interplay in the complex worlds of the patient and doctor.

THEORETICAL FRAMEWORKS TO UNDERSTANDING RENAL NON-ADHERENCE

For the applied psychologist working in the renal setting, it is useful to consider a number of theoretical approaches when dealing with the presenting problems. These include having knowledge of child development from different models (e.g. psychodynamic, humanistic and cognitive-behavioural). Understanding cultural and health beliefs as well as family and systemic models makes for a broader conceptual base.

It is important to understand the person's experience of living with renal disease, and various psychological approaches are useful in attempting to understanding the child's situation. Psychological working may be in the form of counselling or psychotherapy, using any of a number of theoretical perspectives. Taking the position that a person has specific expertise concerning his or her own situation, Ravenette (1980) suggests ways of approaching the child's views, based on Personal Construct Psychology (Kelly, 1955). Gallo, Schultz and Breitmayer (1992) emphasise the importance of taking on board the adolescents' views, language and definitions which can then be used by the health care professionals.

The Health Belief Model (e.g. Becker and Maiman, 1980) as well as the Theory of Reasoned Action (e.g. Ajzen and Fishbein, 1980) are worth bearing in mind. The challenge is in balancing the apparently opposing frameworks; on the one hand the individual, ideographic approach, and on the other hand keeping in touch with the wider systemic material. Ravenette points to the need for balancing objective and subjective perspectives in assessment and therapy.

Mauksch and Roesler (1990) note that social scientists have emphasised the importance of health-care providers pursuing the patient's world view as it relates to health and illness. Issues of health beliefs have been shown to influence adherence to treatment (Becker and Rosenstock, 1984). Rolland (1987) suggests that the clinician should ascertain the family's overall belief system, their views about illness in general, the specific disease in question, and the practical and affective demands of the illness over time. This would clarify issues, as Becker and Maiman (1980) suggest that the patient may possess powerful, well-defined (albeit scientifically erroneous) health beliefs that conflict with the physician's assessment of the problem, and therefore affect adherence with a treatment regime. DiMatteo *et al.* (1993) turn their attention to the physician. They assert that it is physicians' attributes and style of practice that influence patients' adherence to medical treatment. This adds to earlier work on doctor-patient communication (Ley, 1982).

Theoretically, the family should have a major influence on a family member's adherence. In a review of studies relating to the family's impact on health which looks mainly at adherence in adults, Campbell (1986) comments that the family is in a powerful position to influence adherence behaviour, either negatively or positively. The question can be asked about how families influence a child's adherence. Family systems theorists are critical that research has not studied differences between patient and family explanatory models of illness and treatment. Jaber, Steinhardt and Trilling (1991) emphasise the importance of exploring the family's beliefs to avoid problems of non-adherence. Additional factors have been mentioned earlier, such as individual coping style, family environment and the medical context that are likely to affect adherence further. Christ (1982) looks at "dis-synchrony" of coping across children, families, and the treating staff: "Dis-synchrony in coping refers to an occurrence at different points in time of unevenness in specific cognitive appraisals or affective states of parent and patient, parent and parent, patient and sibling, and patient, family and staff."

In this article, Christ acknowledges that there are different representations for each of the participants in terms of goals, values and coping style. However, she does not appear to take into consideration the links between dis-synchrony and the repercussions or effects that such dis-synchrony may have on adherence. Marteau *et al.* (1987) see treatment failure as resulting from a difference in the goals between participants in treatment. In a study investigating children with diabetes, they found significant differences between parents' goals and those of doctors. This matches the view of Masden (1992) who claims that difficulties in treatment arise where the beliefs of family and the health-care provider are different. Such a conceptualisation looks at non-adherence as occurring within a "context of interactions between the patient, family and provider, rather than as a characteristic of the patient, family, or provider" (Masden, 1992; also see Noble, Chapter 3 for a discussion of doctor-patient communication).

An underlying notion here is that of co-evolution within the context of treatment between the patient, family, providers and illness. A useful paradigm is that of General Systems Theory (see Lindegger and Bosman, 1990) as it can be applied to chronic or life-threatening illness. Lindegger and Bosman (1990) consider the application of General Systems Theory to involve the identification of the persons or person systems involved with chronic illness: "as the patient interacts with other people, many of them become an integral part of the illness system, being affected by and in turn affecting the illness [co-evolution]. The personal components most importantly and commonly include the patient, the family and the treatment agency, although other people and groups might also be involved. The disease might be regarded as a participant in this interaction as it is commonly treated in a personified fashion by patients and their families. From a General Systems Theory viewpoint, the chronic illness must be seen as the system involving all these players, with their various interactions."

Hence, within this framework, it is understandable not to simply observe the patient and the role they play in treatment adherence, but also to include in the field of observation the family and professional staff. Bloch (1986) argues further: "it is probably desirable, for example, to study the family and adherence by including in the field of observation issues of *fit* between family and health care system, noting, as well, that the notion of non-compliance is constructed by the health care system".

The focus of investigation into adherence in renal failure clearly needs to entertain different levels of information about the problem, at an individual-based level as well as on interactional aspects whilst holding a systems and meta-view. Psychological work needs to adopt a stance which intervenes at multiple levels. Mullins, Gillman and Harbeck (1992) describe a model which adds a further dimension, the Metasystem Consultation Model (Wynne, McDaniel and Weber, 1986). In this model, the psychologist may view the entire system of the patient, family, and staff from a meta-position and decide which levels need intervention. As Brownbridge and Fielding (1994) point out, psychosocial interventions which occur at different levels and which are focused practically, are important ways of improving adherence to treatment regimes.

A model proposed by Wolff, Theilen and Ehrich (1992), extends the previous frameworks. The Multidimensional Model of Illness Behaviour, takes four levels or dimensions into consideration.

View from the Outside
The observable behaviour.

View from the Inside
The patients'/families' emotional conditions, their feelings and subjective interpretations, which influence behaviour.

Inter-relational View
Influence of interrelations between patients/families and health care providers on feelings/behaviour.

Systemic View
Influence of systemic conditions on the interrelations between patients/families and health care providers.

Figure 1 The Multidimensional Model of Illness Behaviour

Arising out of research looking at the emotional impact of chronic renal failure, this model describes different dimensions of the problem of adherence, and highlights cumulative and interactional effects (Wolff *et al.*, 1996).

The literature on non-adherence to treatments in renal disease identifies this to be a problem for people at all stages in treatment, both for those on dialysis as well as for patients who have had a transplant (Collier and Watson, 1994). Using the theoretical and research foundations available, it is important to offer interventions to assist the child, family and health care providers in dealing with the problems surrounding adherence to treatment. As Brownbridge and Fielding (1994) exhort, future research should aim to develop and evaluate different treatment approaches.

CONCLUSION

This chapter has attempted to highlight some of the current research on adherence in paediatric renal disease and its treatment. The relevance of having a theoretical basis to applied interventions in order to help children and families remains an important consideration.

From the current literature, it would seem that research needs to be advanced by not focusing only on individual characteristics but also on the interplay of a number of factors, including those in the family and medical contexts. DiBlasio *et al.* (1990) claim that, currently, clinical-descriptive studies aim more at obtaining additional information about single phenomena rather than seeing how they differ. La Greca (1988) is critical of research that produces a long list of correlates of medical adherence and comments that most variables that have been investigated have used univariate designs The suggestion is made that research focused on intervention issues could be undertaken to determine what is effective under different conditions and for different people (Patterson, 1988). However, as Rolland (1987) comments, a psychotherapeutic relationship depends on a shared belief system, and it would appear that the fit of values between the patient, family, and the health-care providers is essential.

New approaches to looking at treatment adherence need to take greater account of these systemic and interrelationship dimensions. This provides challenges in terms of methodology and the robustness of measures to assess the different levels of interaction. Both qualitative and quantitative approaches are needed which can assess individuals and systems over time. Within this area the issue of sample size remains a significant issue (La Greca and Varni, 1993), and national or international collaboration in psychosocial research on adherence issues in chronic renal failure would be valuable.

Future directions include the assessment of the views of the participants in treatment and how their understanding affects adherence. Ideas for further study include longitudinal research of adaptation and coping, looking at stress points for the family (e.g. adolescence), personality styles and adherence. Transition points in treatment such as transfer from child to adult services and psychological preparation for this is an under-examined area. Important issues around work environment and stress within the renal team setting and its effect on adherence also needs further investigation.

REFERENCES

Ajzen, I. and Fishbein, M. (1980) *Understanding attitudes and predicting social behaviour.* Englewood Cliffs: Prentice Hall.

Altschuler, J., Black, D., Trompeter, R., Fitzpatrick, M. and Peto, H. (1991) Adolescents in end-stage renal failure: a pilot study of family factors in compliance and treatment considerations. *Family Systems Medicine* **9**, 229–247.

Basch, S., Brown, F. and Cantor, W. (1981) Observations on body image in renal patients. In N.B. Levy (ed.) *Psychonephrology (Part 1): psychological factors in haemodialysis and transplantation.* New York: Plenum.

Becker, M.H. and Maiman, L.A. (1980) Strategies for enhancing patient compliance. *Journal of Community Health* **6**, 113–135.

Becker, M.H. and Rosenstock, I.M. (1984) Compliance with medical advice. In A. Steptoe and A. Matthews (eds.) *Health care and human behaviour.* San Diego, CA: Academic Press.

Bennett, D.S. (1994) Depression among children with chronic medical problems: a meta-analysis. *Journal of Pediatric Psychology* **19,** 149–169.

Bergstein, J.M. (1992) Renal failure. In R.E. Behrman., R.M. Kliegman., W.E. Nelson and V.C. Vaughan III (eds.) *Textbook of pediatrics (14th Edition)*. Philadelphia: Saunders.

Bloch, D.A. (1986) Editoral. *Family Systems Medicine* **4,** 131–133.

Bronfenbrenner, U. (1979) *The ecology of human development.* Cambridge, MA: Harvard University Press.

Brownbridge, G. and Fielding, D.M. (1991) Psychosocial adjustment to end-stage renal failure: comparing haemodialysis, continuous ambulatory peritoneal dialysis and transplantation. *Pediatric Nephrology* **5,** 612–616.

Brownbridge, G. and Fielding, D.M. (1994) Psychosocial adjustment and adherence to dialysis treatment regimes. *Pediatric Nephrology* **8,** 744–749.

Campbell, T.L. (1986) Family's impact on health: a critical review. *Family Systems Medicine* **4,** 135–328.

Christ, G. (1982) "Dis-synchrony" of coping among children with cancer, their families, and the treating staff. In A.E. Christ and K. Flomenhaft (eds.) *Psychosocial family interventions in chronic pediatric illness.* Plenum Press: New York.

Collier, J. and Watson, A.R. (1994) Renal failure in children. In C. Bradley (ed.) *Quality of life following renal failure.* Harwood Academic Publishers.

DiBlasio, P., Molinari, E., Peri, G. and Taverna, A. (1990) Family competence and childhood asthma: a preliminary study. *Family Systems Medicine* **8,** 145–149.

DiMatteo, M.R., Sherborne, C.D., Hays, R.D., Ordway, L., Kravitz, R.L., McGlynn, E.A., Kaplan, S., and Rogers, W.H. (1993) Physicians' characteristics influence patients' adherence to medical treatment: results from the medical outcome study. *Health Psychology* **12,** 93–102.

Donckerwolcke, R.A., Chantler, C. and Broyer, M.J. (1983) Paediatric dialysis. In W. Drukker, F.M. Parsons, and Maher, J.F. (eds.) *Replacement of renal function by dialysis (2nd Edition)*. Boston: Martinus Nijhof.

Erikson, E. (1980) *Identity and the life cycle.* New York: Norton.

Fine, R.N., Salusky, I.B., and Ettenger, R.B. (1987) The therapeutic approach to the infant, child and adolescent with end-stage renal disease. *Pediatric Clinics of North America* **34,** 789–801.

Frey, J. (1984) A family/systems approach to illness maintaining behaviors in chronically ill adolescents. *Family Process,* **23,** 251–260.

Gallo, A.M., Schultz, V.A. and Breitmayer, B.J. (1992) Description of the illness experience by adolescents with chronic renal disease. *ANNA Journal* **19,** 190–193.

Gagnon, D.J., Hudnall, L. and Andrasik, F. (1992) Biofeedback and related procedures in coping with stress. In A.M. La Greca, L.J. Siegel, J.L. Wallander and C.E. Walker (eds.) *Stress and coping in child health.* New York: Guilford Press.

Gorynski, L. and Knight, F. (1992) A peer support group for adolescent dialysis patients. *ANNA Journal* **19,** 262–264.

Hall, D. and Stacey, M. (1979) *Beyond separation: further studies of children in hospital.* London: Routledge and Kegan Paul.

Henning, P., Tomlinson, L., Rigden, S.P.A., Haycock, G.B. and Chantler, C. (1988) *Archives of Disease in Childhood* **63,** 35–40.

Hulstijn-Dirkmaat, G.M. and Damhuis, E.H.W. (1994) Peritoneal dialysis treatment in children and parental stress. *Acta Paediatrica* **83,** 972–976.

Jaber, R., Steinhardt, S. and Trilling, J. (1991) Explanatory models of illness: a pilot study. *Family Systems Medicine* **9,** 39–51.

Kaplan De-Nour, A. and Czaczkes, J.W. (1974) Team-patient interaction in chronic hemodialysis units. *Psychotherapy and Psychosomatics* **24,** 132–136.

Kelly, G.A. (1955) *The psychology of personal constructs.* Norton: New York.

Kuttner, L. (1989) Management of young children's acute pain and anxiety during invasive medical procedures. *Paediatrician* **16,** 39–44.

La Greca, A.M. (1988) Adherence to prescribed medical regimens. In D.K. Routh (ed.) *Handbook of pediatric psychology.* New York: Guilford Press.

La Greca, A.M. and Varni, J.W. (1993) Editorial: interventions in pediatric psychology: a look to the future. *Journal of Pediatric Psychology* **18,** 667–679.

Lansdown, R. and Sokel, B. (1993) Commissioned Review: approaches to pain management in children. *ACPP Review and Newsletter* **15,** 105–111.

Ley, P.(1982) Satisfaction, compliance and communication. *British Journal of Clinical Psychology* **21**, 241–254.

Lindegger, G.C. and Bosman, P. (1990) A systems view of chronic illness and its management. *South African Journal of Psychology* **20**, 32–41.

Marteau, T.M., Johnson, M., Baum, J.D. and Bloch, S. (1987) Goals of treatment in diabetes: A comparison of doctors and parents of children with diabetes. *Journal of Behavioral Medicine* **10**, 33–48.

Masden, W.C. (1992) Problematic treatment: interaction of patient. spouse, and physician beliefs in medical noncompliance. *Family Systems Medicine* **10**, 365–383.

Mauksch, L.B. and Roesler, T. (1990) Expanding the context of the patient's explanatory model using circular questioning. *Family Systems Medicine* **8**, 3–13.

McLoughlin, M. and Hawkins, C. (1994) *Collaborative working between a nurse and social worker at a paediatric renal unit.* Presented at the European Working Group on Psychosocial Aspects of Children with Chronic Renal Failure. Heidelberg, Germany.

Morris, T. and Lawson, A. (1997) *Preparing children for renal dialysis.* Presented at the third research fair in child and adolescent mental health, March, Parkview Clinic, University of Birmingham, UK.

Mullins, L.L., Gillman, J., and Harbeck, C. (1992) Multiple-level interventions in pediatric psychology settings: a behavioural-systems perspective. In A.M. La Greca, L.J. Siegel, J.L. Wallander and C.E. Walker (eds.) *Stress and coping in child health* . New York: Guilford Press.

Patterson, J.M. (1988) Families experiencing stress. *Family Systems Medicine* **6**, 202–237.

Prins, P.J.M. (1994) Anxiety in medical settings. In T.H. Ollendick, N.J. King, and W. Yule (eds) *International handbook of phobic and anxiety disorders in children and adolescents.* New York: Plenum Press.

Ravenette, A.T. (1980) The exploration of consciousness: personal construct intervention with children. In A.W. Landfield and L.M. Leitner (eds.) *Personal construct psychology: psychotherapy and personality.* New York: Wiley.

Reynolds, J.M., Garralda, M.E., Jameson, R.A. and Postlethwaite, R.J. (1988) How parents and families cope with chronic renal failure. *Archives of Disease in Childhood* **63**, 821–826.

Reynolds, J.M., Morton, M.J.S., Garralda, M.E., Postlethwaite, R.J. and Goh, D. (1993) Psychosocial adjustment of adult survivors of a paediatric dialysis and transplant programme. *Archives of Disease in Childhood* **68**, 104–110.

Rissman, R. and Rissman, B.Z. (1987) Compliance. *Family Systems Medicine* **5**, 446–467.

Rolland, J.S. (1987) Family illness paradigms: evolution and significance. *Family Systems Medicine* **5**, 482–503.

Ross, D.M. and Ross, S.A. (1988) *Childhood pain*. Baltimore: Urban and Schwarzenberg.

Rothenberg, M.B. (1982) The effect of a child's chronic illness on the family. In A.E. Christ and K. Flomenhaft (eds.) *Psychosocial family interventions in chronic pediatric illness.* New York: Plenum Press.

Schwartz, A.L., Tegg, S. and Hewerdine, R. (1996) *An evaluation of the Kielder Water independence training experience.* Presented at the European Working Group on Psychosocial Aspects of Children with Chronic Renal Failure, Vienna.

Shulman, S. and Rubinroit, C.I. (1987) The second individuation process in handicapped adolescents. *Journal of Adolescence* **10**, 373–384.

Smith, K.E., Ackerson, J.D. and Blotcky, A.D. (1989) Reducing distress during invasive medical procedures: relating behavioural interventions to preferred coping style in paediatric cancer patients. *Journal of Pediatric Psychology* **14**, 405–419.

Stroebel, E.L. and Stroebel, C.F. (1984) The quieting reflex: a psychophysiological approach for helping children to deal with healthy and unhealthy stress. In J.H. Humphrey (ed.) *Stress in childhood.* New York: AMS Press.

Winkley, L. (1990) Living with chronic illness: consultation to a children's renal dialysis unit. *Journal of Child Psychotherapy* **16**, 49–62.

Wolff, G., Theilen, U. and Ehrich, J.H.H. (1992) The emotional impact of CRF: a study of the interaction of disease, care and coping. *Pediatric Nephrology* **6**, C55.

Wolff, G., Strecker, K., Vester, U., Offner, G., and Brodehl, J. (1996) Non-compliance after transplantation. *Pediatric Nephrology* **10**, C43.

Wynne, L.C., McDaniel, S.H. and Weber, T.T. (1986) *Systems consultation: a new perspective for family therapy.* New York: Guilford Press.

18

Adherence in Hypertension and Coronary Heart Disease

Yori Gidron

Cardiovascular disease is the major cause of mortality in developed countries (Jenkins, 1988). Its most prevalent form is coronary heart disease (CHD), which includes angina pectoris and myocardial infarction (MI). Beyond the physical consequences, CHD causes adverse effects on patients' daily functioning and quality of life (e.g. Kaplan, 1988).

Among the major, but modifiable "traditional" risk factors for developing CHD is elevated blood pressure (BP) or hypertension (HT; Kannel *et al.*, 1986). Essential HT is associated with stable elevated diastolic blood pressure (DBP) and/or systolic blood-pressure (SBP) that is not secondary to another disease. HT is a prevailing disorder, as a recent survey found that 24% of American adults have HT (Burt *et al.*, 1995). Despite the morbidity known to be associated with HT and CHD, non-adherence to prescribed medical treatments in HT and CHD are a prevailing problem. Burt *et al.* (1995) found that only 53% of patients with HT were treated medically for their condition. Non-adherence may account for a certain amount of this percentage, as only 50% of hypertensive patients adhere to their medical recommendations (e.g. Hamilton *et al.*, 1993). Similar estimates have been reported for non-adherence in CHD (e.g. Conn, Taylor and Hayes, 1992). Non-adherence in HT may have adverse long-term effects, as Psaty *et al.* (1990) found that patients with HT who did not fully adhere to prescribed dosages of beta-blockers were at a fourfold increased risk of developing CHD than adhering patients. This suggests an inverse dose-response relationship between the degree of adherence in HT and subsequent development of CHD.

Given the high prevalence of CHD and HT in the population, the morbidity and mortality associated with these disorders, and the high levels of non-adherence and its potential adverse effects, enhancing adherence in HT and CHD is of greatest importance. This chapter will include clinical and empirical perspectives concerning adherence to treatment in HT and CHD. I shall review separately the challenges associated with adherence in HT and CHD, the methods for assessing adherence, the correlates of adherence, and empirical studies examining strategies for enhancing adherence to treatment in HT and CHD. This chapter will conclude with a summary and suggestions for future research.

Among the many definitions of adherence, the one offered by Haynes (1979) will be used: "the extent to which a person's behavior (in terms of taken medication, following diets, or executing life-style changes) coincides with medical or health advice". This definition is flexible and does not specify a fixed percentage of "sufficient" adherence, and it focuses on a broad range of health-behaviours suitable for HT and CHD. Sackett *et al.* (1975) proposed a cut-off of 80% of prescribed medication as an adequate level of adherence, a cut-off associated with systematic reductions in DBP. However, a cut-off may differ dramatically as a function of the medication and individual differences in pharmacokinetics, and may not be easily applied to all forms of treatment (e.g. psychotherapy).

ADHERENCE IN HYPERTENSION

Challenges of Adherence in Hypertension

Several issues unique to hypertension make adhering to its medical regimens a challenge. Kjellgren, Ahlner and Saljo (1995) identified the following issues for consideration in HT. First, unlike other chronic illnesses such as asthma, HT is primarily an asymptomatic disease. Second, HT is a significant CHD risk factor, this "threat" may have serious ramifications for non-adherence and it may be a constant source of anxiety. Third, HT is a chronic disease. This requires persistent and long-term adherence and self-discipline. Developmental (e.g. age-related memory loss), and situational changes (e.g. moving from a relaxed to a time-urgent job) may affect adherence levels. Fourth, antihypertensive medication has side-effects which may seriously affect adherence. Finally, long-term antihypertensive medication is expensive, and this may affect adherence if patients must pay for medication.

Additional challenges include the fact that patients with HT cannot continuously verify their condition, unless they are equipped with ambulatory monitors. This may result in great uncertainty and inability to pacify anxiety concerning BP control, which may lead patients to give up their attempts to adhere adequately. Finally, although adherence in HT can seriously reduce BP levels and risk of CHD (Psaty *et al.*, 1990; Sackett *et al.*, 1975), non-adherence may not affect BP up to a year after termination of treatment (Schmieder, Rockstroh and Messerli, 1991). Thus, from the patient's perspective, HT and its treatment are a continuous challenge requiring self-discipline and persistence.

Rudd (1992) discussed 14 myths physicians may hold about antihypertensive therapy which included: (a) the assumed ease of medication-taking for patients (despite their cost and effect on daily routine); (b) physicians' ability to detect non-adherers (despite evidence to the contrary); (c) that patients can use simple cues for enhancing adherence, (d) that their patients' BP is normal during check-ups (possibly due to adherence prior to check-ups); (e) interpretation of uncontrolled BP as a call for increased doses (though adherence may be adequate and the medication may be ineffective); (f) blaming rather than consulting with non-adhering patients; (g) dangerous minimisation of importance of non-adherence and (h) that in order to increase adherence, patients need only simple regimens (thus neglecting the impact of psychosocial factors on adherence). Physicians and health care providers must recognise the challenges of HT and test the accuracy of their knowledge about adherence when treating patients with HT.

Assessment of Adherence in Hypertension

Several methods have been suggested for assessing adherence in HT, most of which focus on medication intake (see Kjellgren, Ahlner and

Saljo, 1995, and for a general discussion of methods used in measuring adherence, see Myers and Midence, Chapter 1). Dosage counting is a widely used method, measured by pill counting or electronic monitoring. However, dosage counting may only provide information about removal of medication from packages and not about actual medication intake. Additionally, electronic monitoring may have ethical limitations (e.g. invading patients' privacy; patient-doctor trust). Hoelscher, Lichstein and Rosenthal (1986) found that correlations between self-reported and electronically monitored adherence to relaxation-practice in hypertensive patients ranged from .64 to .89, however, patients overestimated their actual practice by 91%. These researchers recommended using objective means for monitoring adherence, and this may be needed particularly in clinical trials (Kjellgren *et al.*, 1995). Serum levels of medications or their metabolites provide information on actual medication intake. However, this method is time-restricted as it depends on the medications' pharmacokinetics. BP control has been used in many studies (e.g. Degoulet *et al.*, 1983). This method assumes that a particular treatment is effective, and that BP control depends directly on adherence levels. However, BP may be unchanged because of reasons unrelated to adherence (e.g. individual pharmacokinetics). Self-report questionnaires, diaries or interviewing the patient may reveal the degree of adherence. Whereas this method is subjective, and may be affected by social desirability and presentation biases, it may reveal patients' difficulties with adherence, and foster improved communication between patients and physicians, which in turn, may improve adherence (Kjellgren *et al.*, 1995). Finally, the number of scheduled appointments kept by patients has been used as an index of adherence (e.g. Degoulet *et al.*, 1983). The validity of this method may be limited as patients may be seeing other health professionals during the same period (Degoulet *et al.*, 1983). A combination of these methods may yield more comprehensive, reliable and valid measures of adherence than any one alone.

Haynes *et al.* (1980) used pill counting as an objective, "gold-standard" taken for all participants, to compare the concurrent validity of different measures (serum levels of potassium, uric acid and antihypertensives, and self-report number of skipped pills/day/week/month). Self-reported number of skipped pills was most strongly correlated with pill counting ($r = .74$), and best differentiated between the adhering ($\geq$ 80% of prescribed dosage) and non-adhering (< 80%) patients. Thus, despite the potential for bias, self-report measures have promising features.

Morisky, Green and Levine (1986) developed a four item interview for assessing medication intake as a feasible, fast to administer, and more valid measure than self-report questionnaires. Utilising patients' tendency to answer "yes" for adhering behaviour, the interview is phrased in such a way that a "yes" response indicates non-adherence. The questions inquire about forgetting, carelessness, stopping after feeling better, and stopping after feeling worse. The scale's internal consistency reliability is sufficient ($r = .61$), and it has a single factor. The correlation between baseline adherence levels and percentage of patients with age-adjusted controlled BP was significant two years later ($r = .43$), and five years later ($r = .58$), supporting the scale's predictive validity. Finally, the scale's sensitivity was .81 and its specificity was .44. However, including another measure of adherence would have enabled a test of the interview's concurrent validity. Although the sensitive phrasing of questions was meant to reduce social desirability, this may be assessed during the interview and added to the final score. Despite these limitations, this brief, reliable and predictive scale is promising.

The Medical Outcomes Study (Sherbourne *et al.*, 1992) employed a comprehensive assessment that included: general adherence (tendency to adhere to doctor's recommendations); degree of adherence to patient-specific recommended behaviours; and degree of adherence to disease-specific measures (for HT: diet, salt-intake, medication intake and physical exercise). Most measures were moderately internally reliable, but their stability over two years was only mild to moderate ($r = .24$ to .58).

Correlates of Adherence in Hypertension

The correlates of adherence may be divided into treatment-related, disease-related, physician-related, patient background and patient trait/state or psychosocial variables. As most of the following data are derived from retrospective correlational designs, one may not infer a causal relationship between these correlates and adherence, unless an experimental design was employed as well. Complexity of treatment regimen, a treatment related variable was investigated by Eisen *et al.*, (1990). They found that patients with HT, who were prescribed three daily doses of antihypertensives, removed from an electronic monitor the prescribed amount of pills on a significantly lower percentage of days (59%) than patients prescribed two and once daily doses (74.9% and 83.6%, respectively). The best predictor of patients' adherence was dose frequency. However, patients were not randomly assigned to dose frequency groups, and it was unclear whether the groups differed on type of antihypertensive. Nevertheless, Eisen *et al.* (1990) recommended that the most important and practical step for health-care providers to increase adherence is to reduce dose-frequency by administering long-acting medications.

Additional treatment-related factors include side-effects and clarity of prescribed regimens (Kjellgren *et al.*, 1995). Although Kjellgren *et al.* (1995) suggest that disease-related variables do not affect adherence, other studies suggest that initial BP levels, previous MI and stroke (Degoulet *et al.*, 1983), presence of heart disease (Sherbourne *et al.*, 1992) and severe illness (DiMatteo *et al.*, 1993) prospectively predict adherence levels on different measures (e.g. appointment keeping, diet and medication intake).

The prospective two year Medical Outcomes Study (DiMatteo *et al.*, 1993) found that after controlling for patient-related variables (e.g. baseline adherence), physicians' job satisfaction predicted patients' general adherence. Doctors' speciality (cardiologists versus others), number of patients per week and making a definite future appointment predicted better adherence to medication. The predictor of adherence to physical exercise was whether doctors answered all of patients' questions, and the predictors of adherence to diet included number of tests ordered. Thus, physicians' working style and personal characteristics affect patient adherence and changes in physicians' working style (e.g. promoting their job-satisfaction, making definite future appointments, answering patients' questions) may increase patient adherence.

Among patient background variables, Eisen *et al.* (1990) found that income, education, living alone and being employed were positively and prospectively related to number of days in which patients removed the prescribed amount of medication. Kjellgren *et al.* (1995) reviewed several studies which suggest that psychosocial factors affect adherence in HT more than socio-demographic factors. Among these psychological factors are hostile feelings, locus of control, patients' perceptions of the duration of their illness and its treatment, patients' beliefs concerning medication taking, and patients' satisfaction with treatment. For example, Hamilton *et al.* (1993) found that patients' perceived severity of illness, perceived benefits from treatment and behavioural intentions significantly predicted the percentage of appointments kept and perceived benefits significantly predicted self-reported adherence. Lee *et al.* (1992) found that skipping weekly doses was associated with significantly higher levels of hostility. Degoulet *et al.* (1983) argued that the profile of patients with HT who dropped out from treatment (i.e. obese, smoking and unmedicated patients) may reflect an unco-operative attitude towards medical recommendations. This mistrusting and unco-operative attitude is a central element in hostility and is manifested by poor health behaviour. Poor health behaviour, in turn, has been suggested as one possible link between hostility and CHD (Houston and Vavak, 1991). Assessing adherence to relaxation-practice with an electronic monitor, Hoelscher *et al.* (1986) found that patients' anticipated benefit and self-efficacy predicted adherence. In contrast, Eisen *et al.* (1990) found that after controlling for dose-frequency and socio-economic status (SES), other psychological variables (e.g. health locus of control) did not predict adherence. The Medical Outcomes Study (Sherbourne *et al.*, 1992) found that baseline adherence levels and less health-related distress predicted more adherence to HT specific recommendations (e.g. diet and medication intake) two years later. These relations remained intact after controlling for social desirability.

Enhancing Adherence in Hypertension

Morisky *et al.* (1986) argued that "the goal of achieving adherence with medical recommendations for hypertensive patients is to improve BP control and ultimately to reduce the risk of premature cardiovascular morbidity and mortality". It appears feasible that this goal can be achieved if empirically based and theoretically-plausible correlates of non-adherence are used to identify non-adhering populations (e.g. initially non-adhering patients; Sherbourne *et al.*, 1992) and if these correlates are treated as therapeutic targets (e.g. hostility; Lee *et al.*, 1992). Thus, for example, hostility reduction treatments (e.g. Gidron and Davidson, 1996) may be useful for enhancing adherence. This may include educating patients about the negative consequences of hostile mistrust towards medical regimens and use of cognitive restructuring and listening skills for altering mistrust and unco-operative behaviour.

Rudd (1992) recommended the following steps for increasing adherence in HT therapy: monitor non-adherers; define goal BP and monitor its achievement; detect adherence obstacles; collaborate with patients about devising treatment plan; simplify regimens; minimise side-effects and patients' fears; consider cheaper alternatives and reinforce adequate adherence. Some of these steps, such as collaborating and planning with patients may be more effective for those with an internal locus of control. Patients with an external locus of control may benefit from more traditional and "authoritative" communication styles. See Horne and Weinman, Chapter 2, for a discussion of locus of control. Future studies may wish to confirm and utilise the locus of control by communication style interaction, an interaction that has been observed in relation to preparation for surgery (e.g. Auerbach *et al.*, 1976).

Kjellgren *et al.* (1995) suggested a reciprocal, co-operation between patients and physicians for enhancing adherence in HT. According to their model, physicians' knowledge, perceptions and attitudes are transmitted to and modified by the patients' knowledge, perceptions and attitudes. Nurses, pharmacists, family and friends mediate this co-operation. Specifically, focusing on short-term rather than long-term goals and observable reinforcements (BP reduction) may be meaningful and helpful to patients. Use of memory enhancing devices (e.g. audio-visual reminders) can enhance adherence. Self-monitoring of adherence and BP is a powerful strategy that provides patients with direct feedback on their adherence behaviour, reinforces successful adherence and provides a sense of responsibility and control. Physicians can support patients by scheduling more appointments, by involving patients in the decisions about their treatment, by providing clear therapeutic regimens that do not impair patients' quality of life, and by adopting an understanding and friendly approach towards patients.

Several clinical trials support these suggestions. Sackett *et al.* (1975) demonstrated that HT and/or treatment convenience were insufficient factors for increasing adherence in HT. In a subsequent trial, Haynes *et al.*, (1976) matched patients with HT on DBP levels and degree of non-adherence and randomly assigned patients either to a supervised experimental or usual care control group. The experimental group included patients self-rating and recording their BP and medication intake, tailoring regimen to patients' daily routines, and supervision and reinforcement. Six months later, experimental participants, but not controls, significantly increased their adherence to medication taking and reduced their DBP compared to base-line levels. Finally, a dose-response relationship emerged between the degree of adherence increases and DBP reduction. However, patients in the experimental group were prescribed more medication by their physicians than controls. Despite this limitation, this study suggests that a simple, cost-effective and patient-oriented *behavioural* intervention enhances adherence and BP reduction in HT.

Testing physicians' role in adherence, Inui *et al.* (1976) assigned doctors either to a single session tutorial or to a no tutorial control condition. The tutorial taught physicians how to detect non-adhering patients and how to devote time to and alter patients' health perceptions based on the Health Belief Model (HBM, e.g. Becker, 1974). Physicians in the tutorial group had more accurate knowledge about non-adherence in HT, wrote significantly more notes about patients' adherence and devoted significantly more time to educating patients than control physicians.

Of greatest importance, significantly more patients of tutored physicians adhered to their drug regimen (took at least 75% of pills), and showed control of their HT than did patients of control physicians. However, randomisation of physicians was not used, and the criterion of DBP < 100 mm Hg for controlled HT was high. Despite these limitations, this study showed how patient adherence is a function of, and can be achieved by, replacing physicians' role as a diagnostician with one as an educator.

Utilising nurses' aid, Hamilton *et al.* (1993) assigned 34 patients with HT to either a special intervention group (SI) or a standard treatment (ST) control group. The SI reminded patients about their appointments, included a 30–40 minute session with a nurse who repeated doctors' instructions, clarified patients' health beliefs, and attempted to modify attitudes incongruent with adherence. After six months, patients in the SI were rated by physicians as more adherent, kept more appointments and showed greater reductions in SBP than controls. However, it was unclear whether physicians were blind to patients' group status.

Several studies investigating the role of spouse support have yielded mixed findings. Wadden (1983) wished to increase patients' adherence to a HT relaxation regimen. Results showed that patients with HT who learned relaxation with their spouses reported practising relaxation significantly more frequently than those who learned relaxation alone. Despite this, the groups were equal at reducing their SBP and DBP over time. Interestingly, among the predictors of BP reduction was degree of adherence to relaxation. Thus, although spouse support may increase patient-adherence to relaxation regimens, this increase may not be responsible for the therapeutic benefits from adhering to relaxation regimens. As baseline hostility was negatively correlated with BP reduction, hostility may have interacted with spouse support. Hostile patients may have reacted with increased BP to spouse support, while the opposite may have occurred with low hostile patients. These trends may have reduced the overall effect on BP reduction of the support group. These interactions, which should be tested, reveal how adherence and health may involve multiple variables that interact in complex ways.

Hoelscher *et al.* (1986) found that a group treatment that was taught relaxation and contingency contracting (e.g. spouse taking patient out for dinner following sufficient adherence) resulted in lower levels of relaxation practice than regular group or individual relaxation treatments. However, the practice of contingency contracting with spouses was not monitored. Hoelscher *et al.* (1986) concluded that more powerful methods for increasing relaxation adherence are needed for patients with HT.

Finally, Friedman *et al.* (1994) tested the efficacy of a behavioural computerised Telephone-Linked Care (TLC) program for enhancing adherence and BP change in HT. Adherence was significantly increased and DBP was significantly reduced in the TLC program compared with a usual care control group, particularly among initially non-adhering patients. These important findings should be replicated in non-American community interventions.

ADHERENCE IN CORONARY HEART DISEASE

Challenges of Adherence in Coronary Heart Disease

While the main challenge of adherence in HT is ensuring that prescribed medication is taken, this is only one of several challenges for

CHD patients. Firstly, patients with CHD are normally treated with a more complex medication regimen than are patients with HT (e.g. aspirin, beta-blockers for myocardial oxygen demand; glyceryl trinitrate for angina pain). Secondly, treatment for CHD may include performance of physical exercises, and dramatic changes in health behaviours such as diet, smoking cessation and stress modification (Owens, McCann and Hutelmyer, 1978), all which attempt to reduce recurrent CHD episodes by targeting CHD risk factors (Jenkins, 1988). Thus, patients with CHD need to adhere to a more complex and personally demanding therapeutic regimen. As patients with CHD are often more ill than those who suffer from HT, CHD-related symptoms and disability may motivate some patients to increase their adherence, and may be a barrier or a source of helplessness for others. The greater challenges in performing the complex medical regimes in CHD and in coping with CHD need to be considered when assessing and planning interventions to enhance adherence in CHD.

Assessment of Adherence in CHD

The comprehensiveness of assessing adherence in CHD follows the complexity of its medical treatment. Thus, to the extent that diet, smoking cessation, physical exercise, stress modification and medication are prescribed, assessing adherence becomes complex as well. Adherence to physical exercises constitutes one measure, and typically includes the number of attended appointments (e.g. Mirotznik, Feldman and Stein, 1995). However, this outcome may not reflect patients' exercising pattern (e.g. the intensity of exercise).

Carney *et al.* (1995) used an unobtrusive electronic monitor for measuring the percentage of days when patients removed medication from the container. Although this measure assesses the date and time each pill is removed, and although its reliability and validity has been supported (Eisen *et al.*, 1990), it measures medication-removal rather than medication intake. More comprehensive measures include the Health Behavior Scale (Miller *et al.*, 1982a). This self-report scale was developed to assess adherence of post-MI patients to their recommended diet, medication, stress modification, smoking reduction and physical exercise. Each behaviour is then assessed in four situations: at home; at work; during social activities and during recreation. The scale's concurrent validity was supported by observing moderately high correlations between self and spouse ratings (Miller *et al.*, 1982b) for diet (r = .85), medication (r = .81) and smoking (r = .62), but not for stress modification (r = .01) or physical activity (r = .25).

Ornish *et al.* (1990) assessed adherence in patients with coronary artery disease (CAD) to a comprehensive lifestyle change program. The assessment included a three-day diary of nutrient intake, self-reported type, frequency and duration of physical exercises and stress-management techniques. Smoking cessation was also tested via plasma-nicotine levels on a random segment sample of their patients. Although the psychometric properties of these measures were not provided, patients in the treatment-group scored significantly higher on total and on each specific prescribed behaviour than controls. Thus, their multidimensional measure of adherence was sensitive to treatment. Ornish *et al.* (1990) also found a strong dose-response relationship between degree of adherence to the lifestyle program and CAD-regression. Thus, this study strongly suggests a *causal* relationship between adherence and disease (CAD) status, an outstanding reason for promoting adherence.

Correlates of Adherence in CHD

The Medical Outcomes Study (Sherbourne *et al.*, 1992) assessed adherence to specific behaviours recommended to patients with heart disease in the same way they did for patients with HT. This included adherence to diet, salt intake, medication intake and physical exercise. This measure was described earlier. Unlike the case with HT, Sherbourne *et al.* (1992) did not find disease-related variables to be predictive of adherence in CHD. However, Daltroy (1985) found that CHD status (e.g. previous MI) predicted greater attendance to physical exercise classes. Sherbourne *et al.* (1992) did find that a treatment-related variable (more dissatisfaction with technical aspects of care), and patient background variables (years of education, age at or above 75, initial adherence levels) predicted greater adherence specifically related to CHD (e.g. medication intake, physical exercise) two years later. As in HT, initial adherence was a good marker of subsequent adherence.

Several studies examined the psychosocial correlates of adherence in CHD. Doherty *et al.* (1983) examined the relationship between spouse support, its determinants and husbands' adherence to behaviours that prevent CHD. The HBM was used as a possible determinant of spouses' supportive behavior. Spouse support as rated by spouses, patients and medical staff was significantly and positively correlated with patients' adherence to medication packet counts. Among highly supported patients (according to the three sources), the mean adherence score (96%) was significantly higher than among patients with low support (70%). Spouses' interest in their husbands' treatment and reminding them to take their medication were positively related to adherence, but "nagging" husbands about their medication or diet was negatively related to adherence. Moreover, highly supported husbands had wives who perceived the treatment as more beneficial than lesser supported husbands. While instrumental support (i.e. how to follow a medical regimen) was assessed, affective support (i.e. whether wife was empathic to husband) was not assessed. Despite this limitation, this study was theoretically based and included valid measures of support and adherence from different sources.

Hilbert (1985) found no relationship between general or health-regimen related support and self-reported general or regimen specific adherence in post MI patients, despite good concurrent validity on most measures of adherence. Hilbert (1985) suggested that certain measures of spouse support may have reflected changes in the home environment which may have been disruptive for patients. In a multiple regression, number of marriages was significantly and negatively related to general adherence. Thus, marital satisfaction or couple interaction style may moderate the effects of spouse support on adherence.

Conn *et al.* (1992) found that self-esteem and social support (i.e. intimacy, reassurance of self-worth and informational, emotional and material support) were significantly and positively related to adherence to exercise post-MI in both males and females. Self-esteem was positively correlated with adherence to diet and stress modification, and social support was positively correlated with medication intake, while neither self-esteem nor social support correlated with smoking-reduction. However, as this was a correlational study using self-report measures alone, self-esteem and social support may have also resulted from patients' adhering levels (Conn *et al.*, 1992).

Nevertheless, the investigators suggest that the components of adherence in CHD should be considered separately, as each component had different correlates, rather than viewing patients as "adherers" or "non-adherers" in general. Additionally, the components of adherence reflected qualitatively different behaviours and processes.

Testing the HBM, Mirotznik *et al.* (1995) found that motivation (i.e. performing special health-care practices) and perceived severity of illness in participants with or at high risk of CHD were positively and independently correlated with number of exercise appointments kept. Unexpectedly, perceived benefits from treatment was negatively correlated with adherence to exercises. However, patients' beliefs were assessed *after* they had attended the exercise sessions, possibly affecting their actual health-beliefs.

A recent study (Burke *et al.*, 1996) found for patients with CHD perceived self-efficacy at implementing a cholesterol free diet was significantly correlated (r=.52) with adherence to a diet. Outcome expectancy regarding dietary management was unrelated to levels of adherence to diet. However, only self-report measures were used, and a conceptual (if not item) overlap existed in the assessment of self-efficacy and actual diet, as both assessed ability to adhere to the recommended diet. Nevertheless, this study suggests that self-efficacy may be a more powerful marker of adherence to diet than outcome expectations (or perceived treatment benefits).

The traits of hostility and depression have been examined in a few studies. As hostility may be related to angina symptoms (e.g. Smith, Follick and Korr, 1984) and to non-adherence (Lee *et al.*, 1992), patients with CHD who score high on hostility may experience more symptoms due to poor adherence. Beaupre *et al.* (1994) found that while hostility and depression were significantly and positively correlated with frequency of angina symptoms in patients with CAD, these traits were unrelated to electronically monitored aspirin-taking. Thus, it is unclear whether poor adherence mediates the relationship between hostility (or depression) and CHD symptoms.

In elderly patients suffering from CAD, diagnosis of clinical depression was associated with a significantly lower percentage of days of adequate medication removal from an electronic counter (45% of days) compared with non-depressed patients (69%) (Carney *et al.*, 1995). The investigators speculated that depression is associated with reduced medication intake via (1) reducing social support, memory and attention and (2) increasing sensitivity to side-effects. In contrast, Skala *et al.* (1994) found that while electronically monitored levels of medication intake were not different in depressed and non-depressed patients with CAD, one aspect of depression (impaired concentration) was significantly associated with poorer adherence. Thus, the cognitive consequences of depression may affect adherence levels in patients with both CAD and CHD. Reduced adherence in depressed patients with CAD may partly account for the relationship between depression and mortality in CHD patients (Frasure-Smith, Lesperance and Talajic, 1993).

Finally, Gallacher (1994) assessed 2100 British men for their attitudes and seven CHD risk factor behaviours. They found significant correlations between attitudes and actual risk-factor behaviours (ranging from r = .30 to .54), with specific attitudes related to specific behaviours (e.g. joy was the strongest correlate of physical activity). Thus, interventions aimed at enhancing adherence should account for and target individuals' specific health-related attitudes (Gallacher, 1994).

Strategies for Enhancing Adherence in CHD

There is a lack of controlled studies investigating enhancement of adherence in CHD. As with HT, strategies for enhancing adherence in CHD are assumed to result in positive health benefits. However, Stegman *et al.* (1987) found that neither positive attitudes toward nor actual adherence to the medical regimen independently predicted fewer recurrent infarcts or less all-cause mortality in post-MI patients.

Hladik and White (1976) tested the acceptability and effectiveness of providing written information concerning medications to low SES cardiovascular patients, in addition to usual oral counselling. The written material included medications' names, purpose, and encouraging full and correct adherence (e.g. not to skip doses). All patients thought the material was useful in answering their questions, 95% read the material, and patients identified correctly 63% and 74% of medications' names and purposes. However, no control group was used, baseline knowledge was not assessed, and a reliable and valid measure of adherence was not employed.

Dapcich-Miura and Hovell (1979) tested the effects of providing tokens for social awards to an 82-year old MI patient for adhering to recommended walking, potassium consumption, and three pre-scribed medications. The intervention was responsible for increasing adherence to all three behaviours and frequency of angina pain and family arguments decreased as well. Although no follow-up was conducted, these results suggest that behavioural reinforcement can enhance an MI patient's adherence to a complex medical regimen. Daltroy (1985) found that counselling patients with CHD over the telephone about the benefits of physical exercise and methods for overcoming its drawbacks, together with a written pamphlet resulted in greater attendance to physical exercise classes than the written pamphlet alone. However, this was found only after controlling for several background measures (e.g. location of exercise classes, CHD status).

The Minnesota Heart Health Program (MHHP; Mittlemark *et al.*, 1986) aimed at increasing awareness and adherence to smoking cessation, preventing HT, reducing salt, fat and alcohol consump-tion, and increasing physical exercise for preventing CHD at the community of Mankato, Minnesota, USA. The MHHP involved community leaders and the media in conducting population-wide screening and education and special educational programs for adults, children and health professionals together with community-based campaigns. There were high participation rates (60.5% of adults visited heart-health centres, 65% of recruited physicians underwent continuing education classes), and there was a signi-ficantly greater awareness of CHD prevention activities in Mankato than in a matched comparison community. Finally, significantly lower rates of smoking and saliva-based tobacco metabolites were found in adolescents in the intervention community during all six years of follow-up than among adolescents from a comparison community (Perry *et al.* 1992). Thus, population-based efforts for increasing adherence to CHD prevention are feasible and effective.

Finally, in a further analysis of a clinical trial that included the Health Behavior Scale (Miller *et al.*, 1982a), patients with CHD, who scored high on hostility and who were undergoing a hostility-reduction intervention reported at post-treatment greater increases in adherence to diet recommendations (significant) and physical activ-ity (a non-significant trend) than controls, after considering baseline adherence levels (Gidron, Davidson and Bata, 1996). Although adherence was assessed with a self-report measure alone, this study suggests that reducing hostility, a significant CHD risk factor (Miller et al, 1996) and a marker of non-adherence (Lee *et al.*, 1992), may enhance adherence in hostile CHD patients in addition to improving certain health outcomes (Gidron *et al.*, 1996). Conceptually, increased adherence reflects reduced hostility, as co-operating more with medical advice is a sign of reduced mistrust and antagonism towards a patient's physician.

CONCLUDING REMARKS

This chapter reviewed the challenges of adhering, the methods for assessing adherence and its correlates and strategies for enhancing it in both HT and CHD. Non-adherence constitutes a problem of epidemic magnitude, with approximately 50% of patients not adhering in different degrees to treatment in either disease (e.g. Conn *et al.*, 1992; Hamilton *et al.*, 1993). Non-adherence in HT increases the risk of CHD (Psaty *et al.*, 1990), as HT is a significant CHD risk factor (Kannel *et al.*, 1986). Among the challenges facing patients with HT are its asymptomatic nature, the lack of constant feedback on BP control, the nature of the treatment (self-administered), the fact that the condition is chronic and may lead to CHD and that the drug treatment has side-effects (Kjellgren *et al.*, 1995). Physicians incorrectly perceive adherence in HT as an easy task, non-adherence as an easily detectable, modifiable and unimportant problem, and that physicians should blame rather than consult their non-adhering patients (Rudd, 1992).

Adherence in HT may be assessed via pill counting, serum levels of medications/metabolites, BP levels (but this method assumes that therapy is effective), number of appointments kept, and self-report questionnaires or interviews. Morisky *et al.*'s (1986) well phrased interview is a valid and sensitive measure which clinicians and future studies may wish to include together with estimates of social desirability to increase its validity. Parameters that are related to adherence in HT include medical background (e.g. low BP, CHD, smoking, obesity; Degoulet, 1983; Sherbourne *et al.*, 1992), initial adherence levels (Sherbourne *et al.*, 1992), treatment complexity (e.g. dosage; Eisen *et al.*, 1990), psychological factors (e.g. hostility, illness distress: Lee *et al.*, 1992; Sherbourne *et al.*, 1992), and physician related factors (e.g. job satisfaction, number of patients per week, answering all patients' questions; DiMatteo *et al.*, 1993).

To enhance adherence in HT, Rudd (1992) suggested that non-adhering patients should be detected, adherence and goal BP should be defined to the patient, treatment plan should be outlined and simplified to the patient, costs and side-effects should be reduced and reinforcements for adherence should be provided. While Sackett *et al.* (1975) found that knowledge alone was insufficient for increasing adherence, Haynes *et al.* (1976) showed that having patients record their BP and adherence, match adherence to their daily routine, and provide reinforcements for adherence, significantly increased adherence and reduced BP levels. Wadden (1983) showed that involving patients' spouses can enhance patients' adherence to prescribed relaxation regimes. Involving nurses in the therapeutic regimen (Hamilton *et al.*, 1993) and teaching physicians to detect non-adherence and devote time to patients' health beliefs can enhance adherence as well (Inui *et al.*, 1976). Finally, use of computers at the community level which are time and cost effective have shown promising results (Friedman *et al.*, 1994).

The challenges of adherence in CHD are greater than in HT as the illness is more severe and prescribed regimens are more complex (multiple medications, diet, exercise, smoking cessation, behavior modification). Accordingly, assessment of adherence in CHD includes several measures such as number of attended or scheduled physical exercise appointments (Mirotznik *et al.*, 1995) and the comprehensive Health-Behavior Scale (Miller *et al.*, 1982a) which assesses adherence to all prescribed regimens in CHD. Additional methods include unobtrusive electronic monitoring of the days when patients removed medication (Carney *et al.*, 1995) and Ornish *et al.*'s (1990) self-report and objective assessment of life-style changes in CAD patients.

Among the correlates of adherence in CHD are initial adherence levels (Sherbourne *et al.*, 1992) and psychological factors such as motivation, perceived illness severity (Mirotznik *et al.*, 1995), self-esteem and social support (Conn *et al.*, 1992), spouse support (Doherty *et al.*, 1983), specific health related attitudes (Gallacher *et al.*, 1994), and depression (particularly impaired concentration; Carney *et al.*, 1995; Skala *et al.*, 1994). Doherty *et al.* (1983) and Hilbert (1985) suggest that marital satisfaction and the style of supporting patient adherence may moderate the impact of spouse support on patients' adherence. These complex interactions should be examined in greater detail in future studies.

To enhance adherence in CHD, Hladik and White (1976) showed that providing a booklet of correct medication usage resulted in high degrees of knowledge concerning treatment. Dapcich-Miura and Hovell (1979) demonstrated that a behavioural intervention was solely responsible for increasing an elderly MI patient's adherence to prescribed walking, diet and medication, and Daltroy (1985) found that counselling CHD patients over the telephone and providing them and their spouses with pamphlets increased patients' attendance at physical exercise classes. Mittlemark *et al.* (1986) and Perry *et al.* (1992) demonstrated reductions in long term cigarette consumption in a community intervention. Finally, Gidron *et al.* (1996) found that a hostility-reduction intervention may have increased levels of adherence in high-hostile CHD patients.

Future research should improve the assessment of adherence to treatment in HT and CHD. Factors which have been found to be significantly correlated with non-adherence (e.g. hostility; Lee *et al.*, 1992 or depression; Carney *et al.*, 1995) should be part of any adherence-enhancing treatment, as an empirically based approach for enhancing adherence. Although some of the findings reported above emerge from European samples (French, Swedish, British), more non-North American research is needed before generalisation of these findings is possible (Kjellgren *et al.*, 1995). Cultural differences and differing health-care systems may affect patients' interpretations, responses to and forms of carrying out medical regimens.

Finally, as a note of caution, Hays *et al.* (1994) concluded that "the relationship between adherence and health outcomes is much more complex than has often been assumed". While some studies show a dose-response relationship between adherence and disease-status (e.g. Ornish *et al.*, 1990), others do not support this assumption (Stegman *et al.*, 1987). Lack of a dose-response relationship may be due to an invalid measure of adherence, an ineffective treatment (Hays *et al.*, 1994), "break-down" of adherence into incorrect dose units, an insensitive/invalid disease-status measure, or a combination of these reasons. This issue has implications for the evaluation of health care in general. Future studies should address the relation between treatment, adherence and health with careful consideration of the complexities involved in these constructs, our basic assumptions about them, their assessment, and other mediators affecting them.

REFERENCES

Auerbach, S.M., Kendall, P.C., Cuttler, H. F. and Levitt, N.R. (1976) Anxiety, locus of control, type of preparatory information, and adjustment to dental surgery. *Journal of Consulting and Clinical Psychology* **44**, 809–818.

Beaupre, P.M., Carney, R.M., Freedland, K.E. and Eisen, S.A. (1994) The relation of depression and hostility to anginal symptoms and medication adherence in patients with coronary artery disease. Presented at The 15th Anniversary Meeting of The Society of Behavioural Medicine, April, Boston, USA.

Becker, M.H. (1974) The health belief model and sick role behavior. *Health Education Monographs* **2**, 409–419.

Burke, L.E., Dunbar-Jacob, J., Sereika, S. and Rohay, J.M. (1996) Outcome expectation versus self efficacy as predictive of dietary adherence in cardiac rehabilitation patients. Presented at The 4th International Conference of Behavioural Medicine, March, Washington, D.C., USA.

Burt, V.L., Whelton, P., Roccella, E.J., Brown, C., Cutler, J.A., Higgins, M., Horan, M.J. and Labarthe, D. (1995) Prevalence of hypertension in the US adult population. Results from the Third National Health and Nutrition Examination Survey, 1988–1991. *Hypertension* **25**, 305–313.

Carney, R.M., Freedland, K.E., Eisen, S.A., Rich, M.W. and Jaffe, A.S. (1995) Major depression and medication adherence in elderly patients with coronary artery disease. *Health Psychology*, **14**, 88–90.

Conn, V.S., Taylor, S.G. and Hayes. V. (1992) Social support, self-esteem, and self-care after myocardial infarction. *Health Values* **16**, 25–31.

Daltroy, L.H. (1985) Improving cardiac patient adherence to exercise regimens: a clinical trial of health education. *Journal of Cardiac Rehabilitation* **5**, 40–49.

Dapcich-Miura, E. and Hovell, M.F. (1979) Contingency management of adherence to a complex medical regimen in an elderly heart patient. *Behavior Therapy* **10,** 193–201.

Degoulet, P., Menard, J., Golmard, J.L., Devries, G., Chatellier, G. and Plouin, P.F. (1983) Factors predictive of attendance at clinic and blood-pressure control in hypertensive patients. *British Medical Journal* **287,** 88–93.

DiMatteo, M.R., Sherbourne, C.D., Hays, R.D., Ordway, L., Kravitz, R.L., McGlynn, E.A., Kaplan, S. and Rogers, W.H. (1993) Physicians' characteristics influence patients' adherence to medical treatment: results from the Medical Outcomes Study. *Health Psychology* **12,** 93–102.

Doherty, W.J., Schrott, H.G., Metcalf, L. and Lasiollo-Vailas, L. (1983) Effect of spouse support and health beliefs on medication adherence. *The Journal of Family Practice* **17,** 837–841.

Eisen, S.A., Miller, D.K., Woodward, R.S., Spitznagel, E. and Przybeck, T.R. (1990) The effect of prescribed daily dose frequency on patient medication compliance. *Archives of Internal Medicine* **150,** 1881–1884.

Frasure-Smith, N., Lesperance, F. and Talajic, M. (1993) Depression following myocardial infarction. Impact on 6-month survival. *Journal of the American Medical Association* **270,** 1819–1825.

Friedman, R.H., Kazis, L.E., Smith, M.B., Stollerman, J. and Torgerson, J. (1994) An automated telephone system to improve medication adherence. Presented at The 15th Anniversary Meeting of The Society of Behavioral Medicine, April, Boston, USA.

Gallacher, J. (1994) Formulative attitudinal research in the development of health promotion programs. Presented at The 15th Anniversary Meeting of The Society of Behavioral Medicine, April, Boston, USA.

Gidron, Y. and Davidson, K. (1996) Development and preliminary testing of a brief intervention for modifying CHD-predictive hostility components. *Journal of Behavioral Medicine* **19,** 203–220.

Gidron, Y., Davidson, K. and Bata, I. (1996) Effects of a brief hostility-reduction treatment on CHD-predictive hostility and health measures of CHD patients. Presented at The 4th International Conference of Behavioral Medicine, March, Washington, DC, USA.

Hamilton, G.A., Roberts, S.J., Johnson, J.M., Tropp, J.R., Anthony-Odgren, D. and Johnson, B. F. (1993) Increasing adherence in patients with primary hypertension: an intervention. *Health Values* **17,** 3–11.

Haynes, R.B. (1979) Determinants of compliance: the disease and the mechanics of treatment. In . R.B. Haynes, D.W. Taylor, and D.L. Sackett (eds.) . *Compliance in health care.* Baltimore: John Hopkins University Press.

Haynes, R.B., Sackett, D.L., Gibson, E.S., Taylor, D.W., Hackett, B.C., Roberts, R.S. and Johnson, A.L. (1976) Improvement of medication compliance in uncontrolled hypertension. *The Lancet* **i,** 1265–1268.

Haynes, R.B., Taylor, D.W., Sackett, D.L., Gibson, E.S., Bernholz, C.D. and Mukherjee, J. (1980) Can simple clinical measurements detect patient noncompliance? *Hypertension* **2,** 757–764.

Hays, R.D., Kravitz, R.L., Mazel, R.M., Sherbourne, C.D., DiMatteo, M.R., Rogers, W.H. and Greenfield, S. (1994) The impact of patient adherence on health outcomes for patients with chronic disease in the Medical Outcomes Study. *Journal of Behavioral Medicine* **17,** 347–360.

Hilbert, G.A. (1985) Spouse support and myocardial infarction patient compliance. *Nursing Research* **34,** 217–220.

Hladik, W.B. and White, S.J. (1976) Evaluation of written reinforcements used in counseling cardiovascular patients. *American Journal of Hospital Pharmacology* **33,** 1277–1280.

Hoelscher, T.J., Lichstein, K.L. and Rosenthal, T.L. (1986) Home relaxation practice in hypertension treatment: Objective assessment and compliance induction. *Journal of Consulting and Clinical Psychology* **54,** 217–221.

Houston, B.K. and Vavak, C.R. (1991) Cynical hostility: developmental factors, psychosocial correlates, and health behaviors. *Health Psychology* **10,** 9–17.

Inui, T.S., Yourtee, E.L. and Williamson, J.W. (1976) Improved outcomes in hypertension after physician tutorials: a controlled trial. *Annals of Internal Medicine* **84,** 646–651.

Jenkins, C. D. (1988). Epidemiology of Cardiovascular Diseases. *Journal of Consulting and Clinical Psychology* **56,** 324–332.

Kannel, W.B., Neaton, J D., Wentworth, D. , Thomas, H.E., Stamler, J., Hulley, S.B. and Kjelsberg, M.O.(1986) Overall and coronary heart disease mortality rates in relation to major risk factors in

325,348 men screened for the MRFIT. *American Heart Journal* **112**, 825–836.

Kaplan, R.M. (1988) Health-related quality of life in cardiovascular disease. *Journal of Consulting and Clinical Psychology* **3**, 382–392.

Kjellgren, K.I., Ahlner, J. and Saljo, R. (1995) Taking antihypertensive medication: controlling or co-operating with patients? *International Journal of Cardiology* **47**, 257–268.

Lee, D., De Leon, C.F.M., Jenkins, C D., Croog, S.H., Levine, S. and Sudilovski, A. (1992) Relation of hostility to medication adherence, symptom complaints, and blood pressure reduction in a clinical field trial of antihypertensive medication. *Journal of Psychosomatic Research* **36**, 181–190.

Miller, P., Johnson. N., Garrett, M.J. Wikoff, R. and McMahon, M. (1982a) Health beliefs of and adherence to the medical regimen by patients with ischemic heart disease. *Heart Lung*, **11**, 332–339.

Miller, P., Wikoff, R., McMahon, M., Garrett, M.J. and Johnson. N. (1982b) Development of a Health Attitude Scale. *Nursing Research* **31**, 132–136.

Miller, T.Q., Smith, T.W., Turner, C.W., Guijarro, M.L. and Hallet, A.J. (1996) A meta-analytic review of research on hostility and physical health. *Psychological Bulletin* **119**, 322–348.

Mirotznik, J., Feldman, L. and Stein, R. (1995) The Health Belief Model and Adherence with a community center-based, supervised coronary heart disease exercise program. *Journal of Community Health* **20**, 233–247.

Mittlemark, M.B., Luepker, R.V., Jacobs, D.R., Bracht, N.F., Carlow, R., Crow, W., Finnegan, J., Grimm, R.H., Jeffery, R.W., Kline, F.G, Mullis, R.M., Murray, D.M., Pechacek, T.F., Perry, C.L., Pirie, P.L. and Blackburn, H. (1986) Community-wide prevention of cardiovascular disease: education strategies of the Minnesota Heart Health Program. *Preventive Medicine* **15**, 1–17.

Morisky, D.E., Green, L.W. and Levine, D.M. (1986) Concurrent and predictive validity of a self-reported measure of medication adherence. *Medical Care* **24**, 67–74.

Ornish, D., Brown, S.E., Scherwitz, L.W., Billings, J.H., Armstrong, W.T., Ports, T.A., McLanahan, S.M., Kirkeedie, R.L., Brand, R.J. and Gould, K.L. (1990) Can lifestyle changes reverse coronary heart disease? *The Lancet* **336**, 129–133.

Owens, O.F., McCann, C.S. and Hutelmyer, C.M. (1978) Cardiac rehabilitation: a patient education program. *Nursing Research* **27**, 148–150.

Perry, C.L., Kelder, S. H., Murray, D.M. and Klepp, K.I. (1992) Community wide smoking prevention: Long-term outcomes of the Minnesota Heart Health Program and the Class of 1989 Study. *American Journal of Public Health* **82**, 1210–1216.

Psaty, B.M., Koepsell, T.D., Wagner, E.H., LoGerfo, J.P. and Inui, T.S. (1990) The relative risk of incident coronary heart disease associated with recently stopping the use of beta-blockers. *Journal of The American Medical Association* **263**, 1653–1657.

Rudd, P. (1992) Maximizing compliance with antihypertensive therapy. *Drug Therapy* **22**, 25–32.

Sackett, D.L., Haynes, R.B., Gibson, E.S., Hackett, B.C., Taylor, D.W., Roberts, R.S. and Johnson, A.L. (1975) Randomized clinical trial of strategies for improving medication compliance in primary hypertension. *The Lancet* **2**, 1205–1207.

Schmieder, R.E., Rockstroh, J.K. and Messerli, F.H. (1991) An antihypertensive therapy: to stop or not to stop? *Journal of the American Medical Association* **265**, 1566–1571.

Sherbourne, C.D., Hays, R.D., Ordway, L., DiMatteo, M.R. and Kravitz, R.L. (1992) Antecedents of adherence to medical recommendations: results from the Medical Outcomes Study. *Journal of Behavioral Medicine* **15**, 447–468.

Skala, J.A., Freedland, K.E., Eisen, S.A. and Carney, R.M. (1994) Depression, concentration, and medication adherence in patients with coronary disease. Presented at the 15th Anniversary Meeting of The Society of Behavioral Medicine, April, Boston, USA.

Smith, T.W., Follick, M.J. and Korr, K.S. (1984) Anger, Neuroticism, Type A behavior and the experience of angina. *British Journal of Medical Psychology,* **57**, 249–252.

Stegman, M.R., Miller, P.J., Hageman, R.K., Irby, D.E., Kositzky-Klutman, A.K. and Rajek, N.J. (1987) Myocardial infarction survival: how important are patients' attitudes and adherence behaviors? *American Journal of Preventative Medicine* **3**, 147–151.

Wadden, T.A. (1983) Predicting treatment response to relaxation therapy for essential hypertension. *The Journal of Nervous and Mental Disease* **171**, 683–689.

19

Adherence Issues in Methadone Treatments for Opiate Dependence

James Elander

Methadone is a synthetic opiate that is used to treat dependence on heroin and related drugs. Its effects are similar to those of heroin in that it will alleviate heroin withdrawal symptoms, but it causes less euphoria, lasts for longer, and can be prescribed as a linctus or syrup that cannot be injected, as well as in tablets or injectable ampoules. It can be used merely to control withdrawal symptoms by providing reducing doses over a short period (detoxification), or on a more extended basis to allow drug users to stabilise their lives, deal with acute health and social problems, and look at the reasons for their use of opiates before attempting in due course to stop using drugs (methadone maintenance, broadly speaking). The distinction between the two is not always exactly clear as many detoxification programmes go on for much longer than would be needed to manage just the physical aspects of withdrawal, and some programmes described as maintenance are expected to end in detoxification after a limited period.

In whatever way methadone is used, treatment outcome depends almost entirely on patients' willingness and ability to follow a treatment plan (this is also true for most treatments for drug addictions that do not use methadone). Therefore, adherence is often very difficult to differentiate from treatment effectiveness, but looking at methadone treatments specifically from the point of view of adherence can help to improve our understanding of the treatment process, and could help with the development of more effective treatment programmes.

One difficulty with considering adherence in methadone programmes is that prescribing a substitute for illicit opiates opens the door to potential conflicts between the intentions of patients and staff, for many drug users enter treatment at times when they do not really want to stop using drugs. Another difficulty arises because poor adherence may be one of the manifestations of drug dependence, for substance abuse has been shown to be related to not following medical advice in treatments other than for drug dependence (e.g. Jankowski and Drum, 1977; Schlaugh, Reich and Kelly, 1979). Theories of how addictive behaviours change provide partial explanations for the typically low levels of adherence in drug programmes. One influential view (the transtheoretical model) sees recovery from addiction as a series of changes from states of "contemplation" through "action" to "maintenance" (e.g. Prochaska, DiClemente and Norcross, 1992). For a description of the model, see Horne and Weinman, Chapter 2. From this perspective, one of the reasons for poor treatment adherence in methadone programmes is that the individuals concerned are not in the appropriate stage of change. However, severity of dependence is by no means the only influence on treatment adherence (Szapocznik and Ladner, 1977), and adherence problems that arose directly from drug dependence would warrant specific consideration in any case, because small improvements in the part of a patient's problem that affects their response to treatment could have disproportionate overall benefits.

In this chapter I consider ways in which a specific focus on adherence in methadone treatments could contribute to better treatment outcomes. The chapter begins by discussing what constitutes adherence in methadone programmes of different types and considering some of the problems with defining and measuring adherence. Evidence about the influences on adherence as they apply to engagement in treatment, detoxification, and methadone maintenance are then examined. The focus is mainly on aspects of treatment rather than patient characteristics. This is partly because treatment factors offer the greatest immediate scope for interventions to improve adherence, but also because the findings on individual differences in adherence among patients are so inconsistent. For example, in Szapocznik and Ladner's (1977) review of evidence

about treatment retention in methadone maintenance, the only characteristics for which there were consistent relationships were those
that are also considered to be general prognostic indicators for
recovery from addiction, such as employment, stable relationships,
and absence of criminality or multiple drug use.

DEFINING AND MEASURING ADHERENCE

In general terms, the behaviours that constitute adherence are those
a patient must follow to make treatment possible. This almost always
means remaining in treatment, and might also include attending for
observation and assessment, co-operating with inpatient admission,
taking medications as prescribed, providing urine samples for drug
testing, and reporting accurately on drug use and withdrawal distress. The relevant behaviours vary from treatment to treatment, but
to be meaningful they should be distinct from those identified as the
aims of treatment (Gordis, 1979). In many cases, the two have been
confounded because treatment programmes may include elements
of the intended outcome (discontinuing drug use, for example)
among the conditions of remaining in treatment, so that patients
may leave treatment *because* they have started to use drugs again
or have not responded to treatment in the intended way. Useful
indicators of adherence should also be behaviours that can clearly
be shown to improve outcomes, so considering adherence in drug
dependence means making a distinction between two closely correlated parts of behaviour. Part of the difficulty arises because treatment outcome is itself so difficult to assess. Many recoveries from
addiction take place over long periods and several treatment episodes, and patients can be difficult to recontact for follow-up evaluations. Because of this, aspects of adherence such as retention in
treatment are often used as convenient surrogate measures of
short-term treatment effectiveness.

The most important and most studied adherence variable is treatment retention, because of the strong link between time spent in
treatment and long-term treatment outcome. Some analyses of relationships between treatment retention and outcome do not take full
account of selective attrition, where those who are doing best are
more likely to be retained in treatment and available for follow-up

evaluations. However, studies that have followed-up very large numbers of drug users several years after entering long-term treatment programmes of different types, including methadone maintenance, have found that time spent in treatment was a better predictor of outcome than type of treatment (Hubbard *et al.*, 1989). In another large study, duration of treatment in methadone maintenance was a better predictor of long-term outcome than whether or not treatment was successfully terminated (Simpson, Savage and Lloyd, 1979).

The link between treatment retention and outcome is much less strong, however, for detoxification, where evaluations have often shown that increases in the length of time spent in treatment did not lead to greater numbers of patients achieving detoxification. Patients admitted under an urgent admission procedure, for example, discharged themselves significantly earlier then those admitted in the normal way, but were no less likely to complete detoxification (Strang and Connell, 1982). Treatment retention data in that case would have appeared to favour one of the groups when there were no real differences in treatment outcome.

Use of non-prescribed drugs during treatment is the next most widely reported aspect of adherence, and patients' own reports and the results of urine testing are the two main sources of information about this. Urine testing has predictable advantages and disadvantages in the clinical situation (Preston, 1996), and methadone is the drug of choice for treating opiate dependence, partly because it can be detected in urine separately from non-prescribed opiates. In theory, this allows the testers to know whether patients have been taking prescribed medication, as well as whether they have been using non-prescribed drugs. Incorporating very low doses of other drugs in the methadone and monitoring plasma levels even allows illicit extra use of methadone to be detected (Wolff *et al.*, 1991; 1993).

Urinalysis data can be a useful supplement to self-reported drug use during treatment, for whereas it is generally in the patient's interest to report their illicit drug use at the time of entry to a treatment programme, there may be strong incentives to conceal it once they are receiving a methadone prescription. In one study, there was high agreement between self-reports and urinalysis results for intake interviews and same day urines but not four weeks later (Sherman and Bigelow, 1992). Discrepancies between self-reported drug use and that revealed by urine testing would also depend on the consequences of disclosing drug use (which would vary from programme to programme), and on the quality of relationships between patients and staff. In Magura *et al.*'s (1987) study, for example, under-reporting of drug use (where patients' urine samples tested positive for illicit drugs but the patient failed to report drug use in interviews) varied from 32% to 61% at four methadone maintenance centres, and under-reporting was higher where the interviews were conducted by professional staff than by "paraprofessionals" (past or present drug treatment clients). Even urinalysis data has to be treated with caution, however, because the relatively short drug clearance times for opiates mean that illicit use of heroin or methadone would be detected only if it had taken place a few days before testing. Patients may also be more likely to provide samples of urine for testing, or to follow the urine testing procedure properly, when they were confident that their sample would not reveal illicit drug use.

ENGAGEMENT IN TREATMENT

Starting treatment could be regarded as an initial act of adherence, for most estimates show that heroin users who attend drugs services are a small minority of the heroin using population (Hartnoll *et al.*, 1985), and engaging drug users in treatment who would otherwise not be there is an important objective in the overall drugs strategy. Groups that have been targeted in this way include younger heroin users, women, and ethnic minorities, as well as those at high risk for HIV (Department of Health and Social Security, 1988). In most cases, such efforts have centred on designing treatment services to be more acceptable to new patients or on removing very concrete obstacles such as access or cost. For example, when coupons for free detoxification were issued in New Jersey, USA, 84% were redeemed for treatment and 28% of the participants continued in treatment after the free detoxification period (Jackson *et al.*, 1989).

Many of the procedures by which patients are referred from one agency to another and assessed for treatment can affect the likelihood of drug users who have initially sought help actually engaging in treatment. Waiting times are the first obvious consideration, and Bucknall, Robertson and Strachan (1986) showed that first appointments at a hospital clinic were more likely to be attended by those who had waited for shorter periods. The engagement rate was 61% for self-referrals, who were seen within one week of presentation, and between 18% and 53% for other types of referral, who waited up to four weeks or more for a first appointment. Treatment evaluations with waiting list controls also show how waiting times can affect engagement and retention rates. In one such study, patients who were randomly assigned to an "interim" clinic were more likely to be in treatment 16 months later than those who had been assigned to stay on the waiting list for a comprehensive treatment programme (Yancovitz *et al.*, 1991).

One reason why potential patients sometimes have to wait for treatment is that full assessment is usually an important part of the treatment protocol. Almost all treatment services involve some element of patient assessment and selection, the aim of which is to assess the individual's ability to benefit from treatment and maximise adherence by preparing patients for treatment. One review concluded that screening or recommendation of patients was the most important predictor of successful detoxification (Milby, 1988), but in several cases where formal comprehensive assessment for treatment was compared with reduced or streamlined assessment procedures, the adherence and outcome data have not favoured the more intensive and time consuming procedures. Strang and Connell (1982), for example, found that there were no differences in the proportions who completed either the detoxification or the rehabilitation phases of inpatient treatment between those admitted under a procedure for urgent admission and those admitted after the standard multidisciplinary outpatient assessment procedure. In one study of assessment procedures for methadone maintenance, patients who had been formally assessed were more likely to use illicit drugs, drop out or be expelled from the programme than those accepted for treatment by a rapid intake procedure. The formal assessment process in that case deterred half the initial applicants yet apparently either selected individuals with a worse prognosis or had a negative effect on treatment adherence (Bell, Caplehorn and McNeil, 1994).

Waiting times for treatment and procedures for assessment and referral offer some scope for improving engagement rates, but there are probably limits to how far effective treatments could be extended to include drug users who would not otherwise have sought treatment. For example, compulsory forms of treatment have been shown to have only modest success rates (Kramer, Bass and Berecochea, 1968), and some authorities have argued against seeking dramatic increases in the numbers of drug users in treatment because of the likelihood of steeply diminishing returns (Drummond *et al.*, 1987).

DETOXIFICATION

Detoxification is usually just one of several phases of treatment for opiate dependence, and is usually intended to be followed by interventions to reduce the risk of relapse to drug use. The aim is to eliminate the acute physical dependence on opiates while providing whatever supportive and therapeutic resources are available. The standard approach of stabilisation on prescribed opiates, usually methadone, and gradual dose reduction has the potential for almost complete effectiveness in the physiological side of the treatment, so that outcomes for particular detoxification episodes depend almost entirely on patients' adherence and their ability to cope with mild to moderate withdrawal symptoms.

Inpatient detoxifications are usually fairly short (10 days in some cases), often involve more intensive psychological interventions, isolate the patient from external influences to a greater extent, and may employ more careful selection of patients. Outpatient programmes often involve longer and more flexible dose reduction schedules but are less intensive and generally produce disappointing results. One comparison reported that only 17% of outpatients compared with 81% of inpatients completed treatment (Gossop, Johns and Green, 1986). Figures like those probably reflect the fact that treatment adherence in detoxification is related only weakly and indirectly to the pharmacological control of withdrawal symptoms and is much more strongly related to the overall intensity of the treatment programme.

Looking first at the evidence about inpatient detoxification programmes, the complicated relationship between withdrawal symptoms and adherence can be illustrated by examining the effects of interventions to reduce the severity of withdrawal symptoms. Where these have been based on physical factors, such as the rate of dose reductions, they have had little effect on treatment retention in spite of successfully reducing withdrawal severity. Gossop *et al.* (1989), for example, compared patients who were detoxified in hospital over 10 days or 21 days. Those who were detoxified over 10 days experienced more intense withdrawal symptoms that peaked earlier, but were no less likely to complete the treatment than those detoxified over the longer period. Strang and Gossop (1990) compared patients whose methadone doses were reduced by the same amount each day to those whose doses were reduced by larger amounts towards the beginning of the 10-day programme. The second group experienced significantly greater withdrawal symptoms, but there were no differences in patient retention or completion of treatment between groups. Non-experimental comparisons between treatment groups also show that differences in intensity of withdrawal symptoms are not necessarily associated with differences in treatment retention. Methadone users experienced more intense withdrawal symptoms than heroin users during a 10-day inpatient detoxification, for example, but were just as successful in completing treatment (Gossop and Strang, 1991).

Withdrawal symptoms are not determined solely by physical factors, however. One study showed that they were related more closely to patients' levels of anxiety and their expectations about withdrawal than the amounts of opiates they had been taking (Phillips, Gossop and Bradley, 1986). Attempts to reduce withdrawal severity that focus on these subjective factors have had greater effects on adherence. In one such study, detoxification patients who were taught in detail about the symptoms they would experience, not only reported milder withdrawal symptoms but were also were more likely to complete treatment than those who were not informed about the withdrawal symptoms they should expect (Green and Gossop, 1988). In other studies of inpatient detoxification, allowing patients to play a role in deciding their rate of dose reduction has led to improved retention and completion rates, decreases in overall methadone consumption, and shorter detoxification periods (Razani *et al.*, 1975; Stern, Edwards and Lerro, 1974).

Similar types of intervention in outpatient detoxification programmes have produced more disappointing results. One study compared patients in a fixed, six-week reduction schedule with those who were allowed to negotiate their rate of reduction over 10 weeks. Those who negotiated their doses achieved smaller reductions but were much less likely to complete detoxification (Dawe *et al.*, 1991). In a similar study, patients who were allowed to regulate their rate of methadone reduction were retained in treatment for longer and used fewer non-prescribed drugs, but reduced their methadone more slowly than those following a physician-regulated detoxification, and were no more likely to complete detoxification (Fulwiler, Hargreaves and Borman, 1979).

Another approach is to provide temporary dose increases, and these have been shown to have positive effects for patients whose adherence was poor and when dose increases were deliberately linked to measures of adherence. In a study with patients whose urine samples had revealed high levels of illicit drug use during the first three weeks of an outpatient programme, treatment retention and clinic attendance were increased by providing extra methadone during the dose reduction phase of detoxification. Illicit opiate use was also reduced, with the fewest opiate-positive urine samples provided by those who received extra methadone only if their most recent urine sample was opiate-free (Higgins *et al.*, 1986). In a similar study, temporary dose increases from 30 mg to 60 mg of methadone had the effect of reducing opiate-positive urine samples and tended to increase the length of time patients were retained in treatment. There was little difference, however, in the numbers who stayed in treatment until the last stage of the detoxification programme (Stitzer *et al.*, 1984).

To sum up the evidence about factors that promote adherence among patients in detoxification programmes, physical influences on the severity of withdrawal seem to affect adherence only marginally affect adherence, whereas psychological influences, like patients' knowledge and expectations about withdrawal, seem to play a more important role. Allowing patients to negotiate their methadone doses or rates of withdrawal has improved adherence in inpatient programmes, but for outpatients most of the effect has been to prolong treatments that ended in failure to complete detoxification. Increasing methadone doses or extending reduction periods may therefore improve adherence in ways that do not improve overall treatment outcomes, whereas addressing the psychological influences on withdrawal distress, or making incentives to remain in treatment contingent on measures of adherence, can improve adherence in ways that make treatment more likely to be effective. A key advantage of inpatient detoxification is that it provides for closer monitoring of patients and for more direct interventions to improve adherence. The greater effectiveness of inpatient detoxification may also be because more intensive psychological contributions to treatment are usually involved, or because patients are more carefully selected for inpatient detoxification.

METHADONE MAINTENANCE

In the earliest form of methadone maintenance, very high doses were used in attempts to remove the incentives for illicit opiate use by establishing a "pharmacological blockade" against their effects (Dole, Nyswander and Kreek, 1966). Maintenance programmes with a more psychotherapeutic or change-oriented rationale have developed since then, and these generally employ lower doses over shorter periods of time, with methadone prescribing combined with different non-pharmacological interventions at different stages of treatment (Moolchan and Hoffman, 1994). Programmes vary considerably in philosophy and practice (Rosenbaum, 1985), but almost all are run on an outpatient basis.

Maintenance approaches to treatment are still controversial, with critics arguing that they can protract addiction and contribute to more general availability of opiates when prescribed methadone is diverted to the illicit market, but most evaluations show fairly clear benefits. One recent review (Bertschy, 1995) concluded that, although results vary, the treatment does have an authentic effect on criminality, HIV risks, mortality and social functioning as well as on illicit drug use, with between 50% and 80% of patients studied not having used heroin in the previous month. Outcomes were to some extent related to patient characteristics, but were much more strongly related to treatment variables. For example, McGlothlin and Anglin (1981) compared two programmes that operated high dose, long retention policies with one that provided low dose, limited duration programmes. Treatment was completed for 12% and 18% of patients in the first two programmes, compared with only 2% of those in the third, and the drop-out rates (where patients themselves stopped attending) were 10% and 16% in the first two compared with 29% in the third. Duration of treatment is a critical influence on long-term outcome, and one extensive review of follow-up studies concluded that "length of time spent in methadone maintenance is related in some way to post methadone maintenance behaviour" and that "more than two to three years of methadone maintenance is necessary before significant behaviour change is observed" (Ward, Mattick and Hall, 1992).

Patients in maintenance programmes probably differ in some ways from those in detoxification programmes. In Bass and Brown's (1973) comparison between patients who chose either maintenance or detoxification, those who chose maintenance were more likely to be living with relatives or a spouse rather than alone or with friends, tended to be older than those who chose detoxification, and were more likely to stay in treatment for six months. This should make for greater adherence in maintenance than detoxification, so far as the two forms of treatment can be compared, and treatment variables are related to adherence in a more encouraging way for methadone maintenance than for outpatient detoxification.

Treatment retention and use of illicit drugs during treatment are the main aspects of adherence to have been examined in methadone maintenance. This is partly because of the clinical significance of those behaviours, but also because other aspects of adherence, such as whether methadone is actually taken as prescribed, are much more difficult to find out about. There is understandably very little systematic evidence about methadone being sold or exchanged for other drugs by patients on methadone programmes. Diversion of methadone to the illicit market is an important aspect of adherence from both a clinical and public health point of view (Greene, Brown and Dupont, 1975), and most maintenance programmes operate sanctions against this as well as illicit drug use, by withdrawing "take home" medication or terminating treatment when it is discovered (Rosenbaum, 1985). A survey of inpatient drug users showed that 43% had previously used methadone illegally, having obtained it in over one-third of those cases from a methadone maintenance patient (Weppner, Stephens and Conrad, 1972), and one trial of heroin maintenance was able to report that 12% of patients were selling part of their prescription every day, whereas none of those in the methadone comparison group were apparently doing so on a regular basis (Hartnoll *et al.*, 1980).

Methadone doses often vary more from one treatment centre to another than between patients at a given centre, and comparisons between strikingly different maintenance approaches are not always easy to interpret. There is probably an upper limit on the gains to be made by increasing doses, but in the low to medium range adherence has been shown to be fairly sensitive to dose. In one analysis, the relative odds of illicit heroin use as revealed by fixed interval urine testing fell steadily for every increase in methadone dose, and were halved at doses of 80 mg by comparison with 40 mg (Caplehorn *et al.*, 1993). Relationships between treatment retention and methadone dose have also been reported (e.g. Joe, Simpson and Hubbard, 1991), but retention is probably less sensitive than illicit drug use to methadone dose levels. In Strain *et al.*'s (1993) randomised, double blind trial in which patients all started treatment with 25 mg of methadone but had their doses adjusted over five weeks and were then maintained for six months on either 0, 20 or 50 mgs of methadone, retention in treatment was significantly better for both the 50mg and 20 mg groups by comparison with the 0 mg group, but only the 50 mg group produced fewer opiate and cocaine positive urines.

Treatment retention is probably influenced more strongly by the way methadone doses are decided than by the dose itself. In one survey of a large number of maintenance programmes, those that operated flexible dosing policies retained patients in treatment for longer, on average, than those where most patients on the programme were maintained on similar doses, whereas the predominant dose level for the programme was not significantly related to patient retention (Brown, Watters and Iglehart, 1982–3). Goldstein, Hansteen and Horns (1975) reported that allowing patients to control their dose levels did not result in widespread increases in doses, with systematic increases only among a small group who also tended to decrease illicit opiate use. Giving patients control over their doses also avoided placing patients and staff in adversarial roles, and was strongly favoured by all of the patients and staff involved in the programme.

However, liberalisations of treatment that go beyond the negotiation of methadone doses have not produced such clear benefits. In one maintenance clinic where policy was changed so that patients were not expelled from treatment for drug use, and take-home medication and negotiation of methadone doses were allowed, retention in treatment was improved but drug use also increased (Hebert and Lauterbach, 1983). Drug users have endorsed in surveys the use of urine testing and expulsion for antisocial behaviour (Jones, Power and Dale, 1994), and in one randomised comparison between a maintenance programme where drug use exceeding set limits resulted in methadone withdrawal and one where there were no consequences for continued drug use, less than a third of those in the more liberal programme completed 12 months treatment, compared with over half of those in the more structured programme (McCarthy and Borders, 1985). Another approach is to make dose *increases* contingent on whether urine samples were drug-free. This was shown to reduce the numbers of patients who supplemented their methadone with illicit drugs, but did not improve treatment retention or completion (Stitzer, Iguchi and Felch, 1992).

Even more direct compromises between treatment goals and acceptability of treatment to patients are raised by the possibility of varying the type of prescription offered in maintenance programmes. Prescribing injectable opiates is the most controversial issue of this kind (Battersby *et al.*, 1992), and at one centre there was intense resistance among patients whose prescriptions were changed from methadone tablets, which can be crushed and injected, to methadone mixture, which cannot (Steels, Hamilton and McLean, 1992). In a trial where drug users seeking heroin maintenance were randomised to maintenance with injectable heroin or oral methadone, the heroin prescription kept more patients in treatment, with 74% compared with 29% still on the programme after 12 months, but led to fewer changes in drug-related behaviours (Hartnoll *et al.*, 1980).

CONCLUSIONS AND DISCUSSION POINTS

The conclusions that can be drawn from this summary of research findings would probably confirm the clinical impressions of those involved in providing methadone-based treatment services for opiate dependence. These are that where patients are more carefully selected and more closely monitored during treatment, adherence can be improved in ways that benefit treatment outcomes by co-operative efforts to involve patients more closely in decisions about treatment. Where methadone is prescribed under more relaxed conditions, as in many outpatient detoxification programmes and some forms of methadone maintenance, more flexible and negotiable treatment approaches have been less successful in promoting adherence, and interventions were effective only where the incentives were conditional on changes in the behaviours that were being targeted.

Most of the interventions that have been tested involved modifications to the treatment that was offered, in the form of increased or extended methadone prescribing. This can sometimes give the appearance of compromising the quality of treatment in order to increase levels of adherence, but opiate dependence differs from most of the other conditions dealt with in this book in ways that make an apparent trade-off like this more reasonable and positive than it would otherwise seem. Firstly, very few single episodes of treatment are successful in their own right, and opiate users typically follow a cycle of repeated treatment and relapse in the process of overcoming dependence. Secondly, many of the benefits to treatment are expected to be felt more widely than by individual patients, in the form of reduced crime, greater public safety and improved public health, especially where the spread of HIV is concerned. Short-term treatment goals can be less important, therefore, than changes either towards eventual individual recovery or towards reductions in the wider social impact of drug use, and the benefits of increased adherence can be greater than the apparent costs of theoretically less desirable outcomes for particular treatment episodes. The approach of compromising treatment goals to achieve other benefits is taken a step further in the philosophy of harm reduction, where attempts are made to reduce the risks associated with drug use rather than treat the patient's drug dependence, but real long-term treatment benefits can result from improvements in adherence at the cost of accepting less ambitious short-term outcomes even where the underlying dependence is the main focus of interventions.

Trade-offs of this kind are not the only way to modify adherence, for there is some limited evidence about interventions that improved adherence by focusing on aspects of treatment other than methadone prescribing. As discussed earlier, Green and Gossop (1988) increased the numbers of patients who completed detoxification by informing them more fully about withdrawal symptoms, and in one community-based methadone programme, attendance at counselling sessions and drug-free urine samples were increased simply by rewarding those behaviours with coupons that could be redeemed for food, fuel or bus travel (Rowan-Szal *et al.*, 1994). Findings like those show that it is possible to improve adherence without modifying the main component of methadone programmes. For treatment interventions that involve modifications either to the methadone regime itself or to the way it is applied, what the evidence from across the range of studies in this area shows is that adherence can be improved in a variety of ways that must vary in effectiveness according to the particular circumstances in which they are applied. However, for best effects it is necessary to focus very closely on the particular behaviours that are involved, and to link the intervention directly to the aspect of adherence that one wishes to promote, rather than simply to make treatment generally more acceptable to the patient or less onerous than it would otherwise be.

REFERENCES

Bass, U.F. and Brown, B.S. (1973) Methadone maintenance and methadone detoxification: a comparison of retention rates and client characteristics. *International Journal of the Addictions* **8**, 889–895.

Battersby, M., Farrell, M., Gossop, M., Robson, P. and Strang, J. (1992) 'Horse Trading': prescribing injectable opiates to opiate addicts. A descriptive study. *Drug and Alcohol Review* **11**, 35–42.

Bell., J., Caplehorn, J.R. and McNeil, D.R. (1994) The effect of intake procedures on performance in methadone maintenance. *Addiction* **89**, 463–471.

Bertschy, G. (1995) Methadone maintenance treatment: an update. *European Archives of Psychiatry and Clinical Neuroscience*, **245** 114–124.

Brown, B.S., Watters, J.K. and Iglehart, A.S. (1982–3) Methadone maintenance dosage levels and program retention. *American Journal of Drug and Alcohol Abuse 9*, 129–139.

Bucknall, A.B.V., Robertson, J.R. and Strachan, T.G. (1986) Use of psychiatric drug treatment services by heroin users from general practice. *British Medical Journal* **292**, 997–999.

Caplehorn, J.R., Bell, J., Kleinbaum, D.G. and Gebski, V.J. (1993) Methadone dose and heroin use during maintenance treatment. *Addiction* **88**, 119–124.

Dawe, S., Griffiths, P., Gossop, M. and Strang, J. (1991) Should opiate addicts be involved in controlling their own detoxification? a comparison of fixed versus negotiable schedules. *British Journal of Addiction* **86**, 977–982.

Department of Health and Social Security (1988) *Aids and Drug Misuse: Part 1. Report of the Advisory Council on the Misuse of Drugs.* London: HMSO.

Dole, V.P., Nyswander, M.E. and Kreek, M.J. (1966) Narcotic blockade. *Archives of Internal Medicine* **118**, 304–309.

Drummond, C., Edwards, G., Glanz, A., Glass, I., Jackson, P., Oppenheimer, E., Sheehan, M., Taylor, C. and Thom, B. (1987) Rethinking drug policies in the context of the acquired immunodeficiency syndrome. *Bulletin on Narcotics* **39**, 29–35.

Fulwiler, R.L., Hargreaves, W.A. and Borman, R.A. (1979) Detoxification from heroin using self vs physician regulation of methadone dose. *International Journal of the Addictions* **14**, 289–298.

Goldstein, A., Hansteen, R.W. and Horns, W.H. (1975) Control of methadone dosage by patients. *Journal of the American Medical Association* **234**, 734–737.

Gordis, L. (1979) Conceptual and methodologic problems in measuring patient compliance. In R.B. Haynes and D.L. Sackett (eds.) *Compliance in health care.* Baltimore, MA: John Hopkins University Press.

Gossop, M., Griffiths, P., Bradley, M. and Strang, J. (1989) Opiate withdrawal symptoms in response to 10-day and 21-day methadone withdrawal programmes. *British Journal of Psychiatry* **154**, 360–363.

Gossop, J., Johns, A. and Green, L. (1986) Opiate withdrawal: in-patient versus out-patient programmes and preferred versus random assignment to treatment. *British Medical Journal* **293**, 103–104.

Gossop, M. and Strang, J. (1991) A comparison of the withdrawal responses of heroin and methadone addicts during detoxification. *British Journal of Psychiatry* **158**, 697–699.

Green, L. and Gossop, M. (1988) Effects of information on the opiate withdrawal syndrome. *British Journal of Addiction* **83**, 305–309.

Greene, M.H., Brown, B.S. and Dupont, R.L. (1975) Controlling the abuse of illicit methadone in Washington, D.C. *Archives of General Psychiatry* **32**, 221–226.

Hartnoll, R.L., Lewis, R., Mitcheson, M. and Bryer, S. (1985) Estimating the prevalence of opioid dependence. *Lancet* **i**, 203–205.

Hartnoll, R.L., Mitcheson, M., Battersby, A., Brown, G., Ellis, M., Fleming, P. and Hedley, N. (1980) Evaluation of heroin maintenance in controlled trial. *Archives of General Psychiatry* **37**, 877–884.

Hebert, S.W. and Lauterbach, E.C. (1983) Methadone maintenance in the small community drug abuse clinic. *International Journal of the Addictions* **18**, 863–874.

Higgins, S.T., Stitzer, M.L., Bigelow, G.E. and Liebson, I.A. (1986) Contingent methadone delivery: effects on illicit opiate use. *Drug and Alcohol Dependence* **17**, 311–322.

Hubbard, R.L., Marsden, M.E., Rachal, J.V., Harwood, H.J., Cavanagh, E.R. and Ginzburg, H.M. (1989) *Drug abuse treatment: a national study of effectiveness.* Chapel Hill, NC: University of North Carolina Press.

Jackson, J.F., Rotkiewicz, L.G., Quinones, M.A. and Passannante, M.R. (1989) A coupon program-drug treatment and AIDS education. *International Journal of the Addictions* **24**, 1035–1051.

Jankowski, C.B. and Drum, D.E. (1977) Diagnostic correlates of discharge against medical advice. *Archives of General Psychiatry* **34**, 153–155.

Joe, G.W., Simpson, D.D. and Hubbard, R.L. (1991) Treatment predictors of tenure in methadone maintenance. *Journal of Substance Abuse* **3**, 73–84.

Jones, S.S., Power, R. and Dale, A. (1994) The patients' charter: drug users' views on the 'ideal' methadone programme. *Addiction Research* **1**, 323–334.

Kramer, J.C., Bass, R.A. and Berecochea, J.E. (1968) Civil commitment for addicts: California program. *American Journal of Psychiatry* **125**, 816–824.

Magura, S., Goldsmith, D., Casriel, C., Goldstein, P.J. and Lipton, D.S. (1987) The validity of methadone clients' self-reported drug use. *International Journal of the Addictions* **22**, 727–749.

McCarthy, J.J. and Borders, O.T. (1985) Limit setting on drug abuse in methadone maintenance patients. *American Journal of Psychiatry* **142**, 1419–1423.

McGlothlin, W.H. and Anglin, M.D. (1981) Long term follow-up of clients of high and low dose methadone programs. *Archives of General Psychiatry* **38**, 1055–1063.

Milby, J.B. (1988) Methadone maintenance to abstinence: how many make it? *Journal of Nervous and Mental Diseases* **176**, 409–422.

Moolchan, E.T. and Hoffman, J.A. (1994) Phases of treatment: a practical approach to methadone maintenance treatment. *International Journal of the Addictions* **29**, 135–160.

Phillips, G., Gossop, M. and Bradley, B. (1986) The influence of psychological factors on the opiate withdrawal syndrome. *British Journal of Psychiatry* **149**, 235–238.

Preston, A. (1996) *The Methadone Briefing.* London: Institute for the Study of Drug Dependence.

Prochaska, J.O., DiClemente, C.C. and Norcross, J.C. (1992) In search of how people change: applications to addictive behaviours. *American Psychologist* **47**, 1102–1114.

Razani, J., Chisholm, D., Glasser, M. and Kappeler, T. (1975) Self-regulated methadone detoxification of heroin addicts, an improved technique in an inpatient setting. *Archives of General Psychiatry* **32**, 909–911.

Rosenbaum, M. (1985) A matter of style: variation among methadone clinics in the control of clients. *Contemporary Drug Problems* **12**, 375–400.

Rowan-Szal, G., Joe, G.W. Chatham, L.R. and Simpson, D.D. (1994) A simple reinforcement system for methadone clients in a community-based treatment program. *Journal of Substance Abuse Treatment* **11**, 217–223.

Schlaugh, R.W., Reich, P. and Kelly, M.J. (1979) Leaving the hospital against medical advice. *New England Journal of Medicine* **300**, 22–24.

Sherman, M.F. and Bigelow, G.E. (1992) Validity of patients' self-reported drug use as a function of treatment status. *Drug and Alcohol Dependence* **30**, 1–11.

Simpson, D.D., Savage, L.J. and Lloyd, M.R. (1979. Follow-up evaluation of drug abuse treatment during 1969 to 1972. *Archives of General Psychiatry* **36**, 772–780.

Steels, M.D., Hamilton, M. and McLean, P.C. (1992) The consequences of a change in formulation of methadone prescribed in a drug clinic. *British Journal of Addiction* **87**, 1549–1554.

Stern, R., Edwards, N.B. and Lerro, F.A. (1974) Methadone on demand as a heroin detoxification procedure. *International Journal of the Addictions* **9**, 863–872.

Stitzer, M.L., McCaul, M.E., Bigelow, G.E. and Liebson, I.A. (1984). Chronic opiate use during methadone detoxification: effects of a dose increase treatment. *Drug and Alcohol Dependence* **14**, 37–44.

Stitzer, M.L., Iguchi, M.Y. and Felch, L.J. (1992). Contingent take home incentives: effects on drug use of methadone maintenance patients. *Journal of Consulting and Clinical Psychology* **60**, 927–934.

Strain, E.C., Stitzer, M.L., Liebson, I.A. and Bigelow, G.E. (1993). Dose-response effects of methadone in the treatment of opioid dependence. *Annals of Internal Medicine* **119**, 23–27.

Strang, J. and Connell, P.H. (1982) Assessment of an urgent admission procedure to an inpatient drug dependence unit. *British Journal of Addiction* **77**, 311–318.

Strang, J. and Gossop, M. (1990). Comparison of linear versus inverse exponential methadone reduction curves in the detoxification of opiate addicts. *Addictive Behaviours* **15**, 541–547.

Szapocznik, J. and Ladner, R. (1977) Factors related to successful retention in methadone maintenance: a review. *International Journal of the Addictions* **12**, 1067–1085.

Ward, J., Mattick, R.P. and Hall, W. (1992). *Key issues in methadone maintenance treatment.* Kensington, New South Wales: New South Wales University Press.

Weppner, R.S., Stephens, R.C., and Conrad, H.T. (1972) Methadone: some aspects of its legal and illegal use. *American Journal of Psychiatry* **129**, 451–455.

Wolff, K., Hay, A.A., Raistrick, D., Calvert, R. and Feely, M. (1991) Measuring compliance in methadone maintenance patients: use of a pharmacological indicator to 'estimate' methadone plasma levels. *Clinical Pharmacology and Therapeutics* **50**, 199–207.

Wolff, K., Hay, A.A., Raistrick, D. and Feely, M. (1993) Use of 'very low-dose phenobarbital' to investigate compliance in patients on reducing doses of methadone (detoxification). *Journal of Substance Abuse Treatment* **10**, 453–458.

Yancovitz, S.R., Des Jarlais, D.C., Peyser, N.P., Drew, A., Friedman, P., Trigg, H.L. and Robinson, J.W. (1991) A randomised trial of an interim methadone clinic. *American Journal of Public Health* **81**, 1185–1191.

Index